Sports Training and Exercise Physiology

Sports Training and Exercise Physiology

Edited by Garrett Cooper

SYRAWOOD
PUBLISHING HOUSE
New York

Published by Syrawood Publishing House,
750 Third Avenue, 9th Floor,
New York, NY 10017, USA
www.syrawoodpublishinghouse.com

Sports Training and Exercise Physiology
Edited by Garrett Cooper

International Standard Book Number: 978-1-68286-498-2 (Hardback)

Cataloging-in-Publication Data

Sports training and exercise physiology / edited by Garrett Cooper.
p. cm.
Includes bibliographical references and index.
ISBN 978-1-68286-498-2
1. Physical education and training. 2. Exercise--Physiological aspects. 3. Sports.
4. Athletes--Nutrition. 5. Sports--Physiological aspects.I. Cooper, Garrett.
GV206 .S76 2017
613.7--dc23

Printed in the United States of America.

TABLE OF CONTENTS

Preface IX

Chapter 1 **Effects of Video-Based Visual Training on Decision-Making and Reactive Agility in Adolescent Football Players** 1
Alfred Nimmerichter, Nikolaus J. R. Weber, Klaus Wirth and Andreas Haller

Chapter 2 **Physiological Characteristics of Incoming Freshmen Field Players in a Men's Division I Collegiate Soccer Team** 10
Robert G. Lockie, DeShaun L. Davis, Samantha A. Birmingham-Babauta, Megan D. Beiley, Jillian M. Hurley, Alyssa A. Stage, John J. Stokes, Tricia M. Tomita, Ibett A. Torne and Adrina Lazar

Chapter 3 **Autonomy Mediates the Relationship between Personality and Physical Activity: An Application of Self-Determination Theory** 27
Meredith L. Ramsey and Eric E. Hall

Chapter 4 **Clinical Assessment of Scapula Motion: Scapula Upward Rotation and Relationship with Injury in Swimmers** 34
Jo Brown, Rebecca Mellifont and Brendan Burkett

Chapter 5 **Cardiac Autonomic and Salivary Responses to a Repeated Training Bout in Elite Swimmers** 44
Rohan Edmonds, Anthony Leicht, Brendan Burkett and Mark McKean

Chapter 6 **"You're Not Born with Talent" Talented Girls' and Boys' Perceptions of their talents as Football Players** 58
Stig Arve Sæther and Ingar Mehus

Chapter 7 **The Effect of Recovery Duration on Technical Proficiency during Small Sided Games of Football** 66
Scott McLean, Hugo Kerhervé, Mitchell Naughton, Geoff P. Lovell, Adam D. Gorman and Colin Solomon

Chapter 8 **Can Fundamental Movement Skill Mastery Be Increased via a Six Week Physical Activity Intervention to have Positive Effects on Physical Activity and Physical Self-Perception?** 76
Elizabeth S. Bryant, Michael J. Duncan, Samantha L. Birch and Rob S. James

Chapter 9 **How Confident can we be in Modelling Female Swimming Performance in Adolescence?** 90
Shilo J. Dormehl, Samuel J. Robertson and Craig A. Williams

Chapter 10 **Martial Arts and Metabolic Diseases** ... 99
Hidetaka Hamasaki

Chapter 11 **Modelling the Progression of Male Swimmers' Performances through Adolescence** ... 111
Shilo J. Dormehl, Samuel J. Robertson and Craig A. Williams

Chapter 12 **The Age in Swimming of Champions in World Championships (1994–2013) and Olympic Games (1992–2012)** ... 120
Beat Knechtle, Nicola Luigi Bragazzi, Stefan König, Pantelis Theodoros Nikolaidis, StefanieWild, Thomas Rosemann and Christoph Alexander Rüst

Chapter 13 **Self-Reported use and Reasons among the General Population for using Sports Nutrition Products and Dietary Supplements** ... 147
FlorisWardenaar, Remko van den Dool, Ingrid Ceelen, Renger Witkamp and Marco Mensink

Chapter 14 **Effects of Short-Term Dynamic Constant External Resistance Training and Subsequent Detraining on Strength of the Trained and Untrained Limbs** ... 158
Pablo B. Costa, Trent J. Herda, Ashley A. Herda and Joel T. Cramer

Chapter 15 **A Description and Comparison of Cardiorespiratory Fitness Measures in Relation to Pitching Performance Among Professional Baseball Pitchers** ... 168
Javair S. Gillett, J. Jay Dawes, Frank J. Spaniol, Matthew R. Rhea, Joe P. Rogowski, Mitchel A. Magrini, Roberto Simao and Derek J. Bunker

Chapter 16 **The Effects of Mental Imagery with Video-Modeling on Self-Efficacy and Maximal Front Squat Ability** ... 176
Daniel J. M. Buck, Jasmin C. Hutchinson, Christa R. Winter and Brian A. Thompson

Chapter 17 **A Comparison between Chocolate Milk and a Raw Milk Honey Solution's Influence on Delayed Onset of Muscle Soreness** ... 186
Andrew Hatchett, Christopher Berry, Claudia Oliva, Douglas Wiley, Jacob St. Hilaire and Alex LaRochelle

Chapter 18 **The Acute Effects of Heavy Deadlifts on Vertical Jump Performance in Men** **193**
Jerry C. Arias, Jared W. Coburn, Lee E. Brown and Andrew J. Galpin

Permissions

List of Contributors

Index

PREFACE

This book aims to highlight the current researches and provides a platform to further the scope of innovations in this area. This book is a product of the combined efforts of many researchers and scientists from different parts of the world. The objective of this book is to provide the readers with the latest information in the field.

This book on sports training deals with the various exercise therapies and routines whose aim is to increase a person's endurance and fitness levels. The book discusses the various requirements that arise when undergoing rigorous training and the techniques and methodologies that are used for measuring a person's fitness levels. Topics included in this book deal with all aspects of sports training and diet and the levels of fitness that is to be maintained. A number of latest researches have been included to keep the readers up-to-date with the global concepts in this area of study. Scientists and students actively engaged in this field will find this book full of crucial and unexplored concepts.

I would like to express my sincere thanks to the authors for their dedicated efforts in the completion of this book. I acknowledge the efforts of the publisher for providing constant support. Lastly, I would like to thank my family for their support in all academic endeavors.

Editor

1

Effects of Video-Based Visual Training on Decision-Making and Reactive Agility in Adolescent Football Players

Alfred Nimmerichter *,†, Nikolaus J. R. Weber †, Klaus Wirth † and Andreas Haller †

Academic Editor: Eling de Bruin

Sport and Exercise Sciences, University of Applied Sciences Wiener Neustadt, Johannes Gutenberg Str. 3, Wiener Neustadt A-2700, Austria; nikolaus.weber@wvnet.at (N.J.R.W.); klaus.wirth@fhwn.ac.at (K.W.); andreas.haller@fhwn.ac.at (A.H.)

* Correspondence: nimmerichter@fhwn.ac.at

† These authors contributed equally to this work.

Abstract: This study investigated the trainability of decision-making and reactive agility via video-based visual training in young athletes. Thirty-four members of a national football academy (age: 14.4 $\pm$ 0.1 years) were randomly assigned to a training (VIS; $n = 18$) or a control group (CON; $n = 16$). In addition to the football training, the VIS completed a video-based visual training twice a week over a period of six weeks during the competition phase. Using the temporal occlusion technique, the players were instructed to react on one-on-one situations shown in 40 videos. The number of successful decisions and the response time were measured with a video-based test. In addition, the reactive-agility sprint test was used. VIS significantly improved the number of successful decisions (22.2 $\pm$ 3.6 s *vs.* 29.8 $\pm$ 4.5 s; $p < 0.001$), response time (0.41 $\pm$ 0.10 s *vs.* 0.31 $\pm$ 0.10 s; $p = 0.006$) and reactive agility (2.22 $\pm$ 0.33 s *vs.* 1.94 $\pm$ 0.11 s; $p = 0.001$) pre- *vs.* post-training. No significant differences were found for CON. The results have shown that video-based visual training improves the time to make decisions as well as reactive agility sprint-time, accompanied by an increase in successful decisions. It remains to be shown whether or not such training can improve simulated or actual game performance.

Keywords: visual training; video-based; decision-making; reactive agility; anticipation; one-on-one; transfer effect; football

---

1. Introduction

Perceptual-cognitive skills such as anticipation and decision-making are crucial performance determinants in team sports such as football, where fast and accurate decisions are required in a complex and rapidly changing environment [1]. Players must pick up information from the ball, teammates and opponents, and the decision-making process occurs under pressure with opponents trying to restrict "time" and "space" available [2]. To initiate quick actions, athletes must focus their attention and visual perception on the most relevant information sources or key events [3]. This is particularly important considering that athletes are constantly confronted with an abundance of environmental and contextual information in every situation.

A number of studies investigated perceptual abilities of high performance athletes and it was shown that there are fundamental perceptual and cognitive differences between experts and novices [4–6]. For instance, better tactical predictions [7], higher anticipation precision [8], and improved situational adaption of eye movement patterns [9] among the experts have been reported. Casanova *et al.* [10] identified four perceptual-cognitive abilities to illustrate the perceptive superiority of experts compared to novices. These are the ability of players to quickly deduce game-relevant key characteristics (advanced cue utilization), knowledge of situations specific to the sport (situational probabilities), recognition of movement patterns (pattern recognition) and visual search strategy. These qualities are also associated with "game intelligence" [11]. Perceptual-cognitive skills have been described as "executive functions", regulating thought and action, and have been suggested to predict the success of ball sport players [12]. Sheppard *et al.* [13] emphasized the importance of perceptive performance for agility, which is a decisive skill in football. In addition, skills such as anticipation, decision-making, reactivity and creativity are considered key elements of reactive agility [11,14].

Eye-tracking studies have been shown that experts possessed a superior perceptual system when compared to non-experts. For instance, analysis of visual search behavior found that experts had more visual fixations of a shorter duration, recognized game scenes quicker, localized relevant objects more precisely and anticipated actions of their opponents earlier [5,15]. The results of the visual movement tracking show that the complexity of situations in game sports requires a deliberate focus of visual attention just on game-relevant information.

Numerous studies addressed the training modalities of perceptual-cognitive skills. Research into video training over the past two decades focused on perceptual-cognitive skills in team sports [16–20] as well as in individual sports [4,8,21]. Sport-specific, video-based perception training has been confirmed to improve perceptual and cognitive skills (for an overview, see [22,23]). The goal of this form of visual perception training is to accelerate the process of performance development, bringing the perceptual abilities of a novice up to expert level as quick as possible [24]. Video-based studies frequently use the temporal occlusion technique [3,8,25–27] where sport-specific video sequences are interrupted at a certain time, leaving subjects to anticipate the actual outcome of the scene. It has been shown that the perspective of the videos shown can affect the learning rate and, therefore, such videos are typically presented from the "first-person" perspective (*i.e.*, perspective of the player) [28].

Although video-based training has been shown to improve perceptual skills, studies on the transferability to sport-specific performance are scarce. Therefore, the aims of this study were to investigate the effects of video-based visual training on decision-making and the transfer to a reactive-agility sprint test in youth football players. It was hypothesized that video-based visual training will improve decision-making and reactive agility sprint-time.

2. Method

2.1. Participants

A total number of 36 male, trained participants from a national football academy were recruited to participate in the study, which was conducted during the competition phase. Two participants from the control group withdrew and thus 34 players completed the study. The players had a training history of 3–5 years and trained 7–10 $h \cdot week^{-1}$. The performance level can be considered high, as the players competed in the highest Austrian youth league and some of them were part of the junior national team. The study was conducted in accordance with the ethical principles of the Declaration of Helsinki and approved by the institutional review board. The participants and their parents were briefed as to the risks of the study and provided written informed consent to participate.

2.2. Study Design

Participants were matched in accordance with their age category (*i.e.*, U15 and U16) and assigned to either the training group (VIS; n = 18; mean ± SD age: 14.4 ± 0.4 years; stature: 171.2 ± 7.2 cm; body mass: 61.8 ± 8.3 kg) or the control group (CON; n = 16; mean ± SD age: 14.4 ± 0.5 years; stature: 169.5 ± 7.8 cm; body mass: 59.7 ± 8.1 kg). In addition to their regular football training, the VIS group completed a six-week intervention program consisting of video-based visual training performed twice a week. The visual training consists of a series of 5–8 s one-on-one video sequences and requires the players to react in response to the video scene (described below). Before and after the training intervention participants were asked to complete a video-based test to assess anticipation and decision-making. In addition, reactive agility was measured using the sprint test described by Sheppard *et al.* [13]. Participants completed two familiarization days before the study, including all training and testing procedures.

2.3. Construction of Training Videos

Prior to commencement, 12 amateur football players were asked to record video sequences of one-on-one situations with a helmet camera (GoPro HD Hero 2; GoPro Inc., San Mateo, CA, USA) from the first-person perspective of the forward. The videos were recorded at a resolution of 1280 × 960 pixels at 48 frames per second and a viewing angle of 170 degrees. The horizontal and vertical image area enables the capturing of both the defending player and the ball.

The attacking behavior of the defenders was pre-arranged and consisted of the four most common defending tackles. These consisted of block tackling, sliding tackling and both front- and back-foot-side tackling, and were chosen on the basis of a video analysis of various national and international football matches.

Before each recording, the defenders were instructed in which way to tackle the forward and to execute the movement in a realistic, dynamic posture to mimic a real one-on-one situation as accurately as possible. Furthermore, defenders were asked to run toward the forward, match his speed and finally attack him. It was also permitted to use feints, but eventually the pre-arranged tackle must be executed.

From a total number of 800 recorded videos, 456 videos were pre-selected and categorized into one of the four defending tackles. Each of the four categories therefore contained 114 videos and the duration of each video was about 5–8 s. To improve the quality of the recordings, video sequences were edited and blurred recordings were stabilized. From every category 20 videos were excluded to be used for the pre- and post-test and were not included in the training intervention. The remaining video sequences were used for the training group during video-based visual training.

2.4. Training Intervention

Over a period of six weeks, two video-based training sessions per week were completed immediately before regular football training between 17 and 19 h. Each training consisted of 32 randomly presented video sequences (eight per defending category) and lasted ~6 min. The videos were individually presented in quiet rooms adjacent to the changing rooms on four laptops (Lenovo ThinkPad T420s) using a commercially available video player (VLC Media Player).

The videos were prepared using the temporal occlusion technique. This time-sensitive sealing technique stops the video at fixed times, in such a way that only certain elements can be perceived, but not the whole movement. The attention should be drawn toward the most informative stimulus, in order to identify the actions of the opponent as soon as possible and optimize their own reaction time.

Using this technique, a 2 s pause was added at the initiation of the defense. During this brief interruption, the participants were asked to mark either "left" or "right" on a prepared form, indicating the direction they believed the forward could successfully pass the defender. After the pause, the video resumed and subjects were made aware of the outcome of the one-on-one situation, thus receiving feedback on their own response. If no answer was marked during the standstill, the answer was considered false.

2.5. Computer Test

The video-based test consisted of 40 videos (10 per defending category), which were shown at the same time of day and place as the training videos and lasted ~12 min. As described above, these videos were exclusively used for the video-based test and not during the training intervention. The videos were prepared with a specialized video player (Utilius® fairplay 5, CCC Software GmbH, Leipzig, German) to include a time marker at the moment the defender initiated his defensive tackle.

This software contains a stopwatch function with an accuracy of 0.01 s. Additionally, the software enabled smooth playback of HD video recordings and could pause precisely at the push of a button.

In contrast to the training videos, test videos were not paused, but subjects stopped the video sequences by pushing a button, along with a stopwatch running in the background. Immediately after stopping the video, subjects had to shout out "left" or "right", again indicating the direction they believed the forward could successfully pass the defender. The direction as well as the time the video was stopped was noted in a prepared computer test report by the supervisor. The number of successful decisions (*i.e.*, direction) and the temporal delay between the time marker and the moment the video was stopped were used to assess the effects of the video-based training on decision-making and anticipation.

2.6. Reactive-Agility Sprint Test

To assess agility in response to a stimulus, the reactive-agility sprint test was used, as it has been shown to provide reliable and valid results. The test-retest intraclass correlation coefficient (ICC) was 0.878 and the technical error of measurement 0.005 s [13]. In the present study the test was conducted on a football field on artificial turf at sea level, at a temperature of 17° and at a wind speed <2 m·s^{-1} using timing gates (Brower TC Timing Systems; Draper, UT, USA) (Figure 1).

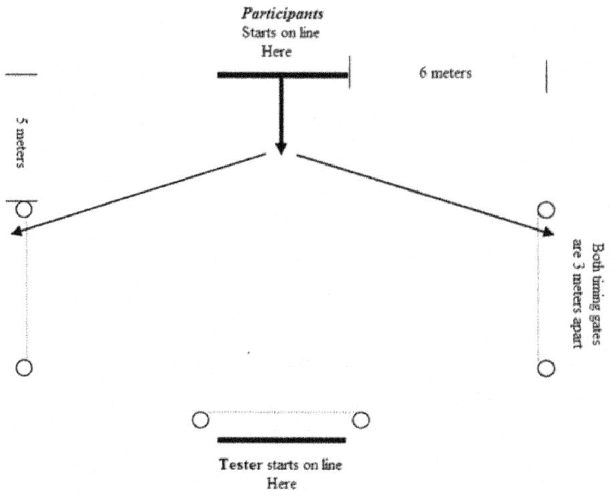

Figure 1. Schematic description of the reactive-agility sprint test [13].

After a standardized warm-up of 15 min, subjects started on the mark opposite to the supervisor and were asked to react as quickly as possible to a tackling stimulus induced by the supervisor by sprinting either to the left or right. The timing was started by the supervisor and stopped by the player by sprinting through the left or right timing gate. Each participant completed six sprints and the average of the sprint times was used to assess reactive agility.

2.7. Statistical Analyses

Statistical analyses were performed with the software SPSS Statistics 21 (IBM Corporation; Armonk, NY, USA). Descriptive data are reported as mean ± standard deviation (SD). After the assumption of normality was verified using the Shapiro-Wilk test, a two-factorial repeated measure analysis of variance with group as the between (VIS *vs.* CON) and time (pre *vs.* post) as the within factor was used to assess the effect of the intervention on response time, response accuracy and sprint time. Significant main effects were followed up with Bonferroni *post-hoc* tests for pairwise comparisons. The level of significance was set at $p < 0.05$.

3. Results

3.1. Computer Test

Response time: There were significant main effects of time ($F_{1,32} = 4.4$; $p = 0.044$) and group ($F_{1,32} = 10.3$; $p = 0.003$). In addition, a significant time × group interaction was observed ($F_{1,32} = 9.8$; $p = 0.004$). The training group significantly improved response time from 0.41 ± 0.10 to 0.31 ± 0.10 s ($p = 0.006$) whereas no significant difference was observed for the control group (0.43 ± 0.09 *vs.* 0.45 ± 0.08 s; $p = 0.297$) (Figure 2).

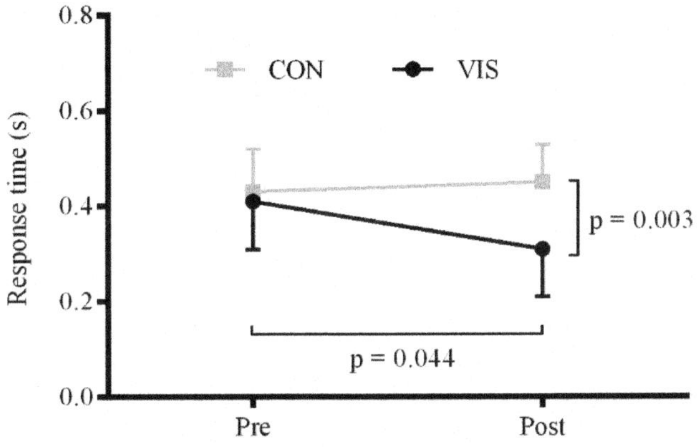

Figure 2. Response time (s) obtained during the computer test. *P*-values for the main effects of time and group are shown. Interactions and *post-hoc* results are presented in the text.

Response accuracy: There were significant main effects of time ($F_{1,32} = 32.9$; $p < 0.001$) and group ($F_{1,32} = 10.0$; $p = 0.003$). In addition, a significant time × group interaction was observed ($F_{1,32} = 12.8$; $p = 0.001$). The training group significantly improved the number of successful decisions from 22.2 ± 3.6 to 29.8 ± 4.5 ($p < 0.001$) whereas no significant difference was observed for the control group (21.6 ± 4.2 *vs.* 23.3 ± 3.8; $p = 0.125$) (Figure 3).

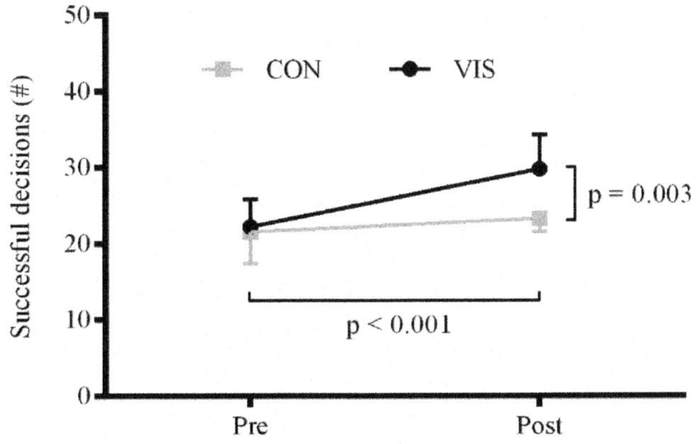

Figure 3. Response accuracy obtained during the computer test. *P*-values for the main effects of time and group are shown. Interactions and *post-hoc* results are presented in the text.

3.2. Reactive-Agility Sprint Test

Sprint time: There was a significant main effect of time ($F_{1,32} = 12.1$; $p = 0.002$) but not of group ($F_{1,32} = 0.5$; $p = 0.495$). A significant time × group interaction was observed ($F_{1,32} = 4.4$; $p = 0.043$).

The training group significantly improved the sprint time from 2.22 ± 0.33 to 1.94 ± 0.11 s (p = 0.001) whereas no significant difference was observed for the control group (2.16 ± 0.24 *vs.* 2.09 ± 0.14 s; p = 0.363) (Figure 4).

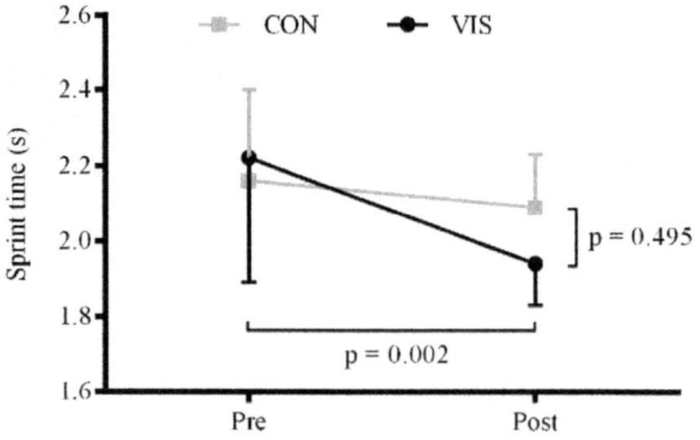

Figure 4. Sprint time (s) obtained during the reactive-agility sprint test. *P*-values for the main effects of time and group are shown. Interactions and *post-hoc* results are presented in the text.

4. Discussion

The aim of this study was to examine the effects of video-based visual training on decision-making and reactive agility in adolescent football players. The main findings were that the visual training group significantly improved response time and response accuracy during the computer test, as well as sprint time obtained from the reactive-agility sprint test. These results suggest that video-based visual training is an appropriate stimulus to train the perception-action coupling in young trained football players.

A number of studies reported differences in perceptual and cognitive skills between experts and novices [4–6] and there is little doubt that experts extract and use the information available (*i.e.*, opponents movement pattern) faster than less-experienced athletes. There is also some evidence of improvements in response time and response accuracy after video-based perceptual training [22,23]. However, there is limited evidence on the transferability into sport performance [25].

The participants in the present study were recruited from a national football academy, had a training history of 3–5 years and underwent the same training during the six-week intervention. The visual training group significantly improved the response time during the computer test by 24% (0.10 s), whereas no significant change (−5% or 0.02 s) was observed in the control group. This result is a 31% difference between the training and the control group after the intervention. Considering the importance of fast decision-making in team sports such as football, this improvement could be a decisive advantage. In addition to fast decision-making, football also requires accurate decisions. In the present study, faster response times did not have negative effects on response accuracy. The visual training group significantly improved the number of successful decisions by 34% (7.56). A small but non-significant change of 8% (1.75) was also found in the control group, resulting in a 28% difference between the training and the control group after the intervention. It could be argued that in a two-choice prediction task (*i.e.*, "left" or "right"), any changes might be the result of guessing. A success rate of approximately 50% (20 successful decisions in the present study) could be expected if a participant is only guessing. However, all but one (–1) participant of the visual training group improved response accuracy. Twelve subjects increased the correct answers by more than five and seven subjects by more than 10 correct answers. In contrast, 10 subjects of the control group improved response accuracy, only two by more than five correct answers. We are therefore confident that our findings are, at least in part, the result of the video-based training.

In addition to the computer-based test, the present study also employed a reactive-agility sprint test to assess the transfer to a field-based performance measure. In accordance with the computer-based test, the visual training group was able to significantly improve sprint time by 13% (0.28 s), while an insignificant change of 3% (0.07 s) was found in the control group. Our results support previous studies in field hockey [29] and rugby [16], showing a transfer from video-based training to field performance. The field test utilized in this study used a semi-specific trigger signal (*i.e.*, tackling stimulus) to induce a more realistic, game-like situation compared with reactive sprint tests that utilize sounds or lights as trigger signals. Given the importance of perception for reactive-agility in football [13], the improvement in reactive-agility sprint time suggests, although does not prove, that video-based training can positively affect game performance. However, reactive-agility is only one of many fitness components in football, thus indicating the complex nature of competitive performance [30]. It should be noted that the participants in our study continued with regular football training during the six-week intervention. However, as the players were from the same national academy and underwent the same training regime, we do not assume a specific effect of athletic training on sprint performance in the visual training group. In addition, the randomization of the groups would minimize such an effect.

In contrast to other studies [17,20,28], where more complex game situations were used to evaluate decision-making, the present study used one-on-one situations recorded from a first-person perspective. The videos were recorded with a helmet camera worn by the forward and therefore represent a dynamic "self-perception" of the playing action. Self-perception has been described as key to mimic the playing action as realistically as possible and to obtain valid and transferable performance effects [28,31]. In accordance with the present study, Hagemann *et al.* [17] found significant improvements in perception-action coupling in three *versus* two game situations.

The training intervention in the present study was conducted over a six-week period, commenced twice a week, and each training session last approximately six minutes. In comparison, previous studies on video-based training used training durations between 10 min and two hours, over time periods up to six weeks [7,16]. It remains to be shown whether or not an increase in training duration and/or number of training sessions could further improve perceptual skills or enhance the transfer into field performance. For example, Williams and Grant [7] reported more pronounced performance improvements in the initial phase compared to the later phase of a video-training intervention. In addition, the longitudinal effects after training cessation need to be further elucidated. Currently, only a few studies reported retained effects in decision-making after two weeks [32] and five months [33], while others did not find such effects after a 32-day retention period [25]. As mentioned above, the participants in our study continued with regular football training during the intervention and it is currently unclear whether or not a video-based visual training alone (e.g., off-season or injury) would improve perceptual-cognitive skills. The efficacy of such training alone without imposing physical strain would further strengthen its practical application.

The study is not without limitations. Firstly, although two familiarization days before the study were conducted to reduce learning effects, we cannot totally exclude such effects associated with the tests. Secondly, this was the first study employing the video-based computer test and, therefore, the test-retest reliability is currently unknown. Thirdly, to increase the ecological validity of the findings, further studies are required to investigate the effects of video-based visual training with the occurrence of fatigue during simulated or actual game situations.

5. Conclusions

In conclusion, the present study showed that video-based visual training results in faster and more accurate decisions during a computer-based test and improves sprint times obtained from a reactive-agility sprint test. It has been shown that youth football players can improve perceptual-cognitive skills with a 6 min video-based training performed twice a week. Therefore, video-based visual training is considered an effective supplement to regular football training. However, further studies are required to investigate the effects in elite-level players, the long-term effects and the efficacy of such training during periods where no specific football training is scheduled.

Acknowledgments: The authors wish to thank the participants for their efforts in this study and the manager and head coaches of the football academy to permit the study.

Author Contributions: Andreas Haller, Nikolaus J. R. Weber and Alfred Nimmerichter designed and conceived the study. Nikolaus J. R. Weber collected the data. Alfred Nimmerichter, Nikolaus J. R. Weber and Andreas Haller analyzed the data. Alfred Nimmerichter, Nikolaus J. R. Weber and Klaus Wirth wrote the original draft of the paper. All authors reviewed and approved the manuscript.

Conflicts of Interest: The authors declare no conflict of interest.

References

1. Ward, P.; Williams, A.M. Perceptual and cognitive skill development in soccer: The multidimensional nature of expert performance. *J. Sport Exerc. Psychol.* **2003**, *25*, 93–111.
2. Williams, A.M. Perceptual skill in soccer: Implications for talent identification and development. *J. Sports Sci.* **2000**, *18*, 737–750. [CrossRef] [PubMed]
3. Cañal-Bruland, R.; Hagemann, N.; Strauß, B. Aufmerksamkeitsbasiertes Wahrnehmungstraining zur taktischen Entscheidungsschulung im Fußball. *Z. für Sportpsychol.* **2005**, *12*, 39–47. [CrossRef]
4. Williams, A.M.; Ward, P.; Smeeton, N.J.; Allen, D. Developing anticipation skills in tennis using on-court instruction: Perception *versus* perception and action. *J. Appl. Sport Psychol.* **2004**, *16*, 350–360. [CrossRef]
5. Williams, A.M.; Davids, K. *Visual Perception and Action in Sport*; E. & F. N. Spon: London, UK, 1999.
6. Mann, D.T.; Williams, A.M.; Ward, P.; Janelle, C.M. Perceptual-cognitive expertise in sport: A meta-analysis. *J. Sport Exerc. Psychol.* **2007**, *29*, 457–478. [PubMed]
7. Williams, A.M.; Grant, A. Training perceptual skill in sport. *Int. J. Sport Psychol.* **1999**, *30*, 194–220.
8. Hagemann, N.; Strauß, B. Perzeptive Expertise von Badmintonspielern. *Z. Psychol.* **2006**, *214*, 37–47. [CrossRef]
9. Abernethy, B.; Zawi, K. Pickup of essential kinematics underpins expert perception of movement patterns. *J. Mot. Behav.* **2007**, *39*, 353–367. [CrossRef] [PubMed]
10. Casanova, F.; Oliveira, J.; Williams, A.M.; Garganta, J. Expertise and perceptual-cognitive performance in soccer: A review. *Rev. Port. De Ciências Do Desporto* **2009**, *9*, 115–122.
11. Roca, A.; Ford, P.R.; Williams, A.M. The processes underlying "game intelligence" skills in soccer players. In *Science and Football VII: The Proceedings of the Seventh World Congress on Science and Football*; Nunome, H., Drust, B., Dawson, B., Eds.; Routledge: London, UK, 2013; pp. 255–260.
12. Vestberg, T.; Gustafson, R.; Maurex, L.; Ingvar, M.; Petrovic, P. Executive functions predict the success of top soccer players. *PLoS ONE* **2012**, *7*, e34731. [CrossRef] [PubMed]
13. Sheppard, J.M.; Young, W.B.; Doyle, T.L.; Sheppard, T.A.; Newton, R.U. An evaluation of a new test of reactive agility and its relationship to sprint speed and change of direction speed. *J. Sci. Med. Sport* **2006**, *9*, 342–349. [CrossRef] [PubMed]
14. Memmert, D. Creativity, expertise, and attention: Exploring their development and their relationships. *J. Sports Sci.* **2010**, *29*, 93–102. [CrossRef] [PubMed]
15. Dicks, M.; Button, C.; Davids, K. Examination of gaze behaviors under *in situ* and video simulation task constraints reveals differences in information pickup for perception and action. *Atten. Percept. Psychophys.* **2010**, *72*, 706–720. [CrossRef] [PubMed]
16. Engelbrecht, L. Sport-specific video-based reactive agility training in rugby union players. Master Thesis, Stellenbosch University, Stellenbosch, South Africa, 2011.
17. Hagemann, N.; Lotz, S.; Canal-Bruland, R. Wahrnehmungs-handlungs-kopplung beim taktischen Entscheidungstraining—Eine exploratorische Studie. *E-J. Beweg. Train.* **2008**, *2*, 17–27.
18. Henry, G.J.; Dawson, B.; Lay, B.S.; Young, W.B. Decision-making accuracy in reactive agility: Quantifying the cost of poor decisions. *J. Strength Cond. Res.* **2013**, *27*, 3190–3196. [CrossRef] [PubMed]
19. Serpell, B.; Young, W.; Ford, M. Are the perceptual and decision-making components of agility trainable? A preliminary investigation. *J. Strength Cond. Res.* **2011**, *25*, 1240–1248. [CrossRef] [PubMed]
20. Vaeyens, R.; Lenoir, M.; Williams, A.M.; Philippaerts, R.M. Mechanisms underpinning successful decision making in skilled youth soccer players: An analysis of visual search behaviors. *J. Mot. Behav.* **2007**, *39*, 395–408. [CrossRef] [PubMed]

21. Hagemann, N.; Schorer, J.; Canal-Bruland, R.; Lotz, S.; Strauss, B. Visual perception in fencing: Do the eye movements of fencers represent their information pickup? *Attent. Percept. Psychophys.* **2010**, *72*, 2204–2214. [CrossRef]
22. Ward, P.; Williams, A.M.; Hancock, P.A. Simulation for performance and training. In *The Cambridge Handbook of Expertise and Expert Performance*; Ericsson, K.A., Charness, N., Feltovich, P.N., Hoffman, R.R., Eds.; Cambridge University Press: New York, NY, USA, 2006; pp. 243–262.
23. Williams, A.M.; Ward, P. Perceptual expertise: Development in sport. In *Expert Performance in Sports*; Starkes, J., Ericsson, K.A., Eds.; Human Kinetics: Chamgaign, IL, USA, 2003; pp. 219–249.
24. Starkes, J.; Lindley, S. Can we hasten expertise by video simulations? *Quest* **1994**, *46*, 211–222. [CrossRef]
25. Farrow, D.; Abernethy, B. Can anticipatory skills be learned through implicit video-based perceptual training? *J. Sports Sci.* **2002**, *20*, 471–485. [CrossRef] [PubMed]
26. Helsen, W.F.; Pauwels, J.M. The relationship between expertise and visual information processing in sport. In *Cognitive Issues in Motor Expertise*; Starkes, J.L., Allard, F., Eds.; Elsevier: Amsterdam, The Netherlands, 1993; pp. 109–134.
27. Schorer, J.; Rienhoff, R.; Fischer, L.; Baker, J. Foveal and peripheral fields of vision influences perceptual skill in anticipating opponents' attacking position in volleyball. *Appl. Psychophysiol. Biofeedback* **2013**, *38*, 185–192. [CrossRef] [PubMed]
28. Roca, A.; Ford, P.R.; McRobert, A.P.; Williams, A.M. Identifying the processes underpinning anticipation and decision-making in a dynamic time-constrained task. *Cogn. Process.* **2011**, *12*, 301–310. [CrossRef] [PubMed]
29. Williams, A.M.; Ward, P.; Chapman, C. Training perceptual skill in field hockey: Is there transfer from the laboratory to the field. *Res. Q. Exerc. Sport* **2003**, *74*, 98–103. [CrossRef] [PubMed]
30. Svensson, M.; Drust, B. Testing soccer players. *J. Sports Sci.* **2005**, *23*, 601–618. [CrossRef] [PubMed]
31. Gibson, J.J. *The Ecological Approach to Visual Perception*; Houghton-Mifflin: Boston, MA, USA, 1979.
32. Gorman, A.; Farrow, D. Perceptual training using explicit and implicit instructional techniques: Does it benefit skilled performers? *Int. J. Sports Sci. Coach.* **2009**, *4*, 193–208. [CrossRef]
33. Abernethy, B.; Schorer, J.; Jackson, R.C.; Hagemann, N. Perceptual training methods compared: The relative efficacy of different approaches to enhancing sport-specific anticipation. *J. Exp. Psychol. Appl.* **2012**, *18*, 143–153. [CrossRef] [PubMed]

2

Physiological Characteristics of Incoming Freshmen Field Players in a Men's Division I Collegiate Soccer Team

Robert G. Lockie *,†, DeShaun L. Davis †, Samantha A. Birmingham-Babauta †, Megan D. Beiley †, Jillian M. Hurley †, Alyssa A. Stage †, John J. Stokes †, Tricia M. Tomita †, Ibett A. Torne † and Adrina Lazar †

Department of Kinesiology, California State University, Northridge, CA 91330, USA;
deshaun.davis.907@my.csun.edu (D.L.D.); samantha.birminghambabauta.162@my.csun.edu (S.A.B.-B.);
megan.beiley.78@my.csun.edu (M.D.B.); jillian.hurley.288@my.csun.edu (J.M.H.);
alyssa.stage.634@my.csun.edu (A.A.S.); john.stokes.91@my.csun.edu (J.J.S.);
tricia.tomita.228@my.csun.edu (T.M.T.); ibett.torne.734@my.csun.edu (I.A.T.);
adrina.lazar.957@my.csun.edu (A.L.)

* Correspondence: robert.lockie@csun.edu

† These authors contributed equally to this work.

Academic Editor: Filipe Manuel Clemente

Abstract: Freshmen college soccer players will have lower training ages than their experienced teammates (sophomores, juniors, seniors). How this is reflected in field test performance is not known. Freshmen ($n = 7$) and experienced ($n = 10$) male field soccer players from the same Division I school completed soccer-specific tests to identify potential differences in incoming freshmen. Testing included: vertical jump (VJ), standing broad jump, and triple hop (TH); 30-m sprint, (0–5, 5–10, 0–10, and 0–30 m intervals); 505 change-of-direction test; Yo-Yo Intermittent Recovery Test Level 2 (YYIRT2); and 6 × 30-m sprints to measure repeated-sprint ability. A MANOVA with Bonferroni *post hoc* was conducted on the performance test data, and effect sizes and z-scores were calculated from the results for magnitude-based inference. There were no significant between-group differences in the performance tests. There were moderate effects for the differences in VJ height, left-leg TH, 0–5, 0–10 and 0–30 m sprint intervals, and YYIRT2 ($d = 0.63$–1.18), with experienced players being superior. According to z-score data, freshmen had meaningful differences below the squad mean in the 30-m sprint, YYIRT2, and jump tests. Freshmen soccer players may need to develop linear speed, high-intensity running, and jump performance upon entering a collegiate program.

Keywords: association football; acceleration; maximal speed; high-intensity running; lower-body power; jump testing; college sports

---

1. Introduction

Participation rates in collegiate men's soccer has increased noticeably from the 1980s and 1990s to the 2000s. In the academic year of 2011–2012, there were over 800 men's teams that featured almost 23,000 players [1]. This volume of players ensures great competition amongst the schools that play collegiate soccer. In order to ensure long-term success for their team in this environment, collegiate coaches from all sports attempt to recruit the best athletes to their respective programs [2]. This will generally involve recruiting players from high school. Once a player is recruited into a soccer program, the coaching and strength and conditioning staff must physically prepare them for the rigors of the collegiate season.

Players straight from high school competing within their first year at university may need more time to positively impact a soccer program. Young athletes will often need to physically mature [3], and will generally have lower training ages in most practice modalities (e.g., high-intensity running and sprinting, strength and power training) when compared to other players on their team [4]. Collegiate athletes are commonly defined by how many years they have been within a program. The general definitions are: freshmen (<2 years); sophomores (3 years); juniors (4 years); and seniors (5 years) [5]. Therefore, freshmen players may be further behind in their physical development when compared to their more experienced teammates.

A further issue for collegiate soccer players is that they will only have a few weeks of pre-season training before they transition into the competitive season [6]. For soccer, this is particularly challenging as this sport places a great demand on a number of different physiological capacities. As a result, field testing batteries for soccer will generally incorporate a range of physiological assessments. This can include assessments of: lower-body power via jump tests, as jumping ability is important for challenging the ball when it is in the air [7], and leg power serves as a foundation for sprinting speed [8]; linear and change-of-direction (COD) speed, which are important skills for attaining ball possession and taking advantage of goal scoring chances [9]; and tests of maximal aerobic capacity and repeated-sprint ability (RSA), which relate to distances covered during a match [10]. These assessments would be useful for the coaching staff in order to understand the characteristics in freshmen soccer players, such that any weaknesses can be targeted during the abbreviated pre-season period.

Therefore, this study investigated the physiological characteristics of freshmen soccer players from a Division I men's program, in order to compare them to experienced players (*i.e.*, sophomores, juniors, and seniors) from the same squad. Only field players were analyzed, due to the dissimilar movement patterns completed by goalkeepers [6,11]. Players were assessed in a bilateral vertical jump (VJ) to indirectly assess leg power in the vertical plane [7,12]; a bilateral and unilateral standing broad jump (SBJ) and triple-hop (TH) from each leg, to indirectly assess leg power in the horizontal plane [13,14]; a 30-m sprint (0–5 m, 0–10 m, and 0–30 m intervals), to assess acceleration and maximum velocity specific to soccer [15–17]; the 505 to measure COD ability [14,15,18]; the Yo-Yo Intermittent Recovery Test level 2 (YYIRT2) to assess soccer-specific aerobic endurance and high-intensity running performance [10,19]; and an RSA test that involved seven 30-m sprints completed on 20-s cycles [20,21]. The hypothesis was that freshmen would perform poorer in each of the field tests when compared to the experienced players. The results from this study will demonstrate those physiological capacities that could be targeted in freshmen soccer players to enhance their development in a Division I collegiate men's team.

2. Materials and Methods

2.1. Subjects

Seventeen field players (age: 20.41 ± 1.54 years; height = 1.81 ± 0.06 m; body mass = 77.54 ± 6.45 kg) from a Division 1 collegiate men's soccer team were recruited for this study. The subjects were required to be: a member of the playing squad and a field player (*i.e.*, defender, midfielder, or forward); over 18 years of age; and injury-free and currently completing full training at the time of testing. As stated, goalkeepers were excluded from this analysis due to dissimilar movement patterns when compared to field players [6,11]. Players were defined by their level of experience and eligibility based on how long they had been in the soccer program, using procedures adapted from Chapman, Whitehead, and Binkert [5]. Two group classifications were used: freshmen (less than two years) and experienced (two years or greater). This resulted in seven players being in the freshmen group (age: 19.21 ± 1.11 years; height = 1.82 ± 0.05 m; body mass = 79.57 ± 8.72 kg), and 10 players in the experienced group (age: 21.20 ± 1.32 years; height = 1.80 ± 0.07 m; body mass = 76.11 ± 4.21 kg). G*Power software (v3.1.9.2, Universität Kiel, Germany) was used to confirm that the sample size of 17 was sufficient for a multivariate analysis of variance (MANOVA), between factors analysis, and ensured the data could be interpreted with a moderate effect level of 0.70 [22–24], and a power level of 0.80 when significance was set at 0.05 [25]. These parameters were set as standardized thresholds for the range of physical performance tests utilized in this research [23,24]. The data used in this study arose as a condition of player monitoring in which player activities were measured over the course of the pre-season [26]. As a result, the institutional ethics committee approved the use and analysis of pre-existing data. The study still conformed to the recommendations of the Declaration of Helsinki, and all subjects received a clear explanation of the study, including the risks and benefits of participation. Each player had also completed the university-mandated physical examination, and read and signed the university consent and medical forms for participation in collegiate athletics.

2.2. Procedures

Testing was incorporated within the team's gym and field sessions that occurred across three weeks in February. All subjects were familiar with the tests performed in this study, as they were consistently used by the team's training staff for general player monitoring. The jump assessments were completed within one gym session, which took approximately 30–45 min to complete. The running assessments were completed prior to field training sessions following the team's usual warm-up. Two field testing sessions were completed, which incorporated the: (1) 30-m sprint, 505 COD speed test, and RSA test; and (2) YYIRT2. The first field session lasted for approximately 60–75 min in duration, while the second field session took approximately 45–60 min. The testing was conducted to fit into the schedule designed by the team's coaching staff, and 48–72 h was provided between each session. In the gym-based session for the jump testing, subjects wore their own athletic trainers, and testing was conducted on a rubber-matted floor. Field testing was conducted on a grass outdoor soccer pitch, and subjects wore their own cleats they used in competition.

Prior to data collection in the first gym testing session, the subject's age, height, and body mass were recorded. Height was measured barefoot using a portable stadiometer (seca, Hamburg, Germany). Body mass was recorded by electronic digital scales (Tanita Corporation, Tokyo, Japan). The gym-based session was preceded by a standardized warm-up designed by the team's coaching staff, consisting of 10 min of jogging, and 10 min of dynamic stretching of the lower limbs. Subjects also completed a standardized warm-up before each field session that was designed by the team's coaching staff, which consisted of 10 min of jogging, 10 min of dynamic stretching of the lower limbs, and linear and lateral runs over 20–30 m that progressively increased in intensity. Examples of the dynamic stretches included walking quadriceps, hamstrings, gluteal, hip flexor, and groin stretches, as well as other dynamic movements, such as running technique drills. This dynamic warm-up followed procedures conducted in previous research that investigated maximal running tests [14,27], thus, the subjects were appropriately prepared for the assessment tasks that were to follow. Subjects completed testing in the order stated in this section, and rotated alphabetically by surname for each test [27], except for the YYIRT2, which was completed as a group. This ensured sufficient recovery periods (*i.e.*, greater than 3 min) between efforts in tests involving multiple trials. A standard metric tape measure was used to measure all distances.

2.3. Vertical Jump (VJ)

The VJ was measured via a jump mat (Just Jump, Probotics Inc., Huntsville, AL, USA) [28]. The subject initially stood on the jump mat keeping their heels on the mat, before completing a countermovement and jumping as high as possible. No preparatory step was used, and no restrictions were placed on the lower-body range of motion during the countermovement. Subjects were free to swing their arms during the jump. This is more practical from a sports perspective, as the arms would generally always be used when jumping during a match to add angular momentum to the jump. Subjects were instructed to maintain straight legs during the flight, before landing on both feet with flexion of the hips, knees, and ankles. Within the software for the mat, jump height was calculated from flight time via the following equation: Jump Height = [$\frac{1}{2}$ × acceleration due to gravity

$(-9.81\ \text{m}\cdot\text{s}^2) \times (\text{total flight time}/2)^2]$ [28]. Each subject completed two trials, and the best trial was used for analysis. The Lewis nomogram was used to calculate the power index [Power ($\text{kg}\cdot\text{m}\cdot\text{s}^{-1}$) = $\sqrt{4.9}$ Body Mass $\sqrt{\text{vertical jump height}}$] [29]. A power index was utilized in this study to standardize for the influence of body mass on VJ height such that heavier subjects would not be penalized [29].

2.4. Standing Broad Jump (SBJ)

The bilateral and unilateral SBJ was performed according to established methods [14]. For the bilateral SBJ, the subject placed the toes of both feet on the back of the starting line, and with a simultaneous arm swing and crouch, then jumped forward as far forward as possible, before finishing with a two-footed landing. Subjects had to execute a correct landing (*i.e.*, "stick" the landing) for the trial to be counted; if not, the trial was disregarded and reattempted. Generally, no more than 1–2 reattempts were required, and the majority of subjects did not need this. No restrictions were placed on the range of the countermovement, or the degree of arm swing used. The distance was measured using a standard tape measure, which was the perpendicular line from the front of the start line to the posterior surface of the back heel at the landing [13,14]. Following the bilateral jumps, subjects completed unilateral jumps in the same manner, for both the left and right legs [14]. Subjects took off from one leg, and then landed on both feet. The distance jumped was measured in the same manner as the bilateral SBJ, and the order of which leg was tested first was randomized. Each subject completed two trials for each jump condition, and the best trial was used.

2.5. Triple Hop (TH)

The TH was used to assess unilateral lower-body functional power [13], and the methods were adapted from Hamilton, Shultz, Schmitz, and Perrin [13]. Similar to the unilateral SBJ, subjects started on one leg with their toes behind the start line. Subjects then completed three consecutive maximal hops, and were required to "stick" the landing on the final hop, and the other leg was not to have any contact with the ground. Failure to do so disqualified the trial, which was reattempted. No more than 1–2 reattempts were generally required for certain subjects. The distance was measured with a standard tape measure from the front of the start line to the posterior surface of the back heel of the leg at the landing [13,14]. Each leg was tested in an alternating order for two trials (four trials total), the order of which was randomized amongst the subjects.

2.6. 30-m Sprint

30-m sprint time was recorded by a timing lights system (Fusion Sports, Coopers Plains, Australia). This timing lights were a single-beam system with microprocessor functionality and error correction processing [30], and previous research has indicated the reliability of sprint testing using this system [31]. Gates were positioned at 0 m, 5 m, 10 m, and 30 m, to measure the 0–5 m, 5–10 m, 0–10 m, and 0–30 m intervals. Sprints over 5 m [15], 10 m [16], and 30 m [17] have been used in the assessment of soccer players. The 0–5 m, 5–10 m, and 0–10 m intervals measured acceleration [8]; the 0–30 m time affords a measure of maximum velocity specific to soccer [17]. Gate height was set at 1.2 m, with a width of 2.5 m, and subjects began the sprint from a standing start 50 cm behind the start line to trigger the first gate. Subjects started at their own time once ready, and they were instructed to run maximally after they initiated their sprint. Subjects completed two trials [3,8], time for each interval was recorded to the nearest 0.001 s, and the fastest trial was used for analysis.

2.7. 505 Change-of-Direction (COD) Speed Test

The methodology for the 505 was used per established methods [14,15,18] with the set-up is shown in Figure 1. Subjects used a standing start with the same body position as the 30-m sprint. The subjects sprinted through the timing gate to the turning line, indicated by a line marked on the grass pitch. Subjects were to place either the left or right foot, depending on the trial, on or behind the turning line, before sprinting back through the gate. Two trials [3,8] were recorded for turns off the left and right side (four trials total), the order of which was randomized amongst the subjects. A researcher was positioned at the turning line, and if the subject changed direction before hitting the turning point, or turned off of the incorrect foot, the trial was disregarded and reattempted after the recovery period. Generally, only 1–2 reattempted trials for those subjects that did miss a trial. Time for each distance was recorded to the nearest 0.001 s, and the fastest trial for each leg was used for analysis.

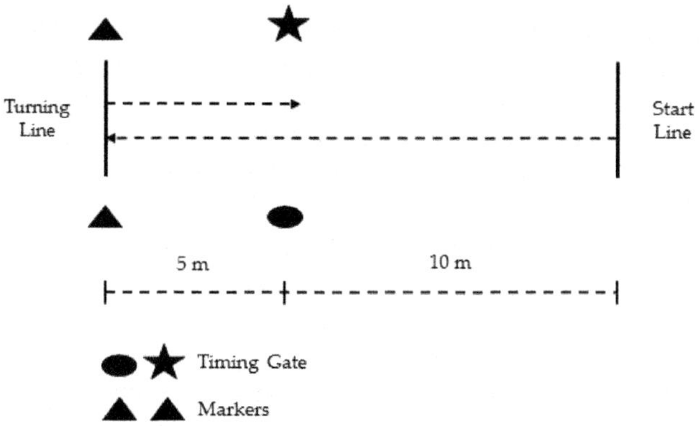

Figure 1. Layout of the 505 COD test. Subjects sprinted over the 10-m distance through the timing gate and over the 5-m distance to the turning line. They then planted either their left or right foot on the turning line to stop and change direction, before sprinting back through the timing gate.

2.8. Yo-Yo Intermittent Recovery Test Level 2 (YYIIRT2)

The YYIRT2 was conducted according to established procedures [10,19]. The test consisted of repeated 2 × 20 m runs at a progressively increased speed. This was controlled by audio beeps from an iPad handheld device (Apple Inc., Cupertino, CA, USA) connected via Bluetooth to a potable speaker (QFX, Inc., Vernon, CA, USA) located immediately adjacent to 20-m long running lanes indicated by markers. Between each running bout, the participants had a 10-s rest period in which they were required to move to a cone 5 m away before returning to the start line. The YYIRT2 started at a speed of 13 kilometers per hour ($km \cdot h^{-1}$), which then increased by 2 $km \cdot h^{-1}$ after the first stage, and 1 $km \cdot h^{-1}$ after the second stage. The test then continued with stepwise 0.5 $km \cdot h^{-1}$ speed increments after every stage until exhaustion. The YYIRT2 was terminated for a subject when they failed to reach the finish line in time on two successive occasions or by volitional exhaustion. This was monitored by the coaching and support staff, and the performance value was recorded as the last completed running bout. All players performed the test within the session. Strong verbal encouragement was provided to players throughout the running of the test.

2.9. Repeated-Sprint Ability (RSA) Test

The RSA test used in this research was adapted from the literature [20,21]. The test consisted of seven 30-m sprints completed on 20-s cycles, shown in Figure 1. Timing lights (Fusion Sports, Coopers Plains, Australia) were used to record the time for each sprint effort to the nearest 0.001 s, and were positioned at the start/finish positions at each end of the sprint zone. The coaches and support staff recorded the recovery intervals with a stopwatch (Accusplit, Pleasanton, CA, USA). After subjects passed through the second timing gate, they decelerated to a marker positioned 10 m past the finish line. This was followed by a 10-m active recovery jog back to the start/finish line for the next sprint (Figure 2). Subjects were required to be stationary at the start position 5 s prior to executing the next sprint, and were provided with feedback as to the progression of the recovery period. Strong verbal encouragement was provided to all subjects by the researchers.

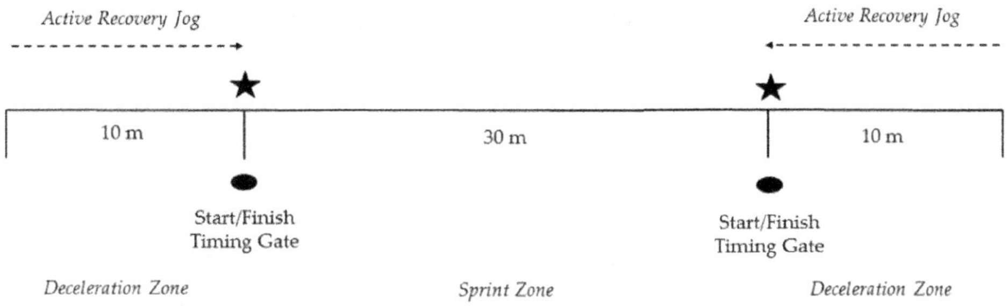

Figure 2. Layout of the RSA test.

Two variables were calculated for the RSA test. They are:

- TT: the sum of all seven sprint times, expressed in s [20,21].
- PD: the decrement in sprint performance was measured as the percent change in sprint time from the first to last sprint [21]. This was calculated via the equation: Percent change (%) = [(last sprint time − first sprint time)/first sprint time] × 100.

2.10. Statistical Analysis

All statistical analyses were computed using the Statistics Package for Social Sciences (Version 22.0; IBM Corporation, New York, NY, USA), and stem-and-leaf plots were used to confirm a normal distribution in the data for each variable. As previously stated, players were placed in groups corresponding to their year of eligibility or experience; freshmen (<2 years' experience) or experienced (≥2 years' experience). Descriptive statistics (mean ± standard deviation [SD]; 95% confidence intervals) were calculated for each test parameter. A MANOVA, with Bonferroni *post hoc* for multiple comparisons, computed any significant differences between age, height, and body mass, the jump assessments, 30-m sprint, 505, YYIRT2, and RSA test measurements. Significance was set at $p < 0.05$. Effect sizes (d) were also calculated for the between-group comparison, where the difference between the means was divided by the pooled SD [32]. In accordance with Hopkins [22], a d less than 0.2 was considered a trivial effect; 0.2 to 0.6 a small effect; 0.6 to 1.2 a moderate effect; 1.2 to 2.0 a large effect; 2.0 to 4.0 a very large effect; and 4.0 and above an extremely large effect. Effect sizes were included in this study to ascertain how much difference existed between the groups irrespective of the p value [23,33], and to provide useful and practical information for the coach and practitioner [23,24].

As significant changes in aspects of athletic performance can be difficult to elicit in trained athletes with longitudinal training [34], this study also incorporated an analysis of worthwhile differences. Buchheit [23] has noted that significance does not inform on magnitude of effects, despite the importance of magnitude. Therefore, this magnitude-based inference analysis was included. The test data for each subject were converted to z-scores, via the formula: z-score = (athlete's test score − average score from the squad)/SD [35]. In accordance with previous recommendations [35] and research [18], the squad mean ($n = 17$) was used in the calculation of the z-score. When appropriate, absolute values for z-scores were derived (e.g., the typical sprint time z-score, where a faster performance equates to a lower sprint time, leads to a negative z-score, so this was converted into an absolute value), such that a positive score above zero represented a superior performance compared to the mean for all tests; a negative score was considered worse than the mean. The mean ± SD for the z-scores were calculated for the freshmen and experienced groups. A worthwhile difference in the z-score was either above or below the squad mean. This was determined by computing the smallest worthwhile change (SWC) in z-score for the test. The SWC for each test was calculated by multiplying the between-subject z-score SD by 0.2, which is the typical small effect [22]. As these were standardized scores, the SD is 1.0, and therefore the SWC is equals 0.2. Thus, those subjects that had a z-score difference (≥0.2 or −0.2) that exceeded the SWC either positively or negatively were deemed to have a meaningful difference in the particular test. These data are important because it also provides useful and practical information for the coach [23,24]. As for the performance test results, a MANOVA with Bonferroni *post hoc* calculated any between-group differences in the z-scores ($p < 0.05$), and effect sizes were calculated. Depending on the results from the z-score data, certain tests were investigated further via individual subject analysis.

3. Results

Table 1 shows the physical characteristics for the freshmen and experienced players. The experienced group were significantly older than the freshmen, although there were no differences in height or body mass.

Table 1. Characteristics (mean ± SD; 95% confidence intervals) of freshmen and experienced players from a Division I collegiate men's soccer team as measured by age, height, and body mass. m: meters; kg: kilograms.

Characteristics	Freshmen (n = 7)	Experienced (n = 10)	p Value	d	d Strength
Age (years)	19.29 ± 1.1 (18.26–20.31)	21.20 ± 1.32 * (20.26–22.14)	0.046	1.57	Large
Height (m)	1.82 ± 0.0 (1.77–1.86)	1.80 ± 0.07 (1.76–1.85)	0.610	0.33	Small
Body Mass (kg)	79.57 ± 8.72 (71.51–87.64)	76.11 ± 4.21 (73.10–79.13)	0.367	0.51	Small

* Significantly different from the freshmen group ($p < 0.05$).

Table 2 displays performance test data. There were no significant differences in any of the jump tests, although there were moderate effects for the greater VJ and left-leg TH for the experienced group. No significant between-group differences were found for the 30-m sprint. There were moderate effects for the 0–5 m, 0–10 m and 0–30 m times, and a trivial effect for the 5–10 m interval. There were also no significant between-group differences in the 505 performed from each leg, nor RSA TT or PD. The greater YYIRT2 distance achieved by the experienced group had a moderate effect, although the difference was not significant.

When considering the z-score analysis for the performance tests (Table 3), there were, again, no significant differences recorded between the experienced and freshmen groups. However, there were numerous examples where a group had a worthwhile difference (z-score $\geqslant 0.2$ or -0.2) above or below the squad mean. The freshmen had a worthwhile difference below the squad mean in each of the jump tests, except VJ power index, the 0–5 m, 0–10 m, and 0–30 m sprint intervals, and the YYIRT2 distance. The experienced group had worthwhile performance differences above the squad mean in the VJ, SBJ, left- and right-leg TH, 0–5 m, 0–10 m, and 0–30 m sprint intervals, and the YYIRT2. The experienced group also had a worthwhile greater PD in the RSA test. Moderate (but non-significant) effects for between-group differences in z-scores were observed for the left-leg TH, the 0–5 m, 0–10 m, and 0–30 m sprint intervals, YYIRT2, and RSA PD. These variables were analyzed further via individual player z-scores.

Table 2. Physiological characteristics (mean ± SD; 95% confidence intervals) of freshmen and experienced players from a Division I collegiate men's soccer team as measured by: vertical jump (VJ); VJ power index (VJ PI); bilateral and unilateral (left and right legs) standing broad jump (SBJ); left- and right-leg triple hop (TH); 30-meter (m) sprint (0–5 m, 0–10 m, and 0–30 m intervals); 505 change-of-direction speed test from the left and right legs; Yo-Yo Intermittent Recovery Test Level 2 (YYIRT2); and total time (TT) and performance decrement from the first to last sprint (PD) from a repeated-sprint ability (RSA) test. kg· m· s^{-1} = kilogram meters per second; s = seconds; %: percentage.

Variables	Freshmen (n = 7)	Experienced (n = 10)	p Value	d	d Strength
VJ (m)	0.62 ± 0.08 (0.55 to 0.70)	0.67 ± 0.08 (0.61 to 0.72)	0.250	0.63	Moderate
VJ PI (kgm· s^{-1})	138.36 ± 13.30 (126.06 to 150.67)	137.38 ± 13.72 (127.56 to 147.19)	0.952	0.07	Trivial
SBJ (m)	2.33 ± 0.26 (2.09 to 2.57)	2.45 ± 0.21 (2.30 to 2.60)	0.324	0.51	Small
SBJ Left (m)	2.10 ± 0.16 (1.95 to 2.24)	2.18 ± 0.21 (1.98 to 2.30)	0.155	0.43	Small
SBJ Right (m)	2.07 ± 0.16 (1.91 to 2.22)	2.14 ± 0.22 (1.98–2.30)	0.082	0.36	Small
TH Left (m)	6.66 ± 0.52 (6.18 to 7.13)	7.04 ± 0.62 (6.51 to 7.56)	0.282	0.66	Moderate
TH Right (m)	6.80 ± 0.72 (6.13 to 7.47)	7.13 ± 0.78 (6.48 to 7.79)	0.244	0.44	Small
0–5 m (s)	1.030 ± 0.040 (0.993 to 1.067)	0.979 ± 0.046 (0.946 to 1.012)	0.060	1.18	Moderate
5–10 m (s)	0.712 ± 0.032 (0.682 to 0.741)	0.711 ± 0.027 (0.692 to 0.730)	0.524	0.03	Trivial
0–10 m (s)	1.742 ± 0.050 (1.696 to 1.788)	1.690 ± 0.059 (1.648 to 1.733)	0.097	0.95	Moderate
0–30 m (s)	4.150 ± 0.149 (4.012 to 4.288)	4.056 ± 0.131 (3.962 to 4.150)	0.157	0.67	Moderate
505 Left (s)	2.245 ± 0.068 (2.182 to 2.308)	2.235 ± 0.198 (2.083 to 2.387)	0.672	0.07	Trivial
505 Right (s)	2.186 ± 0.056 (2.134 to 2.237)	2.210 ± 0.105 (2.129 to 2.291)	0.340	0.29	Small
YYIRT2 (m)	893.33 ± 250.01 (630.96 to 1155.71)	1210.00 ± 379.39 (938.60 to 1481.40)	0.286	0.99	Moderate
RSA TT (s)	32.076 ± 1.310 (30.865 to 33.288)	31.674 ± 0.759 (31.091 to 32.257)	0.279	0.38	Small
RSA PD (%)	3.83 ± 1.93 (2.04 to 5.61)	6.61 ± 5.29 (2.55 to 10.67)	0.083	0.70	Moderate

Table 3. Z-scores (mean ± SD; 95% confidence intervals) and smallest worthwhile change (SWC) above or below the squad mean for freshmen and experienced players from a Division I collegiate men's soccer team as measured by: vertical jump (VJ); bilateral and unilateral (left and right legs) standing broad jump (SBJ); left- and right-leg triple hop (TH); 30-meter (m) sprint (0–5 m, 0–10 m, and 0–30 m intervals); 505 change-of-direction speed test from the left and right legs; Yo-Yo Intermittent Recovery Test Level 2 (YYIRT2); and total time (TT) and performance decrement from the first to last sprint (PD) from a repeated-sprint ability (RSA) test.

Variables	Freshmen (n = 7)	Experienced (n = 10)	p Value	d	d Strength
VJ	−0.32 ± 0.96 § (−1.21 to 0.56)	0.21 ± 1.01 § (−0.51 to 0.94)	0.249	0.54	Small
VJ PI	0.04 ± 1.01 (−0.89 to 0.98)	−0.03 ± 1.04 (−0.78 to 0.71)	0.950	0.07	Trivial
SBJ	−0.28 ± 1.13 § (−1.33 to 0.76)	0.22 ± 0.91 § (−0.43 to 0.87)	0.324	0.49	Small
SBJ Left	−0.29 ± 0.85 § (−1.07 to 0.50)	0.17 ± 1.12 (−0.63 to 0.98)	0.155	0.46	Small
SBJ Right	−0.22 ± 0.82 § (−0.98 to 0.54)	0.14 ± 1.12 (−0.66 to 0.94)	0.082	0.37	Small
TH Left	−0.35 ± 0.85 § (−1.16 to 0.47)	0.30 ± 1.06 § (−0.59 to 1.18)	0.282	0.68	Moderate
TH Right	−0.24 ± 0.96 § (−1.13 to 0.65)	0.21 ± 1.04 § (−0.67 to 1.08)	0.243	0.45	Small
0–5 m	−0.60 ± 0.80 § (−1.34 to 0.14)	0.41 ± 0.93 § (−0.25 to 1.08)	0.060	1.16	Moderate
5–10 m	−0.04 ± 1.14 (−1.09 to 1.02)	0.00 ± 0.97 (−0.69 to 0.69)	0.520	0.04	Trivial
0–10 m	−0.50 ± 0.83 § (−1.27 to 0.26)	0.36 ± 0.99 § (−0.35 to 1.07)	0.096	0.94	Moderate
0–30 m	−0.38 ± 1.04 § (−1.35 to 0.58)	0.28 ± 0.92 § (−0.38 to 0.93)	0.157	0.67	Moderate
505 Left	−0.04 ± 0.45 (−0.45 to 0.37)	0.03 ± 1.31 (−0.98 to 1.04)	0.671	0.07	Trivial
505 Right	0.17 ± 0.66 (−0.44 to 0.78)	−0.12 ± 1.24 (−1.07 to 0.83)	0.342	0.29	Small
YYIRT2	−0.54 ± 0.69 § (−1.26 to 0.18)	0.33 ± 1.04 § (−0.42 to 1.07)	0.286	0.99	Moderate
RSA TT	−0.22 ± 1.29 § (−1.41 to 0.97)	0.17 ± 0.75 (−0.40 to 0.75)	0.280	0.37	Small
RSA PD	0.36 ± 0.45 § (−0.05 to 0.78)	−0.28 ± 1.23 § (−1.23 to 0.66)	0.083	0.69	Moderate

§ SWC greater than 0.2 (superior to squad mean) or less than −0.2 (lower than squad mean).

In the left-leg TH, 6/7 (86%) freshmen were below the squad mean, while 6/10 (60%) of experienced players were above. For the 0–5 m (Figure 3), 0–10 m (Figure 4), and 0–30 m (Figure 5) sprint intervals, 5/7 (71%) of freshmen were below the squad mean. In the experienced players, 6/10 were superior to the mean in the 0–5 m and 0–30 m sprint intervals, while 5/10 (50%) were superior in the 0–10 m interval. In the YYIRT2, 6/7 freshmen performed poorer than the squad mean. 5/10 (50%) experienced players were superior to the mean. Only 2/7 (29%) freshmen were lower than the squad mean in RSA PD, while 7/10 (70%) experienced players were lower.

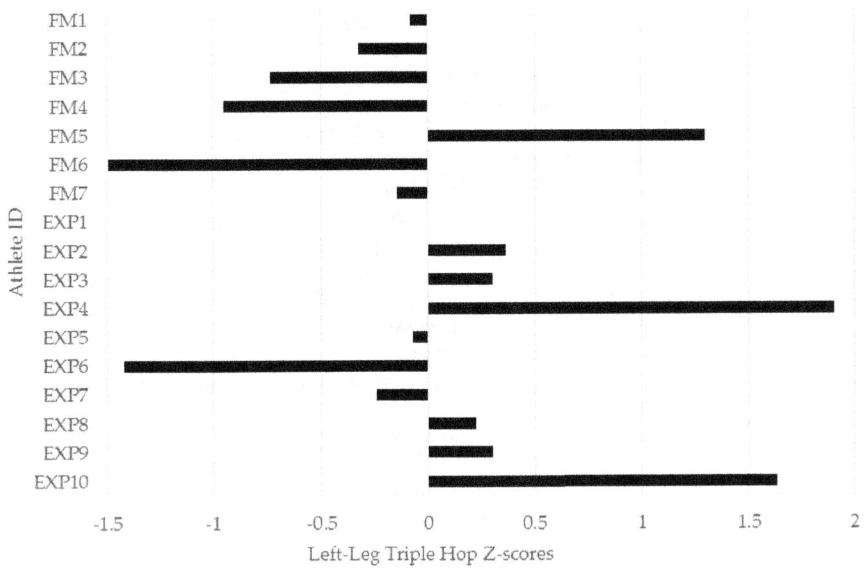

Figure 3. Individual left-leg triple hop z-scores for freshmen (FM) and experienced (EXP) players from a Division I collegiate men's soccer team.

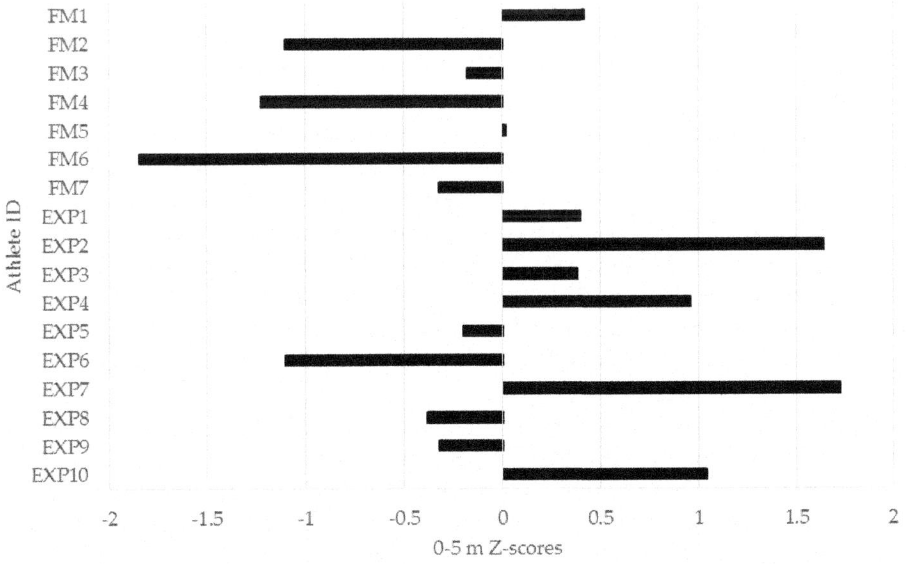

Figure 4. Individual 0–5 meter (m) sprint z-scores for freshmen (FM) and experienced (EXP) players from a Division I collegiate men's soccer team.

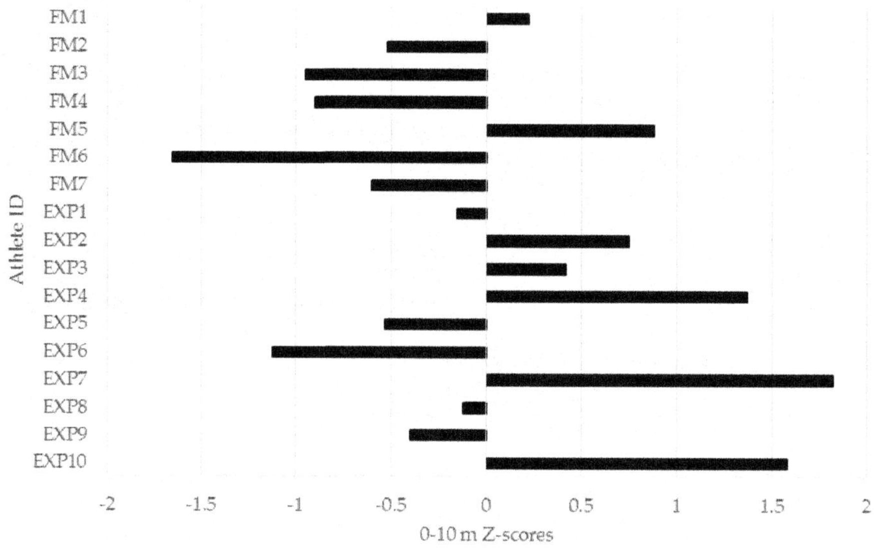

Figure 5. Individual 0–10 meter (m) sprint z-scores for freshmen (FM) and experienced (EXP) players from a Division I collegiate men's soccer team.

4. Discussion

This is the first study to analyze the differences between freshmen and experienced (*i.e.*, sophomores, juniors, and seniors) soccer field players from a Division I men's team in performance tests specific to soccer. The results indicated there were few significant differences between the two groups, which is counter to the study's hypothesis. Experienced players were older (although not taller or heavier; Table 1), and there were no significant differences in the performance tests. Magnitude-based inference analyses indicated some differences in the jump tests, 30-m sprint, YYIRT2, and RSA PD. The z-score analysis also suggested some meaningful differences below the squad mean for the freshmen players in the jump tests (VJ, SBJ, and TH), 30-m sprint, and YYIRT2. In addition to this, the z-score analysis also revealed that, although there was a greater percentage of freshmen players below the squad mean in the 30-m sprint and YYIRT2, there were also experienced players below the standard. The results from this study have implications for collegiate soccer and strength and conditioning coaches.

There were no significant between-group differences in any of the 30-m sprint intervals (Tables 1 and 2). However, it is important to consider magnitudes of difference in sport science research, as this provides the most practical information for a coach [23]. There were moderate effects for the faster 0–5 m, 0–10 m, and 0–30 m sprint intervals for the experienced group (Tables 1 and 2). Additionally, 71% of the freshmen were below the squad mean in the 0–5 m (Figure 4), 0–10 m (Figure 5), and 0–30 m (Figure 6) sprint intervals. Linear speed is a key characteristic for soccer players, as faster running speeds during a match will allow players to position themselves for involvement in play and goal-scoring chances [9]. The results from this study suggest that experienced players from the analyzed squad may have a practically useful difference in linear speed when compared to freshmen [23,24,33]. Nevertheless, what should also be acknowledged is that when considering the individual player data for the 30-m sprint (Figures 4–6), there were still experienced players who were below the squad mean in the different sprint intervals. Although improvements to linear speed could be a focus for incoming freshmen to a men's collegiate soccer team, coaches should carefully monitor the sprinting capacity of experienced players as well.

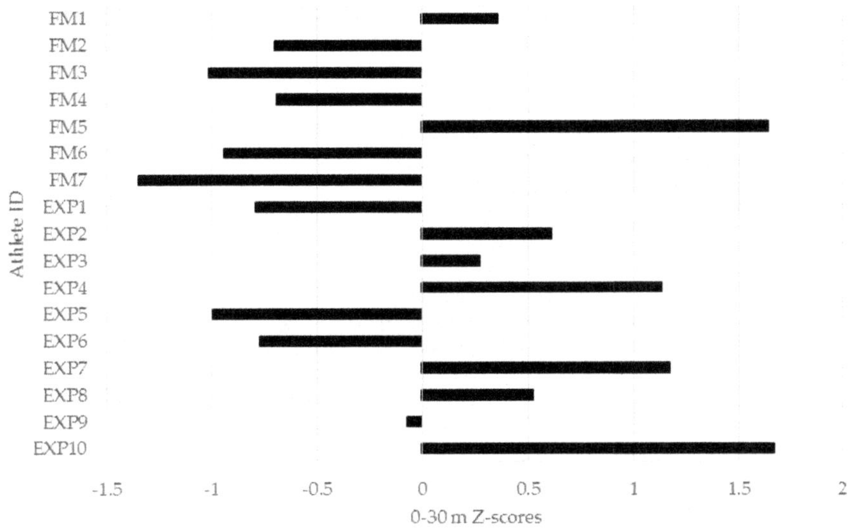

Figure 6. Individual 0–30 meter (m) sprint z-scores for freshmen (FM) and experienced (EXP) players from a Division I collegiate men's soccer team.

The YYIRT2 places great stress on both the aerobic and anaerobic capacity of an athlete, which is shown through reduced levels of creatine phosphate, and high muscle and blood lactate at the end of the test [10]. This provides evidence of the intensity of this assessment, and the YYIRT2 has been validated as a measure of high-intensity running performance in soccer players [19]. In this study, although not significant, there were moderate effects for the greater YYIRT2 distance covered by experienced players when compared to the freshmen group (Tables 2 and 3; Figure 7). The magnitude of this difference [23,24,33] suggests that the experienced collegiate players in this study may have a better ability to tolerate the intensity of the YYIRT2 than the freshmen. Given that international-level soccer players perform better in the YYIRT2 when compared to their lesser counterparts [10], superior performance in the YYIRT2 should also benefit players at the college level. When considering the structure of the test, this could relate to a greater distance covered and more high-intensity running efforts performed during a match [10,19]. These results suggest that high-intensity running training could also be a focus for incoming freshmen to a collegiate men's soccer program. Nevertheless, the individual z-scores for the YYIRT2 illustrated that there were still experienced players meaningfully below the mean for the squad (Figure 7). Strength and conditioning coaches should also ensure that all experienced players are up to standard in high-intensity running performance as measured by the YYIRT2.

Lower-body power, which can be extrapolated from jump testing [8], is also an essential quality for soccer players. An effective VJ is needed when challenging for possession if the ball is in the air [36], while horizontal power, which can be inferred from SBJ and TH performance [13,14], has been linked to faster sprinting speeds in team sport athletes [27]. There were no significant differences between the two groups in any of the jump tests, and VJ power was almost identical between the two groups (Table 2). Nonetheless, magnitude-based inference [23,24,33] indicated meaningful differences below the squad mean in VJ height and the horizontal jump distances in freshmen players, and a moderate difference between the groups in the left-leg TH (Table 3). Indeed, 86% of freshmen performed worse than the squad mean in the left-leg TH (Figure 3). Hamilton, Shultz, Schmitz, and Perrin [13] found that TH distance positively related to both VJ height and isokinetic knee extensor strength in collegiate men's and women's soccer players, providing evidence of its validity as a lower-body performance test. Collectively, the z-score data suggests freshmen soccer players may need to improve jump performance and lower-body power upon their entry into a collegiate program, and this may be more evident in a unilateral jump test such as the TH.

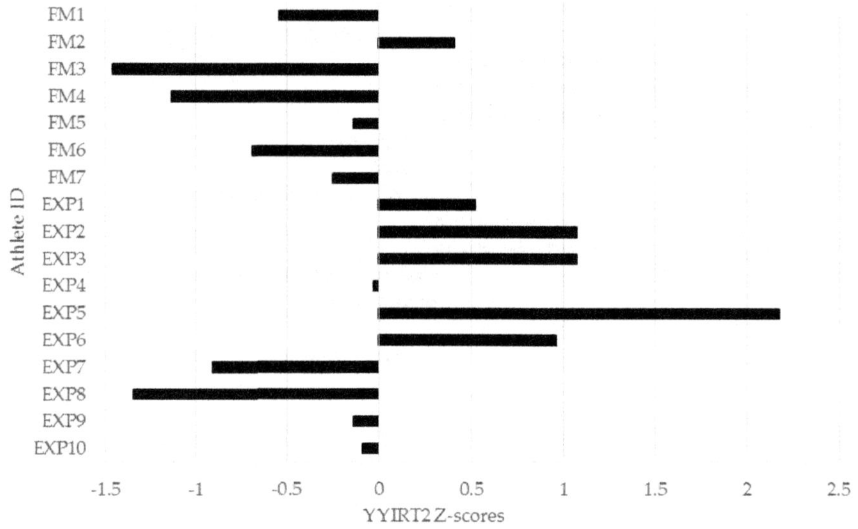

Figure 7. Individual Yo-Yo Intermittent Recovery Test Level 2 (YYIRT2) sprint z-scores for freshmen (FM) and experienced (EXP) players from a Division I collegiate men's soccer team.

There were no significant differences between the freshmen and experienced groups for 505 time from both legs (Table 2), and the z-scores were also close to the squad mean for both groups (Table 3). Within an elite English soccer game, Bloomfield, Polman, and O'Donoghue [11] reported that soccer players perform on average over 700 direction changes. It could be expected that a high volume of COD maneuvers would also occur within soccer matches at lower levels of play, such as high school and collegiate competition. As a result, both the freshmen and experienced players may be effectively conditioned in COD ability from prior training and soccer-playing experience, which could have influenced the study results. Further to this, the 505 only features one, 180° cut [14,15,18]. The number and angle of direction changes can affect how COD ability is assessed [31]. More complex COD tests may present different results in comparisons between freshmen and experienced collegiate men's soccer players, which should be investigated in future research.

Given the results from the 30-m sprint, it could be expected that there would also be differences in the RSA TT when comparing the freshmen and experienced groups. This is because a higher maximal sprinting velocity has been related to lower total times in RSA tests conducted on elite Norwegian [37] and Brazilian [38] male soccer players; however, this was not the case in this research (Tables 2 and 3). The experienced players did have a worthwhile difference above the squad mean for RSA PD (Table 3 and Figure 8), which suggested a greater percentage time drop-off from the first to last sprint. Indeed, one experienced player had a large RSA PD z-score of −2.63. These data could potentially relate to a higher sprinting speed (and, thus, lower sprint time) achieved in the first sprint, which is understandable given the moderately [23,24,33] faster 30-m sprint time achieved by experienced players in the linear speed test (Table 2). Nonetheless, the difference in RSA PD was not significantly different to that from the freshmen group (Tables 2 and 3). The results from this study suggest that the RSA test conducted did not differentiate between freshmen and experienced collegiate men's soccer players from this study.

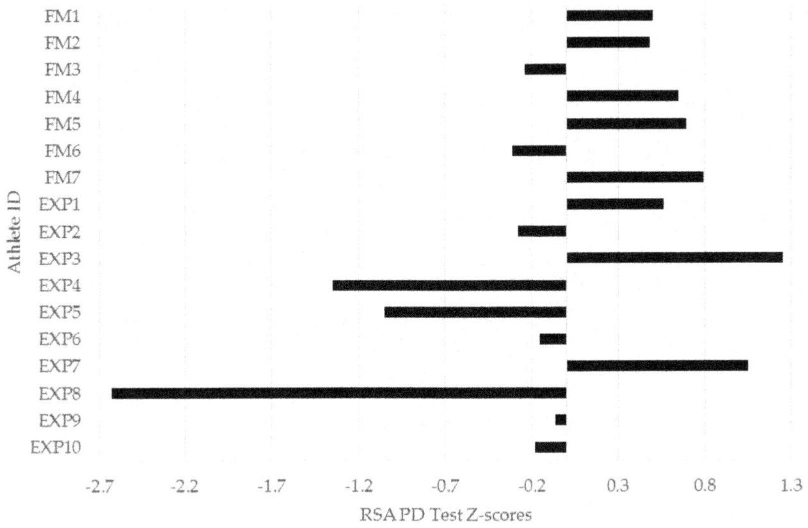

Figure 8. Individual sprint performance decrement from the repeated-sprint ability test (RSA PD) z-scores for freshmen (FM) and experienced (EXP) players from a Division I collegiate men's soccer team.

There are certain limitations with this research that should be discussed. Only one squad was analyzed ($n = 17$), and the sample size dictated using two groups in this study (*i.e.*, freshmen and experienced). A larger sample could have potentially allowed the analysis of players by each year of experience group (*i.e.*, freshmen, sophomores, juniors and seniors). Although analyzing the data via two groups increased the statistical power [25], future research should attempt to increase sample size to investigate any physiological and performance differences between male collegiate soccer players from each year of experience. No measures of lower-body strength were included in this study. The coaching staff for the soccer squad restricted the use of maximum strength testing, due to a perceived risk of injury during testing [39]. As lower-body strength has been related to superior jumping [12,40] and sprinting [40] performance in athletic populations, future research should measure the maximal strength of freshmen and experienced men's collegiate soccer players. Only one form of COD speed (*i.e.*, the 505) and RSA (*i.e.*, 6 × 30-m sprints completed on 20-s cycles) test were measured in this research. There could potentially be a different response by freshmen and collegiate soccer players if other COD speed or RSA tests were used, and this could be elucidated in future studies. Nonetheless, within the context of these limitations, this study demonstrated that there are certain differences (*i.e.*, linear speed measured by a 30-m sprint and high-intensity running measured by the YYIRT2) between freshmen and experienced collegiate soccer players from a Division I men's team.

5. Conclusions

There were no significant differences in soccer-specific performance tests between freshman and experienced collegiate male players. However, magnitude-based inferences indicated some practical disparities in selected assessments that could have implications for freshmen players and their coaches. Linear speed could be targeted for improvement in freshmen soccer players. Additionally, high-intensity running performance, as measured by the YYIRT2, may need to be enhanced early in a freshmen collegiate players' career. There would also likely be experienced players within a squad that need to improve their maximal sprinting and high-intensity running performance, and coaches should be cognizant of this. The study results also suggested that there were meaningfully lower performances in VJ height, and SBJ and TH distance, in addition to the 30-m sprint and YYIRT2, in the freshmen group. Thus, sprinting speed, high-intensity running, and jump performance could be a focus for freshmen male soccer players entering a collegiate program.

Acknowledgments: This research project received no external financial assistance. None of the authors have any conflict of interest. The authors would like to acknowledge the participants for their contribution to the study. Thanks also to Keith West and Jeff Crelling for facilitating this research, and Dominic Giuliano, Matthew Moreno, Ashley Orjalo, and Fabrice Risso for assisting with data collection.

Author Contributions: Robert G. Lockie was involved in study design, data collection, data interpretation, and manuscript writing. DeShaun L. Davis, Samantha A. Birmingham-Babauta, Megan D. Beiley, Jillian M. Hurley, Alyssa A. Stage, John J. Stokes, Tricia M. Tomita, Ibett A. Torne, and Adrina Lazar were involved in data collection, data interpretation, and manuscript editing.

Conflicts of Interest: The authors declare no conflict of interest.

Abbreviations

The following abbreviations are used in this manuscript:

COD	Change-of-direction
RSA	Repeated-sprint ability
VJ	Vertical jump
SBJ	Standing broad jump
TH	Triple hop
m	Meter
YYIRT2	Yo-Yo Intermittent Recovery Test level 2
s	Second
$km \cdot h^{-1}$	Kilometers per hour
RSA TT	sum of all sprint times from the RSA test
PSA PD	sprint time decrement measured as percentage from first to last sprint in RSA test
SD	Standard deviation
p	Significance
d	Effect size
SWC	Smallest worthwhile change
FM	Freshmen
EXP	Experienced

References

1. NCAA. *Ncaa Sports Sponsorship and Participation Rates Report 1981-1982–2010-2011*; NCAA: Indianapolis, IN, USA, 2012.
2. Bergman, S.A.; Logan, T.D. The effect of recruit quality on college football team performance. *J. Sports Econ.* **2014**. [CrossRef]
3. Dupler, T.L.; Amonette, W.E.; Coleman, A.E.; Hoffman, J.R.; Wenzel, T. Anthropometric and performance differences among high-school football players. *J. Strength Cond. Res.* **2010**, *24*, 1975–1982. [CrossRef] [PubMed]
4. Hoffman, J.R.; Ratamess, N.A.; Kang, J. Performance changes during a college playing career in NCAA Division III football athletes. *J. Strength Cond. Res.* **2011**, *25*, 2351–2357. [CrossRef] [PubMed]
5. Stodden, D.F.; Galitski, H.M. Longitudinal effects of a collegiate strength and conditioning program in American football. *J. Strength Cond. Res.* **2011**, *24*, 2300–2308. [CrossRef] [PubMed]
6. Chapman, P.P.; Whitehead, J.R.; Binkert, R.H. The 225-1b reps-to-fatigue test as a submaximal estimate of 1-rm bench press performance in college football players. *J. Strength Cond. Res.* **1998**, *12*, 258–261. [CrossRef]
7. Arent, S.M.; Pellegrino, J.K.; Williams, C.A.; Difabio, D.A.; Greenwood, J.C. Nutritional supplementation, performance, and oxidative stress in college soccer players. *J. Strength Cond. Res.* **2010**, *24*, 1117–1124. [CrossRef] [PubMed]
8. Boone, J.; Vaeyens, R.; Steyaert, A.; Vanden Bossche, L.; Bourgois, J. Physical fitness of elite belgian soccer players by player position. *J. Strength Cond. Res.* **2012**, *26*, 2051–2057. [CrossRef] [PubMed]
9. Lockie, R.G.; Murphy, A.J.; Knight, T.J.; Janse de Jonge, X.A.K. Factors that differentiate acceleration ability in field sport athletes. *J. Strength Cond. Res.* **2011**, *25*, 2704–2714. [CrossRef] [PubMed]
10. Faude, O.; Koch, T.; Meyer, T. Straight sprinting is the most frequent action in goal situations in professional football. *J. Sports Sci.* **2012**, *30*, 625–631. [CrossRef] [PubMed]

11. Krustrup, P.; Mohr, M.; Nybo, L.; Jensen, J.M.; Nielsen, J.J.; Bangsbo, J. The yo-yo ir2 test: Physiological response, reliability, and application to elite soccer. *Med. Sci. Sports Exerc.* **2006**, *38*, 1666–1673. [CrossRef] [PubMed]
12. Bloomfield, J.; Polman, R.; O'Donoghue, P. Physical demands of different positions in fa premier league soccer. *J. Sports Sci. Med.* **2007**, *6*, 63–70. [PubMed]
13. Wisloff, U.; Castagna, C.; Helgerud, J.; Jones, R.; Hoff, J. Strong correlation of maximal squat strength with sprint performance and vertical jump height in elite soccer players. *Br. J. Sports Med.* **2004**, *38*, 285–288. [CrossRef] [PubMed]
14. Hamilton, R.T.; Shultz, S.J.; Schmitz, R.J.; Perrin, D.H. Triple-hop distance as a valid predictor of lower limb strength and power. *J. Athl. Train.* **2008**, *43*, 144–151. [CrossRef] [PubMed]
15. Lockie, R.G.; Schultz, A.B.; Jordan, C.A.; Callaghan, S.J.; Jeffriess, M.D.; Luczo, T.M. Can selected functional movement screen assessments be used to identify movement deficiencies that could affect multidirectional speed and jump performance? *J. Strength Cond. Res.* **2015**, *29*, 195–205. [CrossRef] [PubMed]
16. Maio Alves, J.M.; Rebelo, A.N.; Abrantes, C.; Sampaio, J. Short-term effects of complex and contrast training in soccer players' vertical jump, sprint, and agility abilities. *J. Strength Cond. Res.* **2010**, *24*, 936–941. [CrossRef] [PubMed]
17. Sporis, G.; Jukic, I.; Ostojic, S.M.; Milanovic, D. Fitness profiling in soccer: Physical and physiologic characteristics of elite players. *J. Strength Cond. Res.* **2009**, *23*, 1947–1953. [CrossRef] [PubMed]
18. Magal, M.; Smith, R.T.; Dyer, J.J.; Hoffman, J.R. Seasonal variation in physical performance-related variables in male ncaa division iii soccer players. *J. Strength Cond. Res.* **2009**, *23*, 2555–2559. [CrossRef] [PubMed]
19. Nimphius, S.; Callaghan, S.J.; Sptieri, T.; Lockie, R.G. Change of direction deficit: A more isolated measure of change of direction performance than total 505 time. *J. Strength Cond. Res.* **2016**. in press. [CrossRef] [PubMed]
20. Karakoç, B.; Akalan, C.; Alemdaroğlu, U.; Arslan, E. The relationship between the yo-yo tests, anaerobic performance and aerobic performance in young soccer players. *J. Hum. Kinet.* **2012**, *35*, 81–88. [CrossRef] [PubMed]
21. Chaouachi, A.; Manzi, V.; Wong del, P.; Chaalali, A.; Laurencelle, L.; Chamari, K.; Castagna, C. Intermittent endurance and repeated sprint ability in soccer players. *J. Strength Cond. Res.* **2010**, *24*, 2663–2669. [CrossRef] [PubMed]
22. Pyne, D.B.; Saunders, P.U.; Montgomery, P.G.; Hewitt, A.J.; Sheehan, K. Relationships between repeated sprint testing, speed, and endurance. *J. Strength Cond. Res.* **2008**, *22*, 1633–1637. [CrossRef] [PubMed]
23. Hopkins, W.G. How to interpret changes in an athletic performance test. *Sportscience* **2004**, *8*, 1–7.
24. Buchheit, M. The numbers will love you back in return—I promise. *Int. J. Sports Physiol. Perform.* **2016**, *11*, 551–554. [CrossRef] [PubMed]
25. Winter, E.M.; Abt, G.A.; Nevill, A.M. Metrics of meaningfulness as opposed to sleights of significance. *J. Sports Sci.* **2014**, *32*, 901–902. [CrossRef] [PubMed]
26. Faul, F.; Erdfelder, E.; Lang, A.G.; Buchner, A. G*power 3: A flexible statistical power analysis program for the social, behavioral, and biomedical sciences. *Behav. Res. Methods* **2007**, *39*, 175–191. [CrossRef] [PubMed]
27. Winter, E.M.; Maughan, R.J. Requirements for ethics approvals. *J. Sports Sci.* **2009**, *27*, 985. [CrossRef] [PubMed]
28. Lockie, R.G.; Jeffriess, M.D.; Schultz, A.B.; Callaghan, S.J. Relationship between absolute and relative power with linear and change-of-direction speed in junior american football players from australia. *J. Aust. Strength Cond.* **2012**, *20*, 4–12.
29. McFarland, I.; Dawes, J.J.; Elder, C.; Lockie, R. Relationship of two vertical jumping tests to sprint and change of direction speed among male and female collegiate soccer players. *Sports* **2016**, *4*. [CrossRef]
30. Stockbrugger, B.A.; Haennel, R.G. Contributing factors to performance of a medicine ball explosive power test: A comparison between jump and nonjump athletes. *J. Strength Cond. Res.* **2003**, *17*, 768–774. [CrossRef] [PubMed]
31. Fusion Sport. Timing Accuracy: Are You up to Speed? 2010. Available online: http://www.fusionsport.com/support/product-information/research-tech-specs?download=54:timing-accuracy-research-update (accessed on 23 May 2016).

32. Lockie, R.G.; Schultz, A.B.; Callaghan, S.J.; Jeffriess, M.D.; Berry, S.P. Reliability and validity of a new test of change-of-direction speed for field-based sports: The change-of-direction and acceleration test (codat). *J. Sports Sci. Med.* **2013**, *12*, 88–96. [PubMed]
33. Cohen, J. *Statistical Power Analysis for the Behavioral Sciences*, 2nd ed.; Lawrence Earlbaum Associates: Hillsdale, NJ, USA, 1988; p. 567.
34. Durlak, J.A. How to select, calculate, and interpret effect sizes. *J. Pediatr. Psychol.* **2009**, *34*, 917–928. [CrossRef] [PubMed]
35. McGuigan, M.R.; Cormack, S.J.; Gill, N.D. Strength and power profiling of athletes: Selecting tests and how to use the information for program design. *Strength Cond. J.* **2013**, *35*, 7–14. [CrossRef]
36. Haugen, T.A.; Tonnessen, E.; Seiler, S. Speed and countermovement-jump characteristics of elite female soccer players, 1995–2010. *Int. J. Sports Physiol. Perform.* **2012**, *7*, 340–349. [PubMed]
37. Ingebrigtsen, J.; Brochmann, M.; Castagna, C.; Bradley, P.S.; Ade, J.; Krustrup, P.; Holtermann, A. Relationships between field performance tests in high-level soccer players. *J. Strength Cond. Res.* **2014**, *28*, 942–949. [CrossRef] [PubMed]
38. Da Silva, J.F.; Guglielmo, L.G.; Bishop, D. Relationship between different measures of aerobic fitness and repeated-sprint ability in elite soccer players. *J. Strength Cond. Res.* **2010**, *24*, 2115–2121. [CrossRef] [PubMed]
39. West, D.J.; Owen, N.J.; Jones, M.R.; Bracken, R.M.; Cook, C.J.; Cunningham, D.J.; Shearer, D.A.; Finn, C.V.; Newton, R.U.; Crewther, B.T.; *et al.* Relationships between force-time characteristics of the isometric midthigh pull and dynamic performance in professional rugby league players. *J. Strength Cond. Res.* **2011**, *25*, 3070–3075. [CrossRef] [PubMed]
40. Cronin, J.B.; Hansen, K.T. Strength and power predictors of sports speed. *J. Strength Cond. Res.* **2005**, *19*, 349–357. [CrossRef] [PubMed]

3

Autonomy Mediates the Relationship between Personality and Physical Activity: An Application of Self-Determination Theory

Meredith L. Ramsey and Eric E. Hall *

Department of Exercise Science, Elon University, Elon, NC 27244, USA; mramsey3@elon.edu
* Correspondence: ehall@elon.edu

Academic Editor: Eling de Bruin

Abstract: This study sought to examine tenets of Self-Determination Theory by testing a mediation model of physical activity and personality via autonomy. A total of 290 adults were recruited to complete a one-time online survey of exercise habits and individual characteristics. Surveys assessed personality, autonomy, and physical activity. A measurement model specifying direct effects between personality dimensions and physical activity and indirect effects operating through autonomy provided an excellent fit to the data ($X^2 = 0.66$, $df = 3$, $p = 0.88$, RMSEA(90% CI) = 0.00 (0.00–0.05), CFI = 0.99, SRMR = 0.01). Results indicated significant ($p < 0.05$) effects of Extroversion ($\beta = 0.42$), Conscientiousness ($\beta = 0.96$), and Emotional Stability ($\beta = 0.60$) on autonomy, which in turn, was significantly associated with physical activity ($\beta = 0.55$). No significant effects were observed for Agreeableness or Intellect. None of the personality constructs were found to be directly associated with physical activity. This model accounted for 27% of the variance in physical activity. The results of this study suggest that autonomy is significantly associated with physical activity. Therefore, attempts to improve autonomy in individuals may be a useful intervention strategy in improving physical activity levels.

Keywords: personality; physical activity; autonomy; self-determination

1. Introduction

Despite recent and widespread public health initiatives to increase physical activity, physical inactivity continues to plague today's society [1,2]. The American College of Sports Medicine recommends that adults should engage in at least 150 min of moderate-intensity exercise each week for cardiorespiratory fitness. This can be accomplished by engaging in moderate-intensity exercise for 30 to 60 min 5 days per week or vigorous-intensity exercise 20 to 60 min 3 days per week [3]. Currently only 43.5% of American adults meet this requirement [1]. Living a sedentary lifestyle has shown many negative health implications including increased risk of cardiovascular disease, metabolic disorders, musculoskeletal disorders, psychological disorders, pulmonary diseases, and some cancers [2].

One theory that has been used to examine motivations and their relationship with physical activity behavior is Self-Determination Theory (SDT) [4]. SDT helps to explain affective, cognitive, and behavioral response within an achievement activity and has been used in multiple areas such as academics and athletics; with more recent efforts to examine these principles within the exercise domain [4,5]. SDT suggests that motivation lies on a continuum ranging from amotivation to intrinsic motivation. Amotivation is described as having no motivation to engage in an activity while intrinsic motivation is when an activity is not done for reward or any form of reinforcement, but done for fun, enjoyment or pleasure [5]. Extrinsic motivation falls between the two and is done because the person expects some sort of reward or outcome [5]. When moving across the continuum from amotivation to intrinsic motivation there is a growing amount of autonomy or self-determination [4]. A recent systematic review found there is positive relationship between more autonomous forms of motivation and physical activity behavior and adherence [6]. These consistent findings have led to theory based interventions, using SDT, to improve autonomy and promote physical activity [7].

In addition to SDT, previous research has examined the relationship between personality and physical activity and found that extraversion, conscientiousness, and neuroticism of the five factor model [8,9] are related to exercise behaviors [10–12]. A recent meta-analysis by Wilson and Dishman [13] utilizing 64 studies found small, significant correlations for extraversion, neuroticism and conscientiousness similar to the previous studies mentioned, but also found a relationship with openness. The findings that extraversion and neuroticism are related to physical activity level is consistent with Eysenck's theory of personality which suggests that extraverts will seek out sensory stimulation (e.g., exercise) and people high in neuroticism may avoid stimulation because of higher levels of negative affect and heightened autonomic response [14]. It is possible that conscientiousness is related to physical activity because it may help the individual satisfy their need for competence and self-regulation [15].

Only two known studies have attempted to examine both SDT and personality as they related to physical activity [15,16]. Ingledew and colleagues [15] examined personality and self-determination in relation to exercise for individuals in the maintenance stage of change. The results indicated participants who were less neurotic, more extroverted, and more conscientious were more likely to be self-determined (higher autonomy) in regard to exercise. A limitation of this study was that they did not try to predict physical activity behavior based on the measures of autonomy and personality, and they only used individuals in the maintenance stage in their data analysis. Furthermore, a study conducted by Lewis and Sutton [16] sought to determine the relationship between personality and exercise participation, while also trying to determine if the relationship was mediated by autonomy. The results indicated that more autonomous behavior was positively correlated with exercise participation. Also, extroversion, conscientiousness, and agreeableness were positively related to increased exercise frequency with extroversion and conscientiousness being mediated by intrinsic and external motivation [16].

The purpose of the current study was to determine the relationship between personality, autonomy, and physical activity behavior. It was hypothesized that personality and autonomy would be directly related to physical activity, but the relationships between personality and physical activity may be mediated by autonomy. It is important to examine mediating pathways through autonomy to identify potential mechanisms as well as target points for intervention, autonomy provides a modifiable pathway by which physical activity levels might be impacted in the presence of certain personality traits.

2. Methods

2.1. *Participants*

Two hundred ninety adults were recruited for this study (218 females, 64 males, 8 non-reported; mean age 23.9 ± 9.2 years; mean BMI 23.8 ± 5.0; 91.7% Caucasian). Participants were recruited through postings on the university website as well as through social media postings by the authors. The study was approved by the university's IRB and all participants read and consented to participate in the study.

2.2. *Measures*

The International Personality Item Pool (IPIP) [17] was used to assess personality based on dimensions of extraversion, agreeableness, conscientiousness, emotional stability (opposite of neuroticism), and intellect/imagination [18,19]. There were a total of 50 questions with 10 questions being for each sub-scale and Previous research has found scales generated from the IPIP to be valid and reliable [18,19].

The Behavioral Regulation in Exercise Questionnaire-2 (BREQ-2) [20] was used to measure self-determination and is based on five dimensions including amotivation, external regulation, introjected regulation, identified regulation, and intrinsic regulation. These items from the BREQ-2 are weighed and then aggregated to determine the Relative Autonomy Index with higher scores representing greater autonomy [20]. The Relative Autonomy Index as derived by BREQ-2 has been previously shown to predict physical activity levels [21].

The Godin Leisure-Time Exercise Questionnaire (GLTEQ) was used to assess physical activity habits over a 7-day period [22]. It asks how often individuals engage in light, moderate, and strenuous activities for at least 15 min or more. From these questions a total met score for the past week was determined.

2.3. Procedures

The participants completed a one-time online survey. The survey included the informed consent which they electronically singed as well as the IPIP scale, BREQ-2 and the GLTEQ as well as self-reported demographic questions. At the end of the survey the participants were given the opportunity to enter them into the drawing for a gift card. Participant remuneration was structured such that one out of every 10 participants was randomly selected to receive a $20 gift card.

2.4. Statistical Analysis

Structural equation modeling (SEM) using MPLUS modeling software (V. 5.1) was used to test the fit of the hypothesized physical activity model (Figure 1). This model specified: (a) direct effects of each of the 5 IPIP sub-scales on physical activity; and (b) indirect effects of the 5 IPIP dimensions on physical activity *through* autonomy. SEM, an extension of general linear modeling, was the preferred analytic method for it allows researchers to test a series of regression equations simultaneously, and unlike regression analysis, does so while accounting for measurement error in the model [23]. Another strength of SEM is that it is designed to test direct and indirect (*i.e.*, mediating) effects among variables. However, SEM has the same limitations of any other type of analyses applied to cross-sectional data, namely that it cannot assess causal relationships in such instances. As SEM requires complete data with no missing values on any variable to conduct model testing, the full-information maximum likelihood (FIML) estimator was used to estimate any missing data on model variables. Using the FIML allowed us to minimize the exclusion of participants from the sample. Of the 290 participants who completed questionnaires, 89% (n = 259) provided complete data.

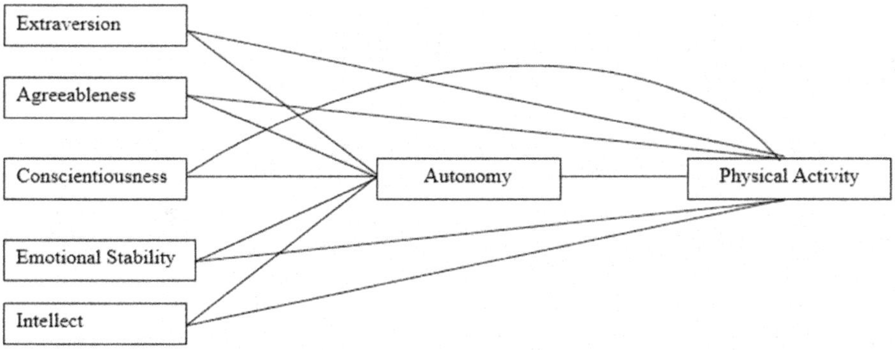

Figure 1. Hypothesized model that was tested with Structural Equation Modeling.

The fit of the model was tested with several standard goodness of fit criteria; the chi-square statistic, root mean square error of approximation (RMSEA), the comparative fit index (CFI), and the standardized root mean residual (SRMR) [24]. A small chi-square with a nonsignificant p value relative to degrees of freedom indicates a good-fitting model. RMSEA reflects the amount of information that is not accounted for by the model. The RMSEA can range from 0 to 1. Values for the RMSEA of .06 or less are indicative of good model fit [24,25]. Similar to RMSEA, the CFI can range from 0 to 1. CFI values of .95 or greater indicate a good model-data fit [24,26]. A value of less than 0.08 for the SRMR indicates an acceptable fit [24].

3. Results

Extraversion ($\beta = 0.42$), conscientiousness ($\beta = 0.96$), and emotional stability ($\beta = 0.60$) were significantly associated ($p < 0.05$) with autonomy. No significant effects on autonomy were observed for agreeableness or intellect. As proposed in the theoretical model, autonomy was positively and significantly associated with physical activity ($\beta = 0.55$). No significant direct effects on physical activity were observed for any of the personality dimensions. The significant indirect effects of extraversion ($\beta = 0.23$), conscientiousness ($\beta = 0.53$), and emotional stability ($\beta = 0.33$) on physical activity through autonomy provide evidence that autonomy partially mediated this relationship. This model provided an excellent fit to the data ($\chi^2 = 2.63$, $df = 5$, $p = 0.76$, RMSEA (90% CI) = 0.00 (0.00–0.06), CFI = 0.99, SRMR = 0.01). The final model, shown in Figure 2, accounted for 27% of the variance in physical activity.

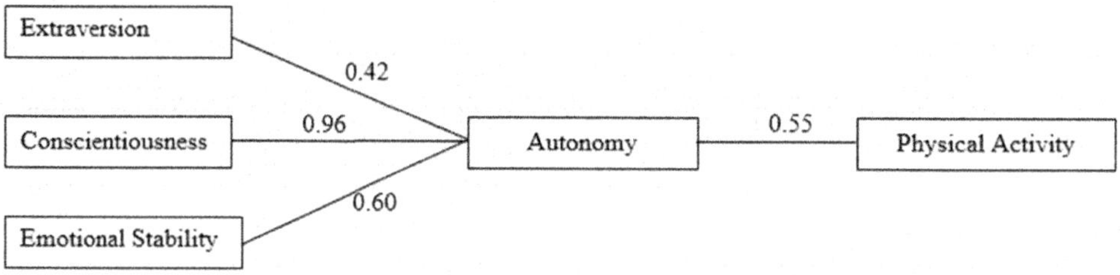

Figure 2. Final Model: only statistically significant ($p < 0.05$) direct paths included in this figure.

4. Discussion

The purpose of this study was to determine the relationship between personality, autonomy, and physical activity behavior. It was hypothesized that autonomy as well as the 5 personality domains would all have a direct relationship to physical activity, and that the 5 personality domains would have a direct relationship to autonomy itself (Figure 1). The results indicated that autonomy ($\beta = 0.55$) was directly related to physical activity indicating a positive relationship. Additionally, extroversion ($\beta = 0.42$), conscientiousness ($\beta = 0.96$), and emotional stability ($\beta = 0.60$) all showed a direct positive relationship to autonomy and an indirect relationship to physical activity via autonomy. Agreeableness and intellect showed no significant relationship to autonomy, and none of the personality domains showed a significant relationship to physical activity directly. Some of these results are inconsistent with research on personality and exercise behavior which has found extroversion, conscientiousness, neuroticism, and sometimes openness were related to physical activity [10–13]. The current study showed that these associations were mediated by autonomy. Previous research has found that extraversion and neuroticism have relationships with affect and this may be one potential way that personality and autonomy may work together to influence physical activity levels [27,28]. Additionally, the self-regulation aspect of conscientiousness may help explain its mediation of autonomy and physical activity [15].

The results of the current study were somewhat consistent with the results of the Ingledew and colleagues [15], which found that individuals who were less neurotic and more extroverted and conscientious had a higher relation to self-determination in regard to exercise. These are consistent with the results of the current study in that extroversion, conscientiousness, and emotional stability (the opposite of neuroticism) were positively correlated to autonomy. The results of the present study went one step further in indicating that autonomy was related to reported exercise participation. This is consistent with the results from the systematic review by Teixeira and colleagues [6] which have shown greater autonomy to be related to physical activity behavior. Moreover, the results of the current study were partially supported by the work of Lewis and Sutton [16], who also found that extroversion and conscientiousness were positively related to exercise frequency and were mediated by self-determination. This is consistent with the current results, but the present study also found an indirect relationship between emotional stability and physical activity behavior. Additionally, Lewis and Sutton [16] found a positive relationship between agreeableness and exercise frequency, which the current study did not.

Understanding the influence of personality on autonomy and physical activity may have unique influences on designing effective physical activity interventions. For persons high in conscientiousness the way to improve autonomy may be through setting proper individualized goals. For those high in extraversion emphasizing possible social interaction in group exercise settings may be helpful for them to find enjoyment in physical activity. For those high in neuroticism, focusing on possible mood improvement may be beneficial. Additionally, attempting to give all participants control over choice of activity and focusing on the experience as opposed to outcomes such as weight loss may help build autonomy and increase physical activity behavior.

This study is not without limitations. One limitation of the study was that the participants were mostly younger adults. There were some participants not within this population, but future research that includes a broader sample in order to have a more generalizable sample of the adult population is warranted. Another limitation of this study is the use of self-report and retrospective measures of physical activity as opposed to monitoring current (objective) physical activity behavior.

5. Conclusion

This study showed that individuals who had high levels of autonomy were more likely to have higher levels of physical activity participation. Additionally, this study concluded that the personality domains of extroversion, conscientiousness, and emotional stability were positively related to autonomy, and that autonomy mediated the relationship between these personality dimensions and exercise participation. This suggests that interventions related to modify and strengthen autonomy may be warranted to promote physical activity. As suggested by Teixeira and colleagues [6], interventions that focus on the experiential rewards of exercise (e.g., enjoyment) or having choices of activities may be a powerful way to reframe thoughts about exercise. However, based on the results of the current study, the role of personality in these interventions should be considered as well, for example the positive affective benefits of exercise might be something those high in neuroticism would embrace [27,28].

Acknowledgments: The authors would like to thank the Elon University Undergraduate Research Program for funding for this study.

Author Contributions: M.R. and E.H. conceived and designed the experiments; M.R. performed the experiments; M.R. and E.H. analyzed the data; M.R. and E.H. wrote the paper.

Conflicts of Interest: The authors declare no conflicts of interest.

References

1. U.S. Department of Health and Human Services. Healthy People 2020. Available online: https://www.healthypeople.gov/2020/topics-objectives/topic/physical-activity/objectives (accessed on 31 December 2015).
2. U.S. Department of Health and Human Services. *2008 Physical Activity Guidelines for Americans*; Health and Human Services: Washington, DC, USA, 2008.

3. Garber, C.E.; Blissmer, B.; Deschenes, M.R.; Franklin, B.A.; Lamonte, M.J.; Lee, I.-M. Quantity and quality of exercise for developing and maintaining cardiorespiratory, musculoskeletal, and neuromotor fitness in apparently healthy adults: Guidance for prescribing exercise. *Med. Sci. Sports Exerc.* **2011**, *43*, 1334–1359. [CrossRef] [PubMed]
4. Hagger, M.S.; Chatzisarantis, N.L.D. *Intrinsic Motivation and Self-Determination in Exercise and Sport*; Human Kinetics: Champaign, IL, USA, 2007.
5. Deci, E.L.; Ryan, R.M. *Intrinsic Motivation and Self-Determination in Human Behavior*; Plenum Press: New York, NY, USA, 1985.
6. Teixeira, P.J.; Carraca, E.V.; Markland, D.; Silva, M.N.; Ryan, R.M. Exercise, physical activity, and self-determination theory: A systematic review. *Int. J. Behav. Nutr. Phys. Act.* **2012**, *9*, 78. [CrossRef] [PubMed]
7. Fortier, M.S.; Duda, J.L.; Guerin, E.; Teixeira, P.J. Promoting physical activity: Development and testing of self-determination theory-based interventions. *Int. J. Behav. Nutr. Phys. Act.* **2012**, *9*, 20. [CrossRef] [PubMed]
8. Costa, P.T.; McCrae, R.R. *The NEO Personality Inventory R: Professional Manual*; Psychological Assessment Resources: Odessa, TX, USA, 1992.
9. McCrae, R.R.; John, O.P. An introduction to the five-factor model and its applications. *J. Pers.* **1992**, *60*, 175–215. [CrossRef] [PubMed]
10. Courneya, K.S.; Bobick, T.M.; Schinke, R.J. Does the theory of planned behavior mediate the relation between personality and exercise behavior? *Basic Appl. Soc. Psych.* **1999**, *21*, 317–324. [CrossRef]
11. Courneya, K.S.; Hellsten, L.M. Personality correlates of exercise behavior, motives, barriers and preferences: An application of the five-factor model. *Pers. Indiv. Diff.* **1998**, *24*, 625–633. [CrossRef]
12. Rhodes, R.E.; Courneya, K.S.; Bobick, T.M. Personality and exercise participation across the breast cancer experience. *Psychooncology* **2001**, *10*, 380–388. [CrossRef] [PubMed]
13. Wilson, K.E.; Dishman, R.K. Personality and physical activity: A systematic review and meta-analysis. *Pers. Indiv. Diff.* **2015**, *72*, 230–242. [CrossRef]
14. Eysenck, H.J.; Nias, D.K.; Cox, D.N. Sport and personality. *Adv. Behav. Res. Ther.* **1982**, *4*, 1–56. [CrossRef]
15. Ingledew, D.K.; Markland, D.; Sheppard, K.E. Personality and self-determination of exercise behaviour. *Pers. Indiv. Diff.* **2004**, *36*, 1921–1932. [CrossRef]
16. Lewis, M.; Sutton, A. Understanding exercise behaviour: Examining the interaction of exercise motivation and personality in predicting exercise frequency. *J. Sport Behav.* **2011**, *34*, 82–97.
17. International Personality Item Pool: A Scientific Collaboratory for the Development of Advanced Measures of Personality Traits and Other Individual Differences. Available online: http://ipip.ori.org/ (accessed on 31 December 2015).
18. Goldberg, L.R. The development of markers for the Big-Five factor structure. *Psychol. Assess.* **1992**, *4*, 26–42. [CrossRef]
19. Goldberg, L.R. A broad-bandwidth, Public-domain, Personality inventory measuring the low-level facets of several five-factor models. *Pers. Psychol. Eur.* **1999**, *7*, 7–28.
20. Markland, D.; Tobin, V. A modification to the Behavioral Regulation in Exercise Questionnaire to include an assessment of amotivation. *J. Sport Exerc. Psychol.* **2004**, *26*, 191–196.
21. Wilson, P.M.; Sabiston, C.M.; Mack, D.E.; Blanchard, C.M. On the nature and function of scoring protocols used in exercise motivation research: an empirical study of the behavioral regulation in exercise questionnaire. *Psychol. Sport Exerc.* **2012**, *13*, 614–622. [CrossRef]
22. Godin, G.; Shephard, R.J. A simple method to assess exercise behavior in the community. *Can. J. Appl. Sport Sci.* **1985**, *10*, 141–146. [PubMed]
23. Hoyle, R.H. *Structural Equation Modeling: Concepts, Issues and Applications*; Sage Publications: Thousand Oaks, CA, USA, 1995.
24. Hu, L.; Bentler, P.M. Cutoff criteria for fit indices in covariance structure analysis: Conventional *versus* new alternatives. *Struct. Equ. Modeling* **1999**, *6*, 1–55. [CrossRef]
25. Browne, M.W.; Cudeck, R. Alternative ways of Assessing Model Fit. In *Testing Structural Equation Models*; Bollen, K.A., Long, J.S., Eds.; Sage: Newbury Park, CA, USA, 1993; pp. 136–162.
26. Bentler, P.M. Comparative fix indexes in structural models. *Psychol. Bull.* **1990**, *107*, 238–246. [CrossRef] [PubMed]

27. Rusting, C.L.; Larsen, R.J. Extraversion, neuroticism, and susceptibility to positive and negative affect: a test of two theoretical models. *Pers. Indiv. Differ.* **1997**, *22*, 607–612. [CrossRef]
28. Smillie, L.D.; DeYoung, C.G.; Hall, P.J. Clarifying the relation between extraversion and positive affect. *J. Pers.* **2015**, *83*, 564–574. [CrossRef] [PubMed]

4

Clinical Assessment of Scapula Motion: Scapula Upward Rotation and Relationship with Injury in Swimmers

Jo Brown †, Rebecca Mellifont † and Brendan Burkett *,†

School of Health and Sport Sciences, University of the Sunshine Coast, Queensland 4552, Australia; jo@physiosync.com.au (J.B.); rebecca.mellifont@usc.edu.au (R.M.)

* Correspondence: bburkett@usc.edu.au

† These authors contributed equally to this work.

Academic Editor: Arno Schmidt-Trucksäss

Abstract: Abnormal scapulothoracic mechanics and scapulohumeral rhythm are implicated in shoulder pathologies, including glenohumeral impingement and rotator cuff tears. Upward scapula rotation, specifically asymmetry of scapula motion and associations of patterns through range with injury, was investigated in dominant and non-dominant limbs of nationally ranked junior and Paralympic swimmers during competition season. The static and throughout phases measures of upward scapula rotation were: Phase I (start position, 45°), Phase II (45° to 90°), Phase III (90° to 135°) and Phase IV (135° to max). Injury was assessed with a validated questionnaire. Differences between side (dominant and non-dominant), group (junior and Paralympic), and phase were examined. Significant differences ($P < 0.05$) between groups were identified for dominant side at rest, 45° and 135°, and in phases II and IV (including range). Scapulohumeral rhythm was higher in the non-dominant limb of Paralympic swimmers but in the dominant limb of junior swimmers. Greatest differences in upward rotation between injured and non-injured swimmers were found in Phase 1: 43.6% (3.3°) Paralympic; 73.1% (8°) junior. Results suggest asymmetry of movement in both limbs, through all phases, and at single points in range, should be investigated for assessing injury and developing preventive strategies and rehabilitation protocols.

Keywords: dominant limb; non-dominant limb; asymmetry of motion; scapula; scapula upward rotation; injury; Paralympic swimmers

---

1. Introduction

The scapula is vital in shoulder function and abnormal scapulothoracic mechanics and scapula–humeral rhythm have been implicated in shoulder pathologies, including glenohumeral impingement and rotator cuff tears. Knowledge of scapulothoracic movements is regarded as crucial in the development of preventative strategies and treatment programs in athletes with shoulder pathology [1]. In swimming, an athlete's scapular musculature plays a pivotal role in stabilizing and preventing impingement because its continuous activation is required throughout the swim stroke [2]. Shoulder injuries have been reported in up to 90% of swimmers [3]. This high prevalence of injury in swimmers has been associated with the inability to maintain a fine balance between strength and instability, in combination with poor endurance of shoulder musculature [4]. These issues are further compounded when the asymmetry between the dominant and non-dominant arms of swimmers are compared [5–7]. Paralympic swimmers have reported the similar shoulder pain/injury issues as able-bodied swimmers [8], with a higher prevalence of upper limb injuries in wheelchair athletes [9].

The challenge for therapists is to accurately identify dysfunctional and/or pathological movement patterns [10], so that appropriate management strategies can be developed [11,12].

Scapula upward rotation is the dominant scapula action throughout shoulder elevation and has been previously implicated in the development of impingement [13,14]. However, inconsistencies exist in reporting the association between upward rotation and injury, particularly as recent literature supports impingement occurring below 90° abduction [11,15]. For example, some studies have found an increase upward rotation in symptomatic subjects [16], other research a decrease [17], or no difference [18,19]. This variation may be accounted for by the measurement protocols adopted, as well as the population size and type, for example, athlete *versus* non-athlete. To better understand this scapulothoracic relationship, the aim of this study was to investigate upward scapula rotation in two distinct swimming populations, with particular interest in asymmetry of scapula motion and associations of patterns through range with injury.

2. Materials and Methods

2.1. Participant Demographics

Human ethics approval was obtained prior to recruitment of participants. Forty-four athletes (22 nationally ranked junior athletes and 22 Paralympic athletes) were tested. Both groups consisted of 11 males and 11 females, and both limbs were tested in each athlete (grouped by arm dominance). The average number of years of athletes' involvement in competitive swimming was 6 years (SD 2.6) in the junior group and 8 years (SD 3.2) in the Paralympic group. For the Paralympic group the IPC swimming class (and impairment) demographics were: S6 (short stature [3]); S7 (cerebral palsy [2], leg amputee [1]); S8 (cerebral palsy [3], leg amputee [2]); S9 (leg amputee [3], arm amputee [3]); S10 (cerebral palsy [4], arm amputee [1]). All participants were tested during the competition phase of the season. Participants were excluded if they had congenital deformity of the scapula or thorax, or had a history of trauma, fracture or surgery of the shoulder girdle.

2.2. Measures of the Shoulder

Two inclinometers (Plurimeter-V gravity referenced inclinometers, Fabrication, White Plains, New York, NY, USA) were used to measure upward scapula rotation, as described previously [20]. A standardized, reliable protocol was followed [21]. Reliability tests were conducted one hour apart and during three consecutive days, producing an Intraclass Correlation Coefficient of 0.95, which was similar to previous studies [22]. One examiner experienced with the use of inclinometers completed all measurements.

The inclinometers measured total shoulder abduction, which involved both glenohumeral and scapula motion within the coronal plane. Measurement required full elbow extension and neural wrist flexion and extension with the thumb leading to ensure consistent vertical alignment. The humeral inclinometer was fixed to the shaft of the humerus with Velcro straps and measured the position of humeral elevation. The scapula inclinometer was aligned along the spine of the scapula and measured upward scapula rotation. Three trials were conducted for each measure and the average score calculated.

The humeral inclinometer was fitted and checked, centered to zero and aligned so the face of the Plurimeter was vertical. The base of the scapula inclinometer was aligned along the spine of the scapula, as per previous protocols [20]. The actual resting position of each participant's humerus relative to the vertical was recorded. Each participant performed a dynamic warm-up with arm-circles for 1 to 2 min. The participant was then asked to externally rotate the arm so that both resting humeral and scapula angles could be measured. Next, the participant was asked to move the arm through the arc of abduction, stopping at 45°, 90°, 135° and maximum shoulder abduction. The point at which motion paused for measurement was determined by the examiner with the humeral inclinometer, and resulted in five positions of abduction. At each position of abduction, the static angle of scapula upward rotation was recorded with the scapular inclinometer. The side measured was randomized and the examiner did not communicate the test results to the participant. Upward rotation was divided into four phases: Phase I (start position of 45°), Phase II (45° to 90°), Phase III (90° to 135°) and Phase IV (135° to max). By dividing the arc of motion into the four phases, the linearity of movement could be determined.

The scapulohumeral rhythm is calculated as a ratio, essentially dividing the glenohumeral elevation or abduction angle by the scapulothoracic angle (amount of upward scapula rotation). This ratio provides information about the scapula rotation, and may indicate muscle imbalance and be related to injury [17].

Shoulder pain (or injury) was defined as an incident (or occurrence) that required altered training, or rest from training, for a week or more. The swimmers who reported a change in their training of a week or more, due to pain or injury, were placed in the injury group as shown in Table 1.

2.3. Statistical Analysis

Means, standard deviations and 95% Confidence Intervals were calculated for all descriptive parameters of upward rotation. Differences between side (dominant and non-dominant), group (junior and Paralympic), and phase were examined with combinations of two-way ANOVA ($P < 0.05$). To provide a practical or clinical measure of any differences between these variables effect statistics were measured using Cohen's d [23]. Both the raw difference (measured in degrees) and percentage difference were calculated so that the differences between injured and non-injured subgroups could be determined.

Table 1. Effect statistics comparing upward rotation measures throughout the phases of movement for injured and non-injured subgroups in junior and Paralympic groups.

Measure	Junior Group				Paralympic Group			
	Injured (°) n = 15	Non-injured (°) n = 7	Raw difference (°)	Percent difference (%)	Injured (°) n = 16	Non-injured (°) n = 6	Raw difference (°)	Percent difference (%)
45°	18.2 (12.6 to 23.3)	19.0 (11.7 to 26.3)	0.7 (−6.6 to 8.1)	0% (−14.1 to 12.3)	27.4 (21 to 33.7)	28.8 (18.9 to 38.3)	2.7 (−0.2 to 14.5)	7.5% (−30.8 to 67.0)
Phase I	12.4 (8.2 to 16.6)	20.1 (13.7 to 28.3)	8.3 (0.4 to 17.2)	73.1% (34.1 to 92.3)	13.4 (9.6 to 19.3)	12.8 (8.7 to 22.3)	3.3 (0.7 to 8.5)	43.6% (11.7 to 96.3)
90°	35.6 (29.8 to 41.4)	33.4 (25.7 to 41.2)	1.4 (−8.2 to 5.3)	5.2% (−16.2 to 12.6)	40.8 (29.6 to 46.5)	41.3 (33.6 to 49.0)	0.7 (−10.8 to 12.2)	2% (−23.0 to 35.1)
Phase II	17.5 (13.5 to 21.4)	19.8 (9.9 to 29.8)	3.6 (−7.5 to 14.7)	15.4% (−33.9 to 28.7)	13.7 (9.1 to 17.6)	12.5 (9.4 to 16.3)	1.2 (−5.3 to 3.0)	0.8% (−33.9 to 48.9)
135°	45.8 (39.6 to 51.2)	43.7 (23.5 to 55.3)	3.8 (−13.9 to 6.6)	5.8% (−27.2 to 22.1)	56.9 (43.6 to 63.1)	53.0 (45.4 to 60.6)	0.7 (−8.0 to 9.4)	1.2% (−14.4 to 19.6)
Phase III	10.2 (7.3 to 13.1)	16.6 (7.3 to 34.9)	7.7 (−7.9 to 23.3)	27.4% (−44.8 to 35.5)	16.1 (10.6 to 19.6)	13.3 (8.9 to 18.3)	1.7 (−7.7 to 11.0)	1% (−30.4 to 40.7)
End of range	61.9 (56.3 to 67.4)	62.6 (55.4 to 69.7)	1.3 (−6.6 to 4.1)	2.2% (−10.0 to 6.3)	66.2 (51.4 to 72.7)	63.7 (59.7 to 67.6)	0.2 (−6.3 to 5.9)	0.3 (−9.3 to 10.8)
Phase IV	19.5 (13.6 to 25.8)	32.6 (13 to 52.1)	12.4 (−2.3 to 27.2)	42% (−5.4 to 25.4)	10.1 (5.5 to 11.9)	10.7 (3.9 to 17.4)	1.2 (−8.1 to 5.8)	4.3% (−25.6 to 17.1)

Note: Values are expressed as mean (95% CI).

3. Results

The influence of dominance on upward scapula upward rotation range and phases was investigated in both groups. Significant differences between junior and Paralympic groups were identified for the dominant side in the resting position and for upward scapula rotation at 45° and 135°, as well as at phases II and IV of the range (Table 2). No significant differences were determined between groups for non-dominant side measures.

Table 2. The influence of dominance on changes in upward scapula upward rotation through the range and phases of motion in junior and Paralympic swimmers.

Measure of Upward Rotation	Dominant Side		Non-Dominant Side	
	Junior (n = 22)	Paralympic (n = 22)	Junior (n = 22)	Paralympic (n = 22)
Rest	6.3 *,a (3.8 to 8.9)	14.6 *,b (10.0 to 18.0)	8.8 a (6.0 to 14.0)	15.9 b (8.0 to 17.1)
45°	18.3 (14.0 to 22.0)	27.8 * (22.0 to 32.0)	24.7 (18.3 to 28.0)	32.5 (20.3 to 34.0)
90°	35.6 (30.6 to 39)	39.0 (32.0 to 45.0)	40.5 (32.0 to 43.3)	43.2 (38.0 to 46.1)
135°	45.8 * (37.9 to 49.7)	53.5 * (43.0 to 60.0)	54.0 (39.0 to 56.6)	56.5 (46.0 to 61.0)
End of range°	62.1 (58.0 to 66.2)	62.5 (54.9 to 70)	67.7 (64.4 to 70.0)	66.5 (55.3 to 70.0)
0 to 45° (Phase I)	12.4 (8.2 to 16.6)	13.3 (10.6 to 16.7)	16.0 (12. 4 to 21.7)	15.0 (10.0 to 18.0)
45 to 90° (Phase II)	17.5 * (13.6 to 21.4)	12.9 * (8.6 to 15.8)	16.5 (12.9 to 20.0)	12.9 (9.0 to 14.4)
90 to 135° (Phase III)	10.2 (7.3 to 13.1)	14.6 (11.3 to 18.5)	13.2 (7.1 to 18.0)	12.8 (12.4 to 19)
135 to max (Phase IV)	19.5* (13.3 to 25.8)	9.7 * (6.5 to 11.9)	14.1 (8.9 to 22.0)	10.1 (6.3 to 13.0)
True arc	56.8 (52.0 to 60.0)	49.2 (43.0 to 55.0)	58.9 (53.2 to 61)	50.5 (44.0 to 56.0)

Notes: values are expressed as mean° (95% CI); significant difference ($p < 0.05$) between groups indicated by paired symbols (*/a/b).

The ranges for Phase II and Phase IV differed significantly between the junior and Paralympic groups in the dominant limb only (Figure 1). In the Paralympic group, the least amount of rotation occurred in Phase IV in both limbs, whilst in the junior group the least amount of rotation occurred in Phase III in both limbs (Figure 1). This difference was reflected in a smaller rate of change of abduction and maximum upward rotation angle in the Paralympic group, and indicated a different scapulohumeral rhythm [24].

The major difference in scapulohumeral rhythm found in the Paralympic group was that the non-dominant limb had a much higher scapulohumeral rhythm than that of the dominant limb (3.5 *vs.* 2.9). However, in the junior group, this relationship was reversed, with the scapulohumeral rhythm of the non-dominant limb lower than that of the dominant limb (3.0 *vs.* 3.4). There were no significant differences between these measures of scapulohumeral rhythm.

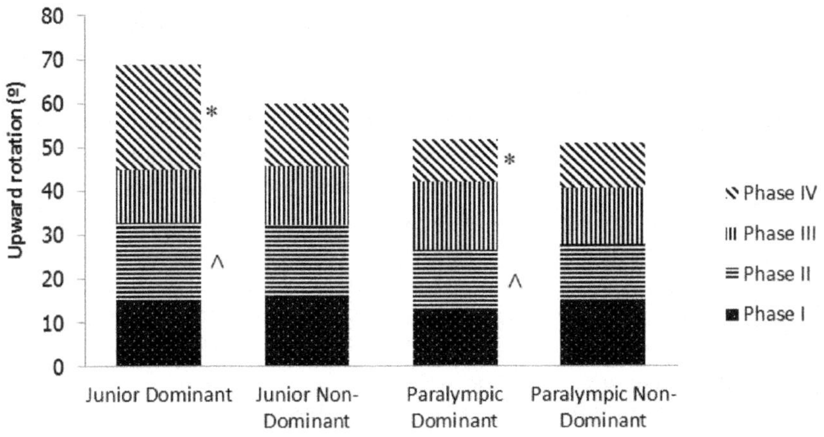

Figure 1. Comparison of phases of upward rotation between dominant and non-dominant limbs for junior and Paralympic swimmers. * and ^ indicate significant differences between groups with matching symbols ($P < 0.05$).

A separate effect analysis to determine the association between injury and both phases and range of scapula upward rotation was also explored in both junior and Paralympic groups, with each group classified into injured and non-injured subgroups (Table 1). The most surprising result was that, in the junior group, a 73.1% (or 8°) difference was found between the injured and non-injured subgroups in Phase I. As there was no difference at 45°, this result most likely reflected the resting position of the scapula. Furthermore, large percentage differences were found between injured and non-injured junior swimmers in the remaining phases, resulting in 42% more range in the non-injured swimmers. For the Paralympic group, the greatest difference between injured and non-injured swimmers was 43.6% (or 3.3°) in Phase 1. For other phases, the differences between the injured and non-injured groups were probably too small for clinical relevance.

4. Discussion

The aim of this study was to investigate upward scapula rotation in two distinct swimming populations, with particular interest in asymmetry of scapula motion and associations of patterns through range with injury. The average total arc of scapula motion for the junior swimmers (dominant side) was 56.8°, and for the Paralympic swimmers 49.2°. These results are consistent with increased ranges of upward scapula rotation described in swimming populations and other overhead athlete populations [25] and are comparable to those found previously in injured swimmers only [20].

In the resting position, significant differences were identified between sides in the junior and Paralympic groups. The mean resting position (dominant side) found in the junior group in this study (6.3°) was similar to a previous value measured in junior swimmers: a scapula resting position angle of 5.4° was found with the arm relaxed at the side [26]. The difference identified between the groups in dominant side resting position suggests that altered scapula resting position may be a compensatory mechanism in the Paralympic group, however this speculated mechanism was not measured or quantified. That is, the altered resting position may be a direct result or influence of each swimmer's disability on scapula mechanics, in order to maximize swim performance or muscle function for activities of daily living. It is noted this small difference between sides could also be attributed to the variability of each individual participant.

A significant difference between dominant and non-dominant sides in the mean resting scapula position (2.5° in junior and 1.3° in Paralympic groups) was found within both groups. Previously, college athletes (of similar age) have presented with values similar to those of the Paralympic group (1.46° difference) [27]. Other studies investigating scapula resting position have found no difference between those with and without impingement symptoms [19,28]. However, differing methods currently limit the usefulness of the relationship between resting scapula position and impingement symptoms. Mounting evidence suggests resting scapula position in isolation is unlikely to detect the difference between symptomatic and asymptomatic athletes [27,29], probably because asymmetry is often present in healthy individuals [30]. This combination of factors highlights the need to consider measurements of dynamic scapula asymmetry through range as part of appropriate clinical reasoning.

In the relatively stable scapula position of 45° abduction of the humerus, the significant difference between groups in upward scapula rotation (approx. 10°) may indicate poor stability resulting from muscle weakness in the Paralympic group. As previously described, surrounding soft tissue and other specific impairments in motor control or strength probably affect scapula position [30]. The significant difference also found between groups at 135° (junior group showed greater upward rotation) is potentially an adaptation to improve stroke mechanics.

Significant differences in rotation were also identified between the phases of both groups. The least amount of upward rotation occurred in Phase IV on the dominant side in the Paralympic group and in Phase III on the dominant side in the junior group. Furthermore, significant differences in upward rotation between groups in both Phase II and Phase IV were identified (Table 2, Figure 1). The largest difference occurred in Phase IV (135° to max.), a range that occupies a high percentage of the swim stroke. This difference reflects increased laxity in the shoulder joint of junior swimmers. The presence of multidirectional instability [31] has been found to cause significantly decreased upward scapula rotation up to 120°, which means that a high percentage of range occurs above this point. In the junior group, the greater rotation in the dominant limbs, with the highest portion of the range and a large between-limb difference in Phase IV (135° to max.), confirms the previous finding (Figure 1). Given established links between scapula dyskinesis and injury [11], these results have clinical implications for identifying functional, relevant dyskinesis, and for developing management strategies in these populations.

In this study the greatest difference identified between injured and non-injured subgroups within the junior group was in Phase I, with the injured subgroup demonstrating an 8.3° (73.1%) smaller range than that of the non-injured subgroup. However, at the 45° position, the range was similar in both subgroups, suggesting that this difference was due to the initial difference in resting position and the influence of soft tissue structures. This finding challenges those of previous studies that have potentially underestimated the impact of resting position in this group [27,30]. The measures of scapulohumeral rhythm (up to 3.5:1 in the Paralympic group) were larger than the common ratio of 2:1, this difference was attributed to the testing of the elite athlete population within the current study and the accepted changes in scapulohumeral rhythm associated with shoulder disorders [24]. As these results have not previously been reported in Paralympic swimming populations, no direct comparisons can be made.

Greater upward scapula rotation at 135° was found in the injured subgroups than in the non-injured subgroups (percentage differences in effect statistics of 5.8% within the junior group and 1.2% within the Paralympic group) (Table 1). However, given the small raw differences, these differences at a point in range are unlikely to be relevant. This finding contrasts with those of Su *et al.* (2004), who found athletes with impingement symptoms have demonstrated less upward rotation at 45°, 90° and 135° post swimming, a finding which is consistent with an induced fatigue effect of scapula stabilizers on the amount of scapula upward rotation. However, the athletes in our study came fresh to the data collection (*i.e.*, were not tested after swimming), and so were not influenced by fatigue, which may account for the difference in the reported results. The results further suggest that the ability to produce a consistent rate of change of scapula rotation through range, even when fatigued, should be considered a goal for swimmers. The identification of asymmetry throughout the range indicates an inability of the athlete to maintain upward scapula rotation.

Moving through the phases, effect statistics consistently showed higher percentages of upward scapula rotation range in phases III and IV in the non-injured subgroup than in the injured subgroup of the junior swimmers (differences of 27% and 42%, respectively). Compared with the injured subgroup, the non-injured subgroup had a better ability to create active range. This difference may result from underlying weakness or inhibition due to pain in the injured group [32], and hence may be a compensatory strategy. These results support the concept that the phase of motion in which the greatest range of rotation occurs, rather than the total range, is of greater clinical relevance, especially given that the range of motion through each phase reflects the balance of scapula–humeral force couples [33].

In Paralympic athletes, the greatest difference between the two subgroups (injured *vs.* non-injured) was also found in the Phase I range (43.6%). Additionally, a significant difference was found at 45°, suggesting that these results truly reflect the differences in movement that are occurring. In contrast to the junior group, a greater Phase I range was found in the injured subgroup of the Paralympic athletes. This finding also contrasts with the results of previous studies that investigated these parameters in able-bodied participants [34], which further supports the need for Paralympic swimmers to be considered as a unique group. The results may indicate use of a compensatory strategy in this group of swimmers, or even that alterations in scapula upward rotation are a transient form of scapula dyskinesis. This notion is supported by studies inducing pain [32] or dysfunction through nerve blocks [35], and by the finding that dyskinesis may be present after a single training session [36]. That 100% of athletes presented with asymmetry of one or more scapula factors in this study suggests that either a certain amount of dyskinesis is transient or that dyskinesis does not depict true dysfunction.

5. Conclusions

To enable an improved understanding of scapula upward rotation, asymmetry of the movement should be investigated through all phases of range, rather than at a single point in range. The phase of movement and comparison with the contra side should be considered in order to determine whether the movement is actually dysfunctional and is related to injury, or is a compensatory strategy signifying weakness of the force couple through range.

The determination of what is normal on an individual athlete basis (especially for Paralympic athletes) may be required for optimum interpretation of results, and to enable the clinician to understand asymmetry and its consequences. In addition, exact movement dysfunction must be determined to develop effective rehabilitation protocols.

Acknowledgments: Editorial assistance was provided by Dr Leigh Findlay (TrueNature Writing and Editing).

Author Contributions: All three authors conceived and designed the experiments; Jo Brown performed the experiments; whilst Jo Brown, Rebecca Mellifont and Brendan Burkett analyzed the data and wrote the paper.

Conflicts of Interest: The authors declare no conflict of interest.

References

1. Von Eisenhart-Rothe, R.; Matsen, F.A.; Eckstein, F.; Vogl, T.; Graichen, H. Pathomechanics in atraumatic shoulder instability: Scapula positioning correlates with humeral head centering. *Clin. Orthop. Relat. Res.* **2005**, *433*, 82–89. [CrossRef] [PubMed]
2. Tate, A.J.; Turner, G.N.; Knab, S.E.; Jorgensen, C.; Strittmatter, A.; Michener, L. Risk factors associated with shoulder pain and disability across the lifespan of competitive swimmers. *J. Athl. Train.* **2012**, *47*, 149–158. [PubMed]
3. Sein, M.L.; Walton, J.; Linklater, J.; Appleyard, R.; Kirkbride, B.; Kuah, D.; Murrell, G.A. Shoulder pain in elite swimmers: Primarily due to swim-volume-induced supraspinatus tendinopathy. *Br. J. Sports Med.* **2010**, *44*, 105–113. [CrossRef] [PubMed]
4. Beach, M.L.; Whitney, S.L.; Dickoff-Hoffman, S. Relationship of shoulder flexibility, strength, and endurance to shoulder pain in competitive swimmers. *J. Orthop. Sports Phys. Ther.* **1992**, *16*, 262–268. [CrossRef] [PubMed]
5. Ozcaldiran, B. A relation between static flexibility and shoulder pain in competitive age-group swimmers. *Pain Clin.* **2002**, *14*, 159–163. [CrossRef]

6. Potts, A.D.; Charlton, J.E.; Smith, H.M. Bilateral arm power imbalance in swim bench exercise to exhaustion. *J. Sports Sci.* **2002**, *20*, 975–979. [CrossRef]
7. Formosa, D.; Mason, B.; Burkett, B. The force-time profile of elite front crawl swimmers. *J. Sport Sci.* **2011**, *29*, 811–819. [CrossRef]
8. Magno e Silva, M.; Bilzon, J.; Duarte, E.; Gorla, J.; Vital, R. Sport injuries in elite paralympic swimmers with visual impairment. *J. Athl. Train.* **2013**, *48*, 493–498. [CrossRef] [PubMed]
9. Fagher, K.; Lexell, J. Sports-related injuries in athletes with disabilities. *Scand. J. Med. Sci. Sports* **2014**, *24*, e320–e331. [CrossRef] [PubMed]
10. Hibberd, E.E.; Oyama, S.; Spang, J.T.; Prentice, W.; Myers, J.B. Effect of a 6-week strengthening program on shoulder and scapular-stabilizer strength and scapular kinematics in division i collegiate swimmers. *J. Sport Rehabil.* **2012**, *21*, 253–265. [PubMed]
11. Ludewig, P.M.; Reynolds, J.F. The association of scapular kinematics and glenohumeral joint pathologies. *J. Orthop. Sports Phys. Ther.* **2009**, *39*, 90–104. [CrossRef] [PubMed]
12. Nijs, J.; Roussel, N.; Struyf, F.; Mottram, S.; Meeusen, R. Clinical assessment of scapula positioning in patients with shoulder pain: State of the art. *J. Manip. Physiol. Ther.* **2007**, *30*, 67–75. [CrossRef] [PubMed]
13. Su, K.P.; Johnson, M.P.; Gracely, E.J.; Karduna, A.R. Scapular rotation in swimmers with and without impingement syndrome: Practice effects. *Med. Sci. Sports Exerc.* **2004**, *36*, 1117–1123. [CrossRef] [PubMed]
14. Yano, Y.; Hamada, J.; Tamai, K.; Yoshizaki, K.; Sahara, R.; Fujiwara, T.; Nohara, Y. Different scapular kinematics in healthy subjects during arm elevation and lowering: Glenohumeral and scapulothoracic patterns. *J. Shoulder Elbow Surg.* **2010**, *19*, 209–215. [CrossRef] [PubMed]
15. Timmons, M.K.; Thigpen, C.A.; Seitz, A.L.; Karduna, A.R.; Arnold, B.L.; Michener, L.A. Scapular kinematics and subacromial-impingement syndrome: A meta-analysis. *J. Sport Rehab.* **2012**, *21*, 354–370.
16. McClure, P.W.; Michener, L.A.; Karduna, A.R. Shoulder function and 3-dimensional scapular kinematics in people with and without shoulder impingement syndrome. *Phys. Ther.* **2006**, *86*, 1075–1090. [PubMed]
17. Ludewig, P.M.; Cook, T.M. Alterations in shoulder kinematics and associated muscle activity in people with symptoms of shoulder impingement. *Phys. Ther.* **2000**, *80*, 276–291. [PubMed]
18. Graichen, H.; Hinterwimmer, S.; von Eisenhart-Rothe, R.; Vogl, T.; Englmeier, K.H.; Eckstein, F. Effect of abducting and adducting muscle activity on glenohumeral translation, scapular kinematics and subacromial space width *in vivo*. *J. Biomech.* **2005**, *38*, 755–760. [CrossRef] [PubMed]
19. Herbert, L.J.; Moffet, H.; McFadyen, B.J.; Dionne, C.E. Scapula behaviour in shoulder impingement syndrome. *Arch. Phys. Med. Rehabil.* **2002**, *83*, 60–79. [CrossRef]
20. Watson, L.; Balster, S.M.; Finch, C.; Dalziel, R. Measurement of scapula upward rotation: A reliable clinical procedure. *Br. J. Sports Med.* **2005**, *39*, 599–603. [CrossRef] [PubMed]
21. Green, S. A standardized protocol for measurement of range of movement of the shoulder using the pluriometer v inclinometer and assessment of its intrarater and interrater reliability. *Arthritis Care Res.* **1998**, 43–52. [CrossRef]
22. Riemann, B.; Witt, J.; Davies, G.J. Glenohumeral joint rotation range of motion in competitive swimmers. *J. Sport Sci.* **2011**, *29*, 1191–1199. [CrossRef] [PubMed]
23. Hopkins, W.G.; Marshall, S.W.; Batterham, A.M.; Hanin, J. Progressive statistics for studies in sports medicine and exercise science. *Med. Sci. Sports Exerc.* **2009**, *41*, 3–13. [CrossRef] [PubMed]
24. Yoshizaki, K.; Hamada, J.; Tamai, K.; Sahara, R.; Fujiwara, A.; Fujimoto, T. Analysis of the scapulohumeral rhythm and electromyography of the shoulder muscles during elevation and lowering: Comparison of dominant and nondominant shoulders. *J. Shoulder Elbow Surg.* **2009**, *18*, 756–763. [CrossRef] [PubMed]
25. Thomas, S.J.; Swanik, K.A.; Swanik, C.; Huxel, K.C. Glenohumeral rotation and scapula position adaptations after a single high school sports season. *J. Athl. Train.* **2009**, *44*, 230–237. [CrossRef] [PubMed]
26. Phadke, V.; Camargo, P.R.; Ludewig, P.M. Scapular and rotator cuff muscle activity during arm elevation: A review of normal function and alterations with shoulder impingement. *Rev. Bras. Fisioter.* **2009**, *13*, 1–9. [CrossRef] [PubMed]
27. Oyama, S.; Myers, J.B.; Wassinger, C.A.; Ricci, R.D.; Lephart, S.M. Asymmetric resting scapular posture in healthy overhead athletes. *J. Athl. Train.* **2008**, *43*, 565–570. [CrossRef] [PubMed]
28. Endo, K.; Ikata, T.; Katoh, S.; Takeda, Y. Radiographic assessment of scapular rotational tilt in chronic shoulder impingement syndrome. *J. Orthop. Sci.* **2001**, *6*, 3–10. [CrossRef] [PubMed]

29. Uhl, T.L.; Kibler, W.B.; Gecewich, B.; Tripp, B.L. Evaluation of clinical assessment methods for scapular dyskinesis. *Arthroscopy* **2009**, *25*, 1240–1248. [CrossRef] [PubMed]
30. Morais, N.V.; Pascoal, A.G. Scapula positioning assessment: Is side-to-side comparsion clinically acceptable? *Man Ther.* **2013**, *18*, 46–56. [CrossRef] [PubMed]
31. Ogston, J.B.; Ludewig, P.M. Differences in 3-dimensional shoulder kinematics between persons with multidirectional instability and asymptomatic controls. *Am. J. Sports Med.* **2007**, *35*, 1361–1370. [CrossRef] [PubMed]
32. Wassinger, C.A.; Sole, G.; Osbourne, H. Clinical measurement of upward scapula rotation in response to acute subacromial pain. *J. Orthop. Sports Phys. Ther.* **2013**, *43*, 199–203. [CrossRef] [PubMed]
33. Joshi, M.; Thigpen, C.A.; Bunn, K.; Karas, S.G.; Padua, D.A. Shoulder external rotation fatigue and scapular muscle activation and kinematics in overhead athletes. *J. Athl. Train.* **2011**, *46*, 349–357. [PubMed]
34. Ludewig, P.M.; Behrens, S.A.; Meyer, S.M.; Spoden, S.M.; Wilson, L.A. Three-dimensional clavicular motion during arm elevation: Reliability and descriptive data. *J. Orthop. Sports Phys. Ther.* **2004**, *34*, 140–149. [CrossRef] [PubMed]
35. McCully, S.P.; Suprak, D.N.; Kosek, P.; Karduna, A.R. Suprascapular nerve block disrupts the normal pattern of scapula kinematics. *Clin. Biomech.* **2006**, *21*, 545–553. [CrossRef] [PubMed]
36. Madsen, P.H.; Bak, K.; Jensen, S.; Welter, U. Training induces scapular dyskinesis in pain-free competitive swimmers: A reliability and observational study. *Clin. J. Sport Med.* **2011**, *21*, 109–113. [CrossRef] [PubMed]

5

Cardiac Autonomic and Salivary Responses to a Repeated Training Bout in Elite Swimmers

Rohan Edmonds [1,†], Anthony Leicht [2,†], Brendan Burkett [1,*,†] and Mark McKean [1,†]

1 School of Health and Sport Sciences, University of the Sunshine Coast, Queensland 4558, Australia; redmonds@skidmore.edu (R.E.); mm@markmckean.com (M.M.)
2 College of Healthcare Sciences, James Cook University, Queensland 4811, Australia; anthony.leicht@jcu.edu.au
* Correspondence: bburkett@usc.edu.au
† These authors contributed equally to this work.

Academic Editor: Arno Schmidt-Trucksäss

Abstract: This study examined the acute training responses of heart rate variability (HRV) and salivary biomarkers (immunoglobulin A and alpha-amylase) following a standardised training bout in Paralympic swimmers. Changes in HRV, sIgA and sAA were documented Monday morning, Monday afternoon and Tuesday morning over a 14-week monitoring period leading into international competition. Magnitude based inferences with effect sizes (ES) were used to assess the practical significance of changes each week. Normal training responses elicited increases in HR, $\alpha 1$, sAA and sIgA, accompanied by decreases in HF(nu), standard deviation of instantaneous RR variability (SD1) and the root mean square of successive differences (RMSSD) from Monday morning to Monday afternoon, and to Tuesday morning with similar week to week responses for most variables. Changes in RMSSD from Monday a.m. to p.m. were likely smaller (less negative) for Week 7 (78/18/3, ES = 0.40) following a competition weekend with similar changes observed from Monday a.m. to Tuesday a.m. (90/5/5, ES = 1.30). In contrast, the change in sAA from Monday a.m. to p.m. was very likely less (more negative) at Week 7 (0/0/99, ES = −2.46), with similar changes observed from Monday a.m. to Tuesday a.m. (0/0/99, ES = −4.69). During the taper period, there were also likely increases in parasympathetic modulations (RMSSD, Weeks 12–14) along with increased immune function (sIgA, Week 13) that demonstrated a favourable state of athlete preparedness. Used together, HRV and sAA provide coaches with valuable information regarding physiological changes in response to training and competition.

Keywords: heart rate variability; Paralympics; alpha-amylase; athlete; stress

---

1. Introduction

Understanding the effect of a given training stimulus on exercise performance is critical for planning training sessions and achieving peak performance. Coaches are constantly working to identify how individual athletes respond to training so they can accurately prescribe an appropriate training load. This ideal load reduces the possibility of negative training responses and enhances positive training adaptations. A range of specific blood variables [1] and psychometric questionnaires [2] have been used to monitor an athlete's response to training loads and quantify athlete fatigue. However, obtaining blood samples can be inconvenient and sometimes painful, especially if used for frequent monitoring. Further, questionnaires can be time consuming and report a subjective measure of fatigue or training load and not internal training load [3]. As a result, there has been increased interest in the monitoring of the autonomic nervous system (ANS) via measures of heart rate (HR), particularly heart rate variability (HRV) [4,5].

Measures of HRV are relatively inexpensive, non-invasive, time efficient and may serve as an important tool for elite athlete populations. With individual changes in cardiac parasympathetic activity proposed as key predictors of improvements in performance [6], the incidence of HRV monitoring of elite athletes has increased due to its ability to document cardiac autonomic responses to training. Understanding the acute HRV responses to regular exercise may help identify ongoing positive or negative training adaptations, allowing coaches to adjust training and recovery protocols with greater accuracy. As a well-recognised marker for assessing training responses in athlete populations, and a marker of predominately cardiac autonomic activity [7], HRV is an important tool used in combination with other physiological markers to comprehensively evaluate an athlete's training status. While HRV has provided guidance with training adaptations [8] the optimal HRV measure and timing of assessment remains unknown with several studies documenting minimal to no change in HRV with regular exercise/training [5,6]. Therefore, HRV measures may be of partial benefit for practical training guidance, especially during complex training programs or with the elite. Use of other markers in combination with HRV may provide a thorough examination of training adaptations and potentially lead to better guidance of training programs for athletes and coaches.

With recent updates in technology, point-of-care analysis of specific salivary biomarkers is now available, providing coaches with additional viable options when assessing recovery and training responses in a quick and easy manner. One such salivary measure is salivary immunoglobulin A (sIgA), a well-recognized indicator of immune function [9]. The majority of immunological studies of elite athletes have concentrated largely on post exercise salivary immune responses [10] with athletes experiencing a transitory decrease in immune function from 3 to 72 h following heavy training or competition [11]. Recently, there has been conjecture as to the influence of exercise on sIgA with studies identifying both increases and decreases [12] in sIgA concentrations following exercise. As proposed by Nieman's 'J shaped' relationship [13] with highly repetitive workloads or strenuous exercise, there is a degree of immunosuppression, which increases the risk of infection for athletes. Therefore, sIgA may help in identifying appropriate immune function and training adaptation, while also highlighting the early signs of illness, a result of excessive workload or insufficient recovery.

In a similar way to sIgA, real-time analysis of salivary alpha-amylase (sAA), a biomarker of stress and sympathetic nervous system activity [14], is now achievable. Used as a marker of neural activity due to its predominant regulation by the sympathetic nervous system, sAA has been successfully applied as an indicator of exercise intensity in well-trained subjects [15]. Previous research has identified significant increases in sAA, ranging from 200% to 265% above baseline following various forms of high intensity exercise and competition [16,17]. However, these responses appear acute in nature with, sAA returning to baseline at 24 h post exercise [16,17]. Subsequently, sAA change has been proposed as an important training response that may provide potential a more precise guide for prescription of training and recovery cycles in athlete populations [18]. While prolonged increases in sympathetic activity were associated with training maladaptation [19,20], further research may extend our understanding of the acute responses of sAA for use during chronic training.

Recognising the importance of acute training responses and their potential to guide training loads, and avoid training maladaptation, the primary aim of this study was to document the acute responses of HRV, sIgA and sAA to daily activities and a standardised high intensity training bout. Secondly, the effects of chronic training on these acute changes were examined to assist coaches for athlete preparation. It was proposed that using HRV, sIgA and sAA in combination would provide a more holistic assessment for a greater understanding of the acute training responses in athlete populations. This knowledge would then contribute to a more accurate prescription of training and recovery cycles, highlighting the early signs of positive and negative training responses during regular periodised training.

2. Materials and Methods

2.1. Participant Demographics

Research approval was granted by the local institutional Human Ethics Research Committee with written consent obtained from all athletes before commencement. Athletes from a high performance Paralympic swimming program were recruited for this study with descriptive statistics and impairment type of each athlete shown in Table 1. All swimmers competed in sprint distance events (<200 m), had competed at the national level in the past 12 months and were ranked in the top 10 worldwide for their main event. Each athlete was classified according to the International Paralympic Committee (IPC) swimming classification code and followed periodised training programs prescribed by the head swimming coach (pool sessions) and strength and conditioning coach (strength sessions).

Table 1. Athlete Characteristics.

Athlete	Sex	Age (years)	Impairment	Athlete (Classification) [a]	National Experience (years) [b]
Athlete 1	F	20	Intellectual	S14	2
Athlete 2	M	29	Amputee	SM10	11
Athlete 3	M	17	Vision	S13	1
Athlete 4	F	15	Cerebral Palsy	S8	1
Athlete 5	M	24	Amputee	S8	6
Athlete 6	M	27	Neuromuscular	S10	11
Athlete 7	M	16	Amputee	S9	1
Athlete 8	M	19	Vision	S13	2

[a] IPC Classification code; [b] Years competing as part of the national Paralympic swimming squad.

2.2. Training Monitoring

Each athlete was monitored during regular periodised training (14 weeks) in the lead up to the 2014 Commonwealth Games and Pan Pacific Para-Swimming Championships [21]. Assessments of resting HR and saliva measures were conducted weekly at 3 time points prior to the start of training (Monday a.m., Monday p.m. and Tuesday a.m.) over the 14-week study period.

2.2.1. Monday a.m. and Tuesday a.m.

Towards the start of each training week, resting HR recordings during the night were acquired (9:00 p.m.–5:00 a.m.) using a Polar RS800CX (Polar Electro Oy, Kuopio, Finland, 1000 Hz). Resting saliva measures were collected at 6:45 a.m. each morning, approximately 10 min before the start of training. These measures were recorded to determine values for HRV, sIgA and sAA prior to the training week and following an afternoon high intensity training session prescribed by the head swimming coach.

2.2.2. Monday p.m.

Resting supine HR and saliva measures were collected at 2:45 p.m. on Monday afternoon, approximately 10 min before the start of training. These measures were recorded to determine values for HRV, sIgA and sAA prior to a high intensity training session prescribed by the head swimming coach. Additionally, these afternoon measures were recorded to examine the influence of daily activity on HRV, sIgA and sAA (*i.e.*, compared to Monday a.m. values).

2.2.3. Training Overview

The training focus of each week varied throughout the 14-week monitoring period with all swimmers following the same training phases that were identified as aerobic maintenance, aerobic capacity, anaerobic capacity, power and speed, and taper (Table 2). As prescribed by the head swimming coach, all athletes trained at a HR below 140 beats per minute (bpm) during the aerobic maintenance phase. The aerobic capacity training phase consisted of low intensity training sessions with a training HR target zone of 140–170 bpm. The anaerobic capacity phase was focussed on high intensity training sessions with a training HR of 170–180 bpm. The power and speed phase included training sessions of higher intensity with moderate recovery periods and no targeted HR zones. The taper training phase consisted of varied intensity training sessions with reduced training volume and no specific HR target zones (Table 2).

Table 2. Average weekly kilometres completed during the 14-week monitoring period.

Training Phase	Week														
	1	2	3	4	5	6	7	8	9	10	11	12	13	14	15
Aerobic Maintenance	28	-	-	-	-	-	-	-	-	-	-	-	-	-	-
Aerobic Capacity	-	34	43	47	48	-	-	-	-	-	-	-	-	-	-
Anaerobic Capacity	-	-	-	-	-	45	48	48	45	47	-	-	-	-	-
Power and Speed	-	-	-	-	-	-	-	-	-	-	46	35	-	-	-
Taper	-	-	-	-	-	-	-	-	-	-	-	-	28	29	-
Competition						X			X				X		X
Swimming Test			X								X				

X indicates competition or swimming test.

The initial training session of each week (*i.e.*, 6:00 a.m. Monday) had an aerobic capacity focus, which did not vary throughout the 14-week monitoring period. The training volume was not controlled for this swim session, however the total swimming distance ranged between 3.5 and 4.5 km during the 14-week monitoring period.

The Monday p.m. (3:00 p.m.) training session was considered the main assessment for the week and the coach used this training session as a gauge of progressive training adaptation. This controlled session was standardised with a consistent volume and swimming activities completed each week across the 14-week monitoring period. The main swimming activities consisted of swimming a total distance of 2.4 km with a 100 m recovery swim (2.5 km total) and was considered a high intensity workload. Volume and intensity of the Monday p.m. training session were consistent throughout the monitoring period, however the training focus shifted according to the training phase (Table 2).

2.3. Procedures

All HR recordings (overnight and resting afternoon) were analysed using Kubios HRV software (v2.1, University of Kuopio, Kuopio, Finland). To ensure a consistent analysis for all athletes, HRV was calculated from the most stable (visually inspected for HR change of less than 10 beats) five minute period (*i.e.*, between 3:00 a.m. and 4:00 a.m. during night time sleep and the last 5 min of the afternoon recording. Ectopic beats and artefact (<5%) were identified and corrected using Kubios' in-built cubic splice interpolation. Along with mean HR, analysis of HRV included time-domain (root mean square of the successive differences (RMSSD)), frequency domain (high frequency normalized units (HFnu)) and non-linear indices (standard deviation of instantaneous RR variability (SD1) and short term fractal scaling exponent (α1)) as previously described [22]. Prior to the commencement of each training session (Monday a.m., Monday p.m. and Tuesday a.m.), saliva samples were obtained from each athlete using an IPRO oral fluid collector (OFC; IPRO Interactive, Oxfordshire, UK). The OFC contains a volume adequacy indicator with a colour change evident (white to dark blue) once 0.5 mL of saliva has been collected. Immediately after collection, each saliva sample was assessed for sIgA and sAA concentrations using an IPRO lateral flow device (IPRO Interactive, Oxfordshire, UK) point of care system as previously described [23]. This method of saliva analysis has previously been validated against ELISA analysis (R^2 = 0.78) [24].

2.4. Data and Statistical Analysis

Comparisons of athlete responses were conducted across two time periods—Monday a.m. to Monday p.m. and Monday a.m. to Tuesday a.m. Acute responses were examined from Monday a.m. to

Monday p.m. to assess the influence of a light training session along with the normal daily influences on HRV, sIgA and sAA. To further examine acute training responses, changes in HRV, sIgA and sAA were examined from Monday a.m. to Tuesday a.m. to identify the influence of a heavy training session, while also accounting for the impact of normal daily influences and a light training session. These comparisons were incorporated to eliminate the impact of diurnal variation and to focus on the effect of high intensity training and its recovery. Acute changes for HRV, sIgA and sAA are presented in relative units (*i.e.*, Monday p.m.—Monday a.m./Monday a.m. × 100 = % change). Weekly comparisons were conducted after transforming the acute change (*i.e.*, +100) and were expressed relative to week one responses.

The practical significance of weekly changes during the monitoring period were assessed via magnitude-based inferences using a downloaded spread sheet [25]. Using standardised differences in means (*i.e.*, Effect Size (ES)) the weekly change was examined with ES threshold values established as small (0.2), moderate (0.6), large (1.2) and very large (2.0) [26]. Magnitude-based inferences were performed using the smallest worthwhile change calculated as 0.2 of the between-subjects standard deviation. Potentially significant positive, trivial or negative changes were identified qualitatively as: almost certainly (>99.5%); very likely (99.5%–95%); likely (95%–75%); possibly (75%–25%); unlikely (25%–5%); very unlikely (5%–0.5%); and almost certainly not (<0.5%). In line with previous research, the true difference was deemed 'unclear' if the chances of having positive and negative changes were both greater than 5% [27].

3. Results

3.1. *Change from Monday a.m. to Monday p.m.*

The percentage change for mean HR at Week 1 was 26.88% (Table 3). Compared to Week 1, changes in mean HR were possibly greater at Week 6, with all other changes unclear during the 14-week monitoring period (Table 3).

The percentage change for HF(nu) at Week 1 was −21.61% (Table 3). Compared to Week 1, changes in HF(nu) were possibly smaller (less negative) at Week 7 and likely smaller (less negative) at Week 10 and Week 13 (Table 3). In contrast, the HF(nu) change was possibly greater (more negative) at Week 6 (Table 3).

The percentage change for SD1 was −26.71% at Week 1 (Table 3). Changes in SD1 compared to Week 1 were likely smaller (less negative) at Week 7 and Week 9 while also possibly smaller (less negative) at Week 13 (Table 3). In contrast, changes in SD1 were possibly greater (more negative) at Week 3 and Week 6, with all other changes trivial or unclear (Table 3).

The percentage change for $\alpha 1$ was 44.64% at Week 1 (Table 3). Compared to Week 1, changes in $\alpha 1$ were unclear except for Weeks 6 and Week 12 which were possibly greater, and Week 7 which was possibly smaller (Table 3).

The percentage change for RMSSD at Week 1 was −28.83% (Figure 1A). Changes for RMSSD were likely smaller (less negative) at Week 7 (78/18/3, ES = 0.40) and Week 9 (83/14/2, ES = 0.44). All other RMSSD changes over the 14-week monitoring period were trivial or unclear (Figure 1A).

For sAA, the percentage change at Week 1 was 15.00% (Figure 1B). Weekly changes for sAA were likely greater for Week 3 (91/6/2, ES = 0.77) and Week 5 (89/7/4, ES = 0.87) while also very likely greater for Weeks 4 (98/2/1, ES = 1.13), 6 (96/2/1, ES = 1.35), 8 (98/1/1, ES = 1.32), 9 (99/1/0, ES = 1.47) and 11 (98/1/0, ES1.35) during the 14-week monitoring period (Figure 1B). In contrast, the sAA change was very likely less (more negative) for Week 7 (0/0/99, ES = −2.46) (Figure 1B).

The percentage change for sIgA was −16.43% at Week 1 (Figure 1C). Weekly changes were mostly trivial or unclear for sIgA when compared to the Week 1 response (Figure 1C). However, sIgA change was likely greater for Week 11 (93/3/4, ES = 1.78), Week 12 (98/1/1, ES = 1.57) and Week 13 (94/4/2, ES = 1.22) (Figure 1C). In contrast, the sIgA change was very likely less for Week 3 (3/3/94, ES = −1.63) (Figure 1C).

Table 3. Monday morning to Tuesday morning change (%) and qualitative inferences for heart rate variability over the 14-week monitoring period.

	Change from Monday a.m. to Monday p.m.													
Week	**1**	**2**	**3**	**4**	**5**	**6**	**7**	**8**	**9**	**10**	**11**	**12**	**13**	**14**
HR	26.88	30.71	32.09	28.12	27.21	35.85	20.74	23.02	23.33	21.90	31.55	30.47	19.80	17.54
(±SD)	(±23.5)	(±29.8)	(±31.5)	(±20.0)	(±20.9)	(±26.4)	(±14.6)	(±13.8)	(±18.0)	(±17.4)	(±19.8)	(±21.0)	(±14.2)	(±11.4)
ES		0.12	0.14	0.07	0.02	0.33	−0.21	−0.11	−0.12	−0.17	0.20	0.15	−0.25	−0.33
QI		Unclear 37/56/7	Unclear 45/38/17	Unclear 32/51/16	Unclear 25/56/19	Possibly +ve 72/24/4	Unclear 12/34/54	Unclear 16/43/41	Unclear 21/36/43	Unclear 7/44/49	Unclear 54/39/7	Unclear 46/45/9	Unclear 12/30/58	Unclear 6/24/70
HF(nu)	−21.61	−13.03	−26.67	−22.27	−22.75	−24.32	−2.84	−7.31	−22.62	−10.00	−18.58	−14.11	2.43	−5.68
(±SD)	(±57.2)	(±53.7)	(±46.1)	(±44.0)	(±35.4)	(±70.2)	(±53.1)	(±86.7)	(±31.9)	(±38.7)	(±33.2)	(±63.3)	(±59.9)	(±74.3)
ES		0.08	−0.03	0.05	0.11	−0.32	0.33	−0.07	0.15	0.34	0.18	0.11	0.39	0.25
QI		Unclear 33/56/12	Unclear 14/65/21	Trivial 11/87/2	Unclear 41/45/15	Possibly −ve 4/25/71	Possibly +ve 71/24/5	Unclear 16/52/32	Unclear 46/35/18	Likely +ve 76/22/3	Unclear 51/44/6	Unclear 37/54/8	Likely +ve 83/16/1	Unclear 60/31/9
SD1	−26.71	−32.74	−32.05	−28.88	−22.10	−36.53	−13.35	−33.77	−10.05	−12.43	−19.65	−22.92	−19.53	−13.65
(±SD)	(±26.6)	(±26.7)	(±33.7)	(±24.1)	(±25.9)	(±24.8)	(±20.2)	(±25.8)	(±21.5)	(±14.2)	(±14.9)	(±27.2)	(±15.9)	(±28.0)
ES		−0.17	−0.23	−0.01	0.16	−0.23	0.38	−0.13	0.44	0.42	0.28	0.16	0.28	0.35
QI		Trivial 1/51/47	Possibly −ve 5/35/59	Unclear 12/73/14	Unclear 48/39/13	Possibly −ve 1/33/66	Likely +ve 77/19/4	Unclear 7/54/40	Likely +ve 79/17/4	Unclear 74/19/7	Unclear 61/28/11	Unclear 48/33/18	Possibly +ve 66/29/5	Unclear 68/23/9
α1	44.64	38.18	50.24	58.37	19.85	65.13	33.21	57.79	35.43	29.47	49.97	71.56	33.13	33.07
(±SD)	(±55.4)	(±53.6)	(±47.8)	(±60.7)	(±34.6)	(±85.3)	(±84.0)	(±78.8)	(±57.2)	(±55.3)	(±61.9)	(±91.4)	(±87.5)	(±53.6)
ES		−0.08	0.13	0.21	−0.35	0.21	−0.32	0.10	−0.13	−0.27	0.08	0.28	−0.31	−0.17
QI		Unclear 7/64/28	Unclear 43/46/11	Unclear 55/39/6	Unclear 8/24/69	Possibly +ve 57/39/5	Possibly −ve 5/26/69	Unclear 38/48/15	Unclear 17/39/44	Unclear 11/28/61	Unclear 36/47/17	Possibly +ve 68/29/3	Unclear 8/26/66	Unclear 9/41/49

Heart rate = HR; High frequency normalised units = HF(nu); standard deviation of instantaneous RR variability = SD1; short term fractal scaling exponent = α1; SD = Standard Deviation; ES = Effect Size; QI = Qualitative Inference; +ve = Positive; −ve = Negative.

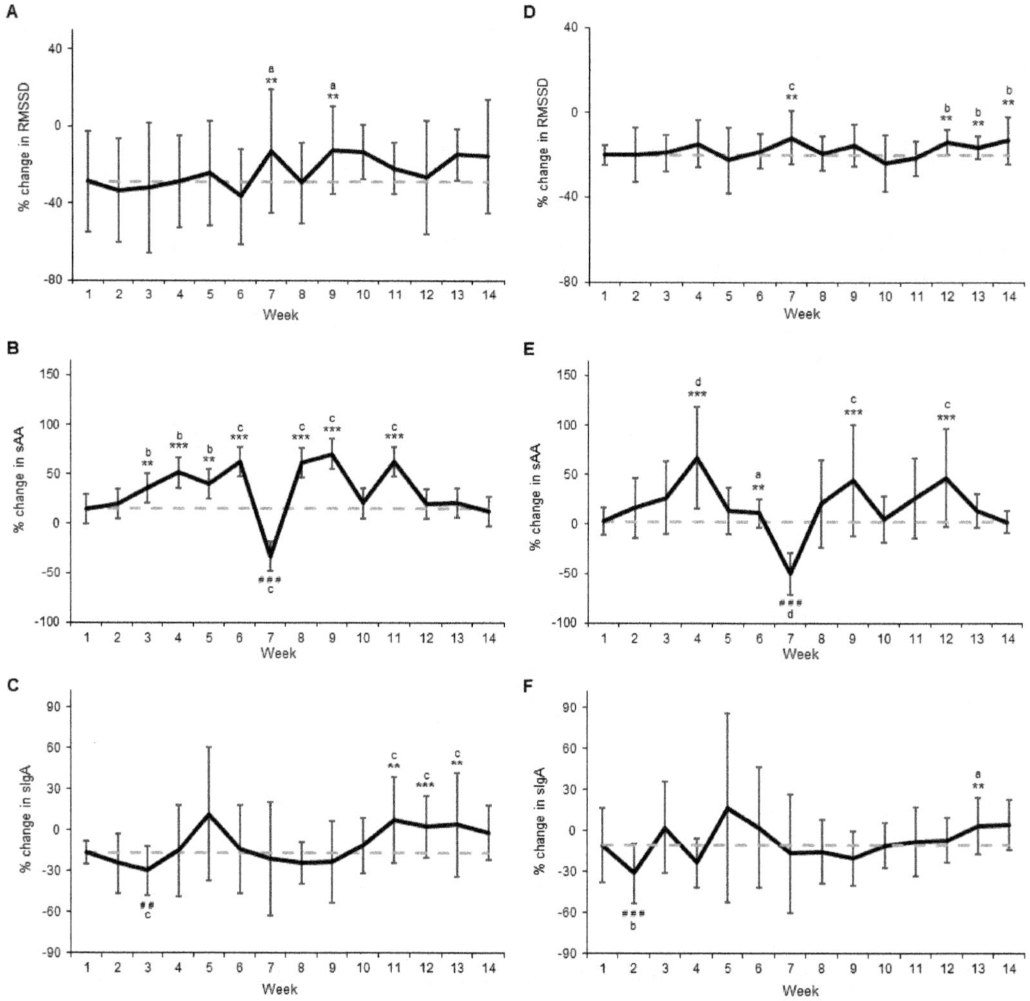

Figure 1. Percentage change (±SD) from Monday a.m. to Monday p.m. for: (**a**) RMSSD (**b**) sAA; (**c**) sIgA; and percentage change from Monday a.m. to Tuesday a.m. for (**d**) RMSSD (**e**) sAA; and (**f**) sIgA over the 14-week monitoring period. SD = Standard Deviation, RMSSD = square root of the mean squared difference of successive RR intervals, sAA = salivary alpha amylase, sIgA = salivary immunoglobulin A. Dashed line represents Week 1 response for comparison. ** likely greater; *** very likely greater; # # likely lower; # # # very likely lower; a indicates small effect size; b indicates moderate effect size; c indicates large effect sizeA.

3.2. Change from Monday a.m. to Tuesday a.m.

The percentage change for mean HR was 5.45% at Week 1 (Table 4) with all changes during the 14-week monitoring period being trivial or unclear (Table 4).

The percentage change at Week 1 was −2.10% for HF(nu) (Table 4) with all changes being trivial or unclear during the 14-week monitoring period (Table 4).

For SD1, the percentage change was −18.67% at Week 1 (Table 4). Changes for SD1 were likely smaller (less negative) for Week 12 and Week 14 (Table 4). In contrast, the change in SD1 at Week 10 was very likely greater (more negative), with all other changes unclear during the 14-week monitoring period (Table 4).

Table 4. Monday morning to Tuesday morning change (%) and qualitative inferences for heart rate variability over the 14-week monitoring period.

	Change from Monday a.m. to Tuesday a.m.													
Week	**1**	**2**	**3**	**4**	**5**	**6**	**7**	**8**	**9**	**10**	**11**	**12**	**13**	**14**
HR	5.45	6.86	6.16	7.73	3.98	9.44	7.75	7.10	6.29	9.26	8.34	6.43	3.56	5.28
(±SD)	(±12.3)	(±8.5)	(±9.9)	(±7.6)	(±13.9)	(±10.7)	(±16.1)	(±9.1)	(±12.9)	(±7.6)	(±8.5)	(±10.0)	(±6.6)	(±5.8)
ES		0.12	0.07	0.18	−0.12	0.28	0.14	0.13	0.06	0.29	0.22	0.08	−0.10	0.03
QI		Trivial 34/63/3	Unclear 39/33/28	Unclear 51/40/9	Unclear 20/37/43	Unclear 60/26/14	Unclear 47/29/25	Unclear 46/30/24	Unclear 40/29/31	Unclear 62/27/11	Unclear 54/28/18	Unclear 30/62/8	Unclear 25/33/42	Unclear 31/43/26
HF(nu)	−2.10	−8.38	−11.94	−5.20	−7.40	11.80	18.43	−13.91	−6.62	−19.42	−18.04	−15.17	7.55	11.17
(±SD)	(±40.3)	(±35.4)	(±34.5)	(±39.8)	(±35.6)	(±40.4)	(±55.4)	(±22.4)	(±39.5)	(±25.9)	(±20.3)	(±29.3)	(±46.4)	(±79.8)
ES		−0.03	−0.07	0.02	−0.04	0.26	0.33	−0.06	−0.02	−0.21	−0.14	−0.14	0.21	0.10
QI		Unclear 25/44/31	Unclear 18/47/34	Unclear 28/49/23	Unclear 34/26/39	Unclear 60/30/10	Unclear 69/24/6	Unclear 20/47/33	Unclear 34/28/38	Unclear 9/37/55	Unclear 11/46/43	Trivial 3/59/38	Unclear 53/27/20	Unclear 41/37/22
SD1	−18.67	−21.80	−19.03	−14.80	−17.52	−18.08	−2.83	−19.83	−15.03	−23.81	−20.00	−13.11	−16.04	−11.61
(±SD)	(±6.4)	(±11.9)	(±8.7)	(±11.1)	(±25.5)	(±8.1)	(±26.6)	(±8.7)	(±9.6)	(±13.3)	(±8.8)	(±6.5)	(±5.5)	(±10.8)
ES		−0.53	−0.08	0.47	−0.25	0.06	1.70	−0.19	0.46	−0.86	−0.22	0.74	0.36	0.89
QI		Unclear 10/15/74	Unclear 29/30/41	Unclear 67/16/17	Unclear 33/14/53	Unclear 39/32/29	Unclear 90/4/6	Unclear 23/26/51	Unclear 70/17/13	Likely −ve 5/8/88	Unclear 16/30/54	Likely +ve 88/8/4	Unclear 67/22/11	Likely +ve 92/6/3
α1	12.34	4.18	19.60	18.61	9.45	22.15	4.08	46.60	4.67	17.58	29.94	22.26	11.40	20.91
(±SD)	(±41.5)	(±33.7)	(±29.1)	(±25.2)	(±39.3)	(±58.2)	(±49.0)	(±43.3)	(±24.3)	(±28.3)	(±29.8)	(±40.3)	(±23.7)	(±56.1)
ES		−0.17	0.23	0.23	−0.09	0.14	−0.28	0.75	−0.12	0.20	0.47	0.25	0.07	0.14
QI		Unclear 7/45/48	Unclear 56/31/13	Unclear 56/29/15	Unclear 31/25/44	Unclear 47/31/22	Unclear 10/28/62	Likely +ve 94/5/1	Unclear 24/31/45	Unclear 54/37/10	Likely +ve 80/16/4	Possibly +ve 65/33/2	Unclear 38/38/25	Unclear 46/34/20

Heart rate = HR; High frequency normalised units = HF(nu); standard deviation of instantaneous RR variability = SD1; short term fractal scaling exponent = α1; SD = Standard Deviation; ES = Effect Size; QI = Qualitative Inference; +ve = Positive; −ve = Negative.

The percentage change for α1 was 12.34% at Week 1 (Table 4). Compared to Week 1, changes in α1 were unclear except for Weeks 8, 11 and 12, which were likely and possibly greater, respectively (Table 4).

The percentage change for RMSSD at Week 1 was −20.09% (Figure 1D). Changes in RMSSD were likely smaller (less negative) for Week 7 (90/5/5, ES = 1.30), Week 12 (93/4/2, ES = 1.01), Week 13 (83/11/5, ES = 0.63) and Week 14 (92/5/3, ES = 1.11) (Figure 1D). All other changes during the 14-week monitoring period were trivial or unclear (Figure 1D).

The percentage change at Week 1 for sAA was 2.95% (Figure 1E). The change in sAA was likely greater at Week 6 (83/14/3, ES = 0.49), while also very likely greater for Week 4 (99/0/0, ES = 2.70), Week 9 (99/1/0, ES = 1.79) and Week 12 (96/2/2, ES = 1.91) (Figure 1E). In contrast, the change in sAA was very likely less (more negative) at Week 7 (0/0/99, ES = −4.69) (Figure 1E). All other changes in sAA were unclear during the 14-week monitoring period (Figure 1E).

The percentage change for sIgA was −10.87% at Week 1 (Figure 1F). The majority of changes for sIgA were trivial or unclear during the 14-week monitoring period (Figure 1F). However, sIgA was likely greater for Week 13 (86/11/2, ES = 0.53) while also very likely less for Week 2 (0/1/99, ES = −0.85) (Figure 1F).

4. Discussion

For the first time, the present study examined cardiac autonomic activity and salivary responses in relation to normal daily influences (Monday a.m. to Monday p.m.) while also examining acute (<24 h, Monday a.m. to Tuesday a.m.) responses to a standardised swimming, training bout. Additionally, this study highlighted the chronic training responses of acute changes in HRV, sIgA and sAA over a 14-week monitoring period, leading into a major international competition.

4.1. Change from Monday a.m. to Monday p.m.

The current study demonstrated the acute increases of HR, α1 and sAA with corresponding decreases in RMSSD, HF(nu), SD1 and sIgA from Monday morning to Monday afternoon.

The increase in mean HR and α1 along with the reciprocal decrease in RMSSD, HF(nu) and SD1 was likely a result of the circadian changes in cardiac autonomic activity and normal daily activities [28,29]. Earlier studies have reported that parasympathetic activity is typically elevated in the morning while sympathetic modulation increases throughout the day as a result of circadian changes in neural discharge and daily activities [28,29]. However, these prior studies were conducted at rest and did not include the impact of daily activities. While the current athletes did not partake in any strenuous physical activity during the day, all athletes were studying at high school or university and as such did not rest all day between training sessions. For the current study, athletes undertook a morning training session that likely increased HR and reduced HRV, though this change was likely to be short-acting due to the low intensity nature of the training session. A previous study has shown that cardiac parasympathetic activity typically returns to baseline within 15 min following low intensity aerobic exercise [7] with the current daily change in HRV likely to be a normal result of daily activities and autonomic nervous system circadian rhythm.

Similar to the change in HRV mentioned above, there was also a consistent increase in sAA from Monday morning to Monday afternoon for most weeks of the 14-week monitoring period. As all training sessions on Monday morning were completed at a low intensity with acute elevations in sAA reported to be short [30,31], the increase in sAA during Monday was likely due to the typical diurnal pattern in this measure. Through examination of hourly levels of sAA in 76 healthy adults (44 women and 32 men), Nater and colleagues [32] identified an average daily increase of approximately 35%. A slightly lower daily increase in sAA (average increase of 18%) was observed for athletes in the current study, suggesting that athletes may display a lower than normal daily variance in sAA. However, of note was the significantly greater sAA increases for most weeks between Week 3 and 11 (average increase of 55%). This response was greater than the observed average daily increase reported by

Nater and colleagues [32] and may represent an accumulated stress response from weekly training for athletes. Remarkably, none of the HRV parameters exhibited this trend for Weeks 3–11 indicating that HRV and sAA may reflect different training responses with sAA potentially more sensitive to the combined stress of training and daily activities. For examples, during Week 6, athletes experienced a greater increase in HR and $\alpha 1$ with corresponding decrease in HF(nu) and SD1 suggesting that athletes were more stimulated over the day. No noticeable changes in training volume or intensity were noted for athletes, with these greater than normal (Week 1) responses potentially a result of an increase in daily activities.

Regardless, the reported Monday a.m. to p.m. changes in HRV and sAA in the current study provide coaches and athletes with normative data to assist in the monitoring of training.

Another key observation from the present study was the negative change in sAA from Monday morning to Monday afternoon at the beginning of Week 7. This assessment was done following a competitive weekend of races with a subsequent elevation in sAA levels Monday morning and a negative change by Monday afternoon. A recent study has shown that elite level competition produces a sustained increase in sAA for up to 48 h after a national swimming grand prix competition similar to that in the current study [21]. Increased levels of cortisol have also been reported after a rugby league match [33] further supporting that high-level competition induces a prolonged stress response, which may influence subsequent training and performance. The current study extends these previous findings and indicates that competition maintains stress responses (*i.e.*, sAA) for some time after the event. Further, this stress response was not altered by a light training session soon after the competition (<24 h) and highlights the need for rest to return athletes to pre competition homeostasis [34].

Accompanying this heightened stress response at the beginning of Week 7, there were smaller a.m. to p.m. responses for HF(nu), SD1 and RMSSD (*i.e.*, smaller negative changes) compared to Week 1. This Week-7 response reflected heightened sympathetic and/or attenuated parasympathetic modulations (*i.e.*, HFnu, SD1 and RMSSD) at Monday a.m. from the lasting effects of the weekend competition, which were altered to a lesser degree during the day. Previous research has highlighted the sustained impact of competition on HRV with a significant reduction in HRV for 48 h after a rugby league match [22] and following a national swimming grand prix [21] being reported. The current study provides further evidence of important physiological changes (*i.e.*, HRV and sAA) in response to severe effort (competition) [21,22,33]. Interestingly, changes in mean HR and the salivary marker of immune function (sIgA) were not different at Week 7 compared to Week 1 indicating that these measures may be insensitive to the stress responses in the days following competition. Subsequently, the monitoring of HRV (HFnu, SD1, and RMSSD) and sAA may provide sound indicators of stress response to training and high level competition for coaches to better manage training workloads of their athletes [21].

4.2. Change from Monday a.m. to Tuesday a.m.

Examining the change in HRV, sIgA and sAA from Monday morning to Tuesday morning highlighted a number of key findings. Similar to the observed change for Monday a.m. to Monday p.m. responses, there were comparable Monday a.m. to Tuesday a.m. changes in mean HR and HRV for most weeks over the monitoring period. The a.m. to a.m. changes though were of a smaller magnitude compared to the a.m. to p.m. changes (see Tables 3 and 4) and likely reflected a similar morning level of cardiac autonomic activity and recovery from the p.m. training session. However, at the beginning of Week 7 (post-competition weekend) there was a greater a.m. to a.m. response (*i.e.*, smaller absolute change) in RMSSD compared to Week 1 that was accompanied by changes in sAA. As described before, the Week 7 response was likely a result of lower HRV and parasympathetic modulations (RMSSD) and greater stress levels (sAA) at Monday a.m. following the competition weekend. Importantly, the overnight response for HRV and sAA in Week 7 did not appear to be altered as a result of the p.m. training session and further highlights the acute effects of training [7] and importance of rest to restore homeostatic balance [34].

Another significant finding from the current study was the greater a.m. to a.m. response for RMSSD towards the end of the monitoring period (*i.e.*, Weeks 12–14). Earlier studies have shown that cardiac autonomic activity may "rebound" from acute training sessions to levels above pre-training, resting values [25,35], similar to that observed in the current study. Interestingly, this response was not evident in the early stages of the monitoring period (Weeks 1–11), suggesting the rebound in cardiac vagal activity observed in Weeks 12–14 was a result of the reduction in training load during the taper training phase. Earlier studies have reported increases in RMSSD during periods of reduced training load [36,37] with this increase related to gains in performance [36]. The current study extends these previous results and indicates that cardiac parasympathetic activity increases in response to training, during periods of reduced training load. This greater training response for RMSSD may further indicate an increased readiness for athlete's to deal with stressors. Future research may identify whether assessing changes in HRV in response to a standardized training bout, as opposed to measuring the absolute change in HRV over time, provides a more detailed understanding of training responses in elite athlete populations.

Curiously, there were likely greater increase in sAA for some Weeks (4, 6, 9 and 12) but not others. There was no apparent trend for these responses and they did not coincide with commencement/end of training phases or with HRV measures. Speculatively, these results may indicate aftereffects of the high intensity training bout on Monday afternoon in combination with the stress responses associated with daily activities previously discussed however, this response was inconsistent. Further investigation may elaborate on the mechanisms and practical implications for such responses.

Lastly, a greater increase in sIgA was noted for Week 13, a taper phase. Earlier studies have reported decreases in sIgA following high intensity exercise bouts, which may alter immune function for up to 72 h and increase an athlete's susceptibility to illness [38–40]. However, previous research has also observed increases in sIgA following various forms of high intensity exercise [41–43]. In the current study the increase in sIgA was reported at 14 h post exercise and as such may not have been the peak value. Therefore the current results highlight a prolonged increase in sIgA, contrary to previous studies [44,45]. No athletes reported any signs of illness during the taper period suggesting that the high intensity training session had no negative influence on the athlete's immune function in the lead up to competition. Additionally, the greater response for sIgA was only observed in Week 13, with greater responses also noted for RMSSD in the week before, during and after sIgA increase (*i.e.*, Weeks 12–14). Subsequently, the reduction in training load, typical during a taper period, may result in heightened parasympathetic modulations along with increased immune function, and provide an appropriate strategy to minimize fatigue and optimize the health status of athletes prior to competition. Further, RMSSD may provide a more sensitive and early indication of the positive training responses during periods of reduced training load. Future studies are encouraged to examine performance measures to substantiate the potential application of sIgA monitoring during long-term training in athletic populations.

While the current results are based on a small sample size (n = 8), numbers of this size are typical of this athlete population, and common in research using elite athlete populations [21,46,47]. Furthermore, statistical analysis was adjusted accordingly with data analysed using magnitude-based inferences to account for individual variations in HRV and saliva variables and to best examine the practical significance of the data when investigating smaller populations. Additionally, the use of nocturnal HRV measures may have limited the current results. Seated HRV measurements have been shown to potentially limit the effect of HRV saturation and as such may provide more beneficial information when compared to nocturnal HRV measures.

5. Conclusions

This unique study has documented the impact of daily activities on HRV and saliva (sIgA and sAA) responses with and without a standardized training bout repeated over a 14-week monitoring period. The current study has identified that cardiac autonomic activity and salivary markers of immune function and stress responded consistently to daily activities and training, likely a result of the effective training and recovery prescription. Additionally, the study highlighted important physiological changes (*i.e.*, HRV and sAA) in response to competition and subsequent rest/recovery. Lastly, HRV appears to be more a sensitive indicator of positive training responses during periods of reduced training load when compared with sIgA. Gaining a better understanding of how these physiological markers respond to various forms of training intensity will lead to an improved understanding of training responses and recovery cycles along with highlighting the early signs of positive and negative training responses in elite athlete populations.

Author Contributions: All authors contributed equally to this paper.

Conflicts of Interest: The authors declare no conflict of interest.

References

1. Heisterberg, M.F.; Fahrenkrug, J.; Krustrup, P.; Storskov, A.; Kjaer, M.; Andersen, J.L. Extensive monitoring through multiple blood samples in professional soccer players. *J. Strength Cond. Res.* **2013**, *27*, 1260–1271. [CrossRef] [PubMed]
2. Borresen, J.; Lambert, M.I. The quantification of training load, the training response and the effect on performance. *Sports Med.* **2009**, *39*, 779–795. [CrossRef] [PubMed]
3. Taylor, K.-L.; Chapman, D.W.; Cronin, J.B.; Newton, M.J.; Gill, N. Fatigue monitoring in high performance sport: A survey of current trends. *J. Aust. Strength Cond.* **2012**, *20*, 12–23.
4. Boullosa, D.A.; Abreu, L.; Nakamura, F.Y.; Munoz, V.E.; Dominguez, E.; Leicht, A.S. Cardiac autonomic adaptations in elite spanish soccer players during preseason. *Int. J. Sports Physiol. Perform.* **2013**, *8*, 400–409. [PubMed]
5. Edmonds, R.; Leicht, A.; McKean, M.; Burkett, B. Daily heart rate variability of paralympic gold medallist swimmers: A 17-week investigation. *J. Sport Health Sci.* **2014**. in press. [CrossRef]
6. Atlaoui, D.; Pichot, V.; Lacoste, L.; Barale, F.; Lacour, J.R.; Chatard, J.C. Heart rate variability, training variation and performance in elite swimmers. *Int. J. Sports Med.* **2007**, *28*, 394–400. [CrossRef] [PubMed]
7. Stanley, J.; Peake, J.M.; Buchheit, M. Cardiac parasympathetic reactivation following exercise: Implications for training prescription. *Sports Med.* **2013**, *43*, 1259–1277. [CrossRef] [PubMed]
8. Plews, D.J.; Laursen, P.B.; Stanley, J.; Kilding, A.E.; Buchheit, M. Training adaptation and heart rate variability in elite endurance athletes: Opening the door to effective monitoring. *Sports Med.* **2013**, *43*, 773–781. [CrossRef] [PubMed]
9. Moreira, A.; de Moura, N.R.; Coutts, A.; Costa, E.C.; Kempton, T.; Aoki, M.S. Monitoring internal training load and mucosal immune responses in futsal athletes. *J. Strength Cond. Res.* **2013**, *27*, 1253–1259. [CrossRef] [PubMed]
10. Pedersen, B.K.; Kappel, M.; Klokker, M.; Nielsen, H.B.; Secher, N.H. The immune system during exposure to extreme physiologic conditions. *Int. J. Sports Med.* **1994**, *15* (Suppl. 3), S116–S121. [CrossRef] [PubMed]
11. Nieman, D.C.; Pedersen, B.K. Exercise and immune function. Recent developments. *Sports Med.* **1999**, *27*, 73–80. [CrossRef] [PubMed]
12. Mackinnon, L.T.; Ginn, E.; Seymour, G.J. Decreased salivary immunoglobulin a secretion rate after intense interval exercise in elite kayakers. *Eur. J. Appl. Physiol. Occup. Physiol.* **1993**, *67*, 180–184. [CrossRef] [PubMed]
13. Nieman, D.C. Exercise, infection, and immunity. *Int. J. Sports Med.* **1994**, *15* (Suppl. 3), S131–S141. [CrossRef] [PubMed]
14. Nater, U.M.; Rohleder, N. Salivary alpha-amylase as a non-invasive biomarker for the sympathetic nervous system: Current state of research. *Psychoneuroendocrinology* **2009**, *34*, 486–496. [CrossRef] [PubMed]
15. Bocanegra, O.L.; Diaz, M.M.; Teixeira, R.R.; Soares, S.S.; Espindola, F.S. Determination of the lactate threshold by means of salivary biomarkers: Chromogranin a as novel marker of exercise intensity. *Eur. J. Appl. Physiol.* **2012**, *112*, 3195–3203. [CrossRef] [PubMed]
16. Steerenberg, P.A.; van Asperen, I.A.; van Nieuw Amerongen, A.; Biewenga, A.; Mol, D.; Medema, G.J. Salivary levels of immunoglobulin a in triathletes. *Eur. J. Oral. Sci.* **1997**, *105*, 305–309. [CrossRef] [PubMed]

17. Walsh, N.P.; Blannin, A.K.; Clark, A.M.; Cook, L.; Robson, P.J.; Gleeson, M. The effects of high-intensity intermittent exercise on saliva iga, total protein and alpha-amylase. *J. Sports Sci.* **1999**, *17*, 129–134. [CrossRef] [PubMed]
18. Papacosta, E.; Nassis, G.P. Saliva as a tool for monitoring steroid, peptide and immune markers in sport and exercise science. *J. Sci. Med. Sport* **2011**, *14*, 424–434. [CrossRef] [PubMed]
19. Hedelin, R.; Wiklund, U.; Bjerle, P.; Henriksson-Larsen, K. Cardiac autonomic imbalance in an overtrained athlete. *Med. Sci. Sports Exerc.* **2000**, *32*, 1531–1533. [CrossRef] [PubMed]
20. Mourot, L.; Bouhaddi, M.; Perrey, S.; Cappelle, S.; Henriet, M.T.; Wolf, J.P.; Rouillon, J.D.; Regnard, J. Decrease in heart rate variability with overtraining: Assessment by the poincare plot analysis. *Clin. Physiol. Funct. Imaging* **2004**, *24*, 10–18. [CrossRef] [PubMed]
21. Edmonds, R.; Burkett, B.; Leicht, A.; McKean, M. Effect of chronic training on heart rate variability, salivary iga and salivary alpha-amylase in elite swimmers with a disability. *PLoS One* **2015**, *10*, e0127749. [CrossRef] [PubMed]
22. Edmonds, R.C.; Sinclair, W.H.; Leicht, A.S. Effect of a training week on heart rate variability in elite youth rugby league players. *Int. J. Sports Med.* **2013**, *34*, 1087–1092. [CrossRef] [PubMed]
23. Dunbar, J.; Armitage, M.; Jehanli, A.; Browne, A. Mucosal immunity and self-reported upper respiratory symptoms in a cohort of premier league academy soccer players. *Int. J. Exerc. Sci. Conf. Proc.* **2013**, *10*, Article 45.
24. Dunbar, J.; Jehanli, A.; Skelhorn, S. Investigating the use of a point of care siga test in the sporting environment. In Proceedings of the 10th International Society of Exercise Immunology, Oxford, UK, 11–13 July 2011; p. 85.
25. Buchheit, M.; Laursen, P.B.; Al Haddad, H.; Ahmaidi, S. Exercise-induced plasma volume expansion and post-exercise parasympathetic reactivation. *Eur. J. Appl. Physiol.* **2009**, *105*, 471–481. [CrossRef] [PubMed]
26. Stanley, J.; Halliday, A.; D'Auria, S.; Buchheit, M.; Leicht, A.S. Effect of sauna-based heat acclimation on plasma volume and heart rate variability. *Eur. J. Appl. Physiol.* **2015**, *115*, 785–794. [CrossRef] [PubMed]
27. Hopkins, W.G.; Marshall, S.W.; Batterham, A.M.; Hanin, J. Progressive statistics for studies in sports medicine and exercise science. *Med. Sci. Sports Exerc.* **2009**, *41*, 3–13. [CrossRef] [PubMed]
28. Massin, M.M.; Maeyns, K.; Withofs, N.; Ravet, F.; Gerard, P. Circadian rhythm of heart rate and heart rate variability. *Arch. Dis. Child.* **2000**, *83*, 179–182. [CrossRef] [PubMed]
29. Hayano, J.; Sakakibara, Y.; Yamada, M.; Kamiya, T.; Fujinami, T.; Yokoyama, K.; Watanabe, Y.; Takata, K. Diurnal variations in vagal and sympathetic cardiac control. *Am. J. Physiol.* **1990**, *258*, H642–H646. [PubMed]
30. Chatterton, R.T., Jr.; Vogelsong, K.M.; Lu, Y.C.; Ellman, A.B.; Hudgens, G.A. Salivary alpha-amylase as a measure of endogenous adrenergic activity. *Clin. Physiol.* **1996**, *16*, 433–448. [CrossRef] [PubMed]
31. Ljungberg, G.; Ericson, T.; Ekblom, B.; Birkhed, D. Saliva and marathon running. *Scand. J. Med. Sci. Sports* **1997**, *7*, 214–219. [CrossRef] [PubMed]
32. Nater, U.M.; Rohleder, N.; Schlotz, W.; Ehlert, U.; Kirschbaum, C. Determinants of the diurnal course of salivary alpha-amylase. *Psychoneuroendocrinology* **2007**, *32*, 392–401. [CrossRef] [PubMed]
33. McLean, B.D.; Coutts, A.J.; Kelly, V.; McGuigan, M.R.; Cormack, S.J. Neuromuscular, endocrine, and perceptual fatigue responses during different length between-match microcycles in professional rugby league players. *Int. J. Sports Physiol. Perform.* **2010**, *5*, 367–383. [PubMed]
34. Carvalho Leme, L.; Milanez, V.; Oliveira, R.; de Paulo Ramos, S.; Leicht, A.; Nakamura, F. The influence of a weekend with passive rest on the psychological and autonomic recovery in professional handball players. *Kinesiology* **2015**, *47*, 44–52.
35. Hautala, A.; Tulppo, M.P.; Makikallio, T.H.; Laukkanen, R.; Nissila, S.; Huikuri, H.V. Changes in cardiac autonomic regulation after prolonged maximal exercise. *Clin. Physiol.* **2001**, *21*, 238–245. [CrossRef] [PubMed]
36. Garet, M.; Tournaire, N.; Roche, F.; Laurent, R.; Lacour, J.R.; Barthelemy, J.C.; Pichot, V. Individual interdependence between nocturnal ans activity and performance in swimmers. *Med. Sci. Sports Exerc.* **2004**, *36*, 2112–2118. [CrossRef] [PubMed]
37. Pichot, V.; Roche, F.; Gaspoz, J.M.; Enjolras, F.; Antoniadis, A.; Minini, P.; Costes, F.; Busso, T.; Lacour, J.R.; Barthelemy, J.C. Relation between heart rate variability and training load in middle-distance runners. *Med. Sci. Sports Exerc.* **2000**, *32*, 1729–1736. [CrossRef] [PubMed]
38. Nieman, D.C. Immune response to heavy exertion. *J. Appl. Physiol.* **1997**, *82*, 1385–1394. [PubMed]

39. Hoffman-Goetz, L.; Pedersen, B.K. Exercise and the immune system: A model of the stress response? *Immunol. Today* **1994**, *15*, 382–387. [CrossRef]
40. Nieman, D.C. Exercise immunology: Practical applications. *Int. J. Sports Med.* **1997**, *18* (Suppl. 1), S91–S100. [CrossRef] [PubMed]
41. Blannin, A.K.; Robson, P.J.; Walsh, N.P.; Clark, A.M.; Glennon, L.; Gleeson, M. The effect of exercising to exhaustion at different intensities on saliva immunoglobulin a, protein and electrolyte secretion. *Int. J. Sports Med.* **1998**, *19*, 547–552. [CrossRef] [PubMed]
42. Sari-Sarraf, V.; Reilly, T.; Doran, D.A.; Atkinson, G. The effects of single and repeated bouts of soccer-specific exercise on salivary iga. *Arch. Oral. Biol.* **2007**, *52*, 526–532. [CrossRef] [PubMed]
43. Nehlsen-Cannarella, S.L.; Nieman, D.C.; Fagoaga, O.R.; Kelln, W.J.; Henson, D.A.; Shannon, M.; Davis, J.M. Saliva immunoglobulins in elite women rowers. *Eur. J. Appl. Physiol.* **2000**, *81*, 222–228. [CrossRef] [PubMed]
44. Allgrove, J.E.; Gomes, E.; Hough, J.; Gleeson, M. Effects of exercise intensity on salivary antimicrobial proteins and markers of stress in active men. *J. Sports Sci.* **2008**, *26*, 653–661. [CrossRef] [PubMed]
45. Sari-Sarraf, V.; Reilly, T.; Doran, D.A. Salivary iga response to intermittent and continuous exercise. *Int. J. Sports Med.* **2006**, *27*, 849–855. [CrossRef] [PubMed]
46. Edmonds, R.C.; Leicht, A.S.; McKean, M.; Burkett, B. Daily heart rate variability during an 18-day staging camp in paralympic medallist swimmers. *J. Exerc. Physiol.* **2014**, *17*, 84–92.
47. Plews, D.J.; Laursen, P.B.; Kilding, A.E.; Buchheit, M. Heart rate variability in elite triathletes, is variation in variability the key to effective training? A case comparison. *Eur. J. Appl. Physiol.* **2012**, *112*, 3729–3741. [CrossRef] [PubMed]

6

"You're Not Born with Talent" Talented Girls' and Boys' Perceptions of Their Talents as Football Players

Stig Arve Sæther * and Ingar Mehus

Department of Sociology and Political Science, Norwegian University of Science and Technology, Dragvoll, Trondheim 7491, Norway; ingar.mehus@svt.ntnu.no
* Correspondence: stigarve@ntnu.no

Academic Editor: Eling de Bruin

Abstract: Generally in sports, there is a strong assumption of a connection between skill level in young age and adulthood. Studies have mainly focused on the coaches' understanding and role in identifying and developing talent. In this article we turn our attention towards the athletes' perspectives, interviewing talented young football players (five boys and five girls) about their perceptions of their own talent and development. The objective of the article is to investigate how boys and girls perceive their talent and to discuss how various perceptions influence coaching practice in talent development. We introduce the following questions: (a) do the players use a static or dynamic perception of their own talent and (b) do the players consider specific or general skills to be most important in their skill development? Results show that the boys have a more static perception of talent compared to the girls. Furthermore, the boys in this study stress the importance of highly specified skills. The girls have a more balanced view on what is important, but tend to stress the importance of basic skills. The study suggests two potential implications. First, the coaches should be aware of the possible vulnerability following players' static perception of talent. Second, an exclusive focus on specified skills might make for less optimal preparation for the changing demands young players meet when moving through the different levels of play on their way to high level football. In future research it would be interesting to investigate how players with a lower skill level, not yet regarded as talent, perceive their talent and skill development.

Keywords: football; talent development; youth sports; skills; perception of talent

---

1. Introduction

Most top-level clubs in European football are looking for the most talented boys and girls. The players who, compared with their peers, have skills that are recognized and highlighted as important and are described as potential professional football players [1]. The value and reasoning for the clubs' and coaches' focus on identifying the most talented players rest on several basic assumptions regarding talent development. Some well-established assumptions are that talent is hereditary, that talent is domain-specific, that a trained eye can identify talent at an early age, and that such early indicators predict future success [2].

Talented football players are obviously part of selection systems where the benefits of being among the selected are clear [3], even though there are many obstacles in this process [4]. However, focusing on identifying and selecting the most talented players could impact both the players' assessments of their own skills, and which skills they think are preferable for being defined as talented players. From a player perspective, they are dependent on understanding which skills to develop to increase the likelihood of becoming a professional football player. They are confronted with many of the basic assumptions that underlie the selection process, coloring their understanding of the value of their own talent. Abbott and Collins [5] distinguish between static and dynamic perception of skill development. The static perception focuses on skills as congenital and less trainable. This perspective basically focuses on identifying the most talented players, where the players must prove their skills to the coaches and clubs. The dynamic perception highlights skills to be largely dependent on efforts to improve, and sees talent as something players achieve through training. It should be noted that talent identification and talent development are not necessarily experienced as separate processes for all football coaches, but rather are reflexively aligned [6]. Interestingly though, research has shown that top-level coaches have problems defining the criteria used when identifying talented players [7].

2. Context

Even if previous research on factors affecting talent development has been extensive among male players [8–10], research has not been able to confirm most of the basic assumptions [8,11]. Research investigating female players' talent development has been less extensive, with a lack of research targeting the development process from a longitudinal perspective [12,13]. A factor indicating that the selection process among female players is less essential compared to male players is the less pronounced relative age effect [14]. This effect is described as the tendency of selecting talented players by an early birth month, especially the first three months of the year [15–17]. These results could indicate that female players could regard their skills as less dependent on talent, which could suggest that they will lean on a more dynamic perception of talent.

Partly based on the basic assumptions of talent development, there are different models and theoretical frameworks aiming to understand talent development. The focus on training volume has been highlighted [18], introducing the term deliberate practice, indicating a linear relationship between training volume and skill level. Deliberate practice is characterized by being controlled by a coach, giving instructions and guidelines, as well as the training session having clear goals. This perspective has, however, been challenged by Côté and Fraser-Thomas [19], introducing deliberate play as an alternative to deliberate practice, where deliberate play is characterized by being self-organized and does not necessarily include a clear goal for every training session. These two perspectives on talent development also indicate the difference between focusing on highly specific skills compared to more general football skills. While some players tend to focus on developing highly specific skills, others focus on more general skills, compensating for deficiencies in one area by strengthening others [20]. The complexity of developing expertise in football is an argument for not needing extraordinary capacities within all of the various technical, psychological and physical demands [21]. Even so, Haugaasen and Jordet [22] highlighted that football-specific practice is essential in talent development.

The coach is of great importance for the development of young players [23], and coaches' understanding of player development impacts the players' development [24,25]. If one accepts the strong focus on the identification and selective targeting of the few "chosen" talented players as a strong paradigm in football, one can also imagine that the players' perceptions of their own talent is essential for their own development. In spite of this paradigm, previous research has, to a small extent, studied how talented footballers perceive their own talent and what factors have made an impact on their development.

The Current Study

This study is designed as a focus group interview with talented football players in order to investigate their perceptions of talent and how their development has been dependent on their own talent. The objective of the article is to investigate how boys and girls perceive their talent and to discuss how various perceptions influence coaching practice in talent development. We introduce the following questions: (a) do the players use a static or dynamic perception of their own talent and (b) do the players consider specific or general skills most important in their skill development?

3. Method

3.1. Participants

The respondents are a selection of 10 Norwegian players (five boys and five girls) aged 14–16 years. Participants were recruited to participate in this study if they met the following inclusion criteria: Participants must have been selected to a district, region or age-specific national team, within the last 12 months. Representatives from the regional football association selected the players.

3.2. Data Collection Procedure

The first author was the moderator of two focus group interviews in September (three girls and one boy) and November 2013 (four boys and two girls). Focus group interviews were conducted in the office of the local football association, with chairs arranged in a circular manner around a boardroom table. A tape recorder was set up in the center of the table. The two sessions lasted 37 and 45 min.

Focus groups have proven valuable in similar settings, involving Danish talented young football players [26]. Focus groups as a method for data collection emphasize the relatively "non-hierarchical" relationship between moderator and participants [27], encouraging an informal atmosphere in which participants speak freely about all included topics without straying from the subject [28]. Another major advantage is that focus groups allow researchers to observe interactions and discussions. Statements and arguments from participants in the group could be analyzed through consensus and dissensus [29]. According to Berg and Lune [28], some important disadvantages of focus groups are: (a) only group, not individual, responses are obtained in the results; (b) dominant personalities may overpower and steer the group's responses unless the moderator is sufficiently active; and (c) focus group data does not offer the same depth of information as a long semi-structured interview. Hence, the moderator's guide was made with the purpose of providing players with the opportunity to elaborate on the various topics that were raised, while the moderator had the opportunity to follow up "tracks" in the conversation. All players were systematically asked to answer all questions, which they did, ensuring that all players got to speak their opinions on the matter. Examples of questions from the moderators guide include: "is talent trainable?", "do you consider specific skills more important than general skills?" and "what are your thoughts on explaining how you have reach this skill level?".

3.3. Analytical Process

The interviews were transcribed verbatim, analyzed through content analysis and coded in two categories: perceived talent and general *vs.* specific skills. The data material was sorted by these two categories, searching for patterns of consensus and dissensus. During the focus group interviews the moderator took notes of interactionary cues including headshakes, interrupting each other's sentences and side comments. These observations were also coded and used as a supplement in our analysis.

4. Results and Discussion

Results show that the boys have a more static perception of talent compared to the girls. Furthermore, the boys in this study stress the importance of highly specified skills. The girls have a more balanced view on what is important, but tend to stress the importance of basic skills.

4.1. The Girls' and Boys' Understandings of Talent

The girls and boys in this study have already been identified and selected as talented football players. It is thus interesting to investigate how the players themselves understand both their own talent and talent in general. Do they perceive talent in terms of being static, meaning hereditary, or in terms of being dynamic, meaning the result of targeted training over time? When asked directly about the importance of heritage, two of the girls gave the following answers:

"I do not think there is much (heredity)" (G2).

"One is not born with a talent . . . One gets better; we are after all not born with skills" (G4).

In other words, there was consensus among the girls in the two focus groups, indicating a weak link between talent and heritage. Instead they perceive talent as something they must train for, and thus have a dynamic perception of skill:

"(. . .) We have worked for it, many believe that, or that, many may say that a talent, you've got it, you've inherited things and stuff, but I think that we have also trained for it, we want to accomplish something, it does not come by itself" (G3).

Among males, however, there is a more widespread belief that talent is something innate:

"There are many that are good from the start somehow. That just has it in him" (B5).

"One cannot start without having good genes. You cannot start as completely miserable" (B3).

The boys in the study connect their talent to genes and something they just "have in them", and thus seem to have a more static perception of the skill concept. It may therefore seem that boys partially agree with the basic assumptions that are often associated with talent, with talent being understood as hereditary [2]. This does not necessarily imply that one is born to be a footballer, but talent can just as easily be related to inherited ability to handle high amounts of training or mental strength:

"It is possible to have a talent for training too. They just train themselves good" (B2).

"Either you have the will and the mental strength or you do not" (B5).

Results show a clear gender dimension in how players perceive their talent. Girls have a more dynamic perception of talent, which basically means that talent is a result of training [5]. Boys, on the other hand, have a more static perception of talent, understanding talent to be largely inherited. The static understanding of talent holds true for both football talent and training talent, leading to an understanding of targeted training having a limited effect. However, this does not imply that talent is taken for granted for the foreseeable future. As some of the players stated:

"The talent can stop anytime. Perhaps at this time, now (15–16 years)" (B2).

"Many people say that we float on a talent, but that it's maybe at a young age" (G1).

Regardless of the importance of the genetic component of talent, several players highlight the importance of developing skills, and not only relying on their current skills, especially since they consider their current age as a turning point in their potential professional career. A potential explanation for the players' difficulties in defining which skills they should develop could be seen in line with the difficulties even top-level coaches have when asked to define which criteria they use to identify the most talented players [7].

A talent is something you can "lose", according to several of the players. One example mentioned by one of the players was the importance of training, and the fact that players not defined as talented could have a higher training load and thus achieve a higher skill level based on training. According to Ericsson and his colleagues [18], players' skills come as a direct result of their training load, and could thus explain why some players "catch up" in terms of skill level. Even so, training load has not been found to be a significant indicator to predict future skills [19]. Overall, several players describe their talent as something short-term, confined to a young age, that can be lost if you take a breather in your development as a player. On one hand, this is in agreement with the dynamic perception of talent [5]. On the other hand, it does not seem like the players think they can retrieve a talent if first lost, which fits better into a static perception of talent.

Compared with the girls in this study and earlier studies on elite coaches [7], the boys in this study appear to embrace a more static perception of talent. One explanation could be that boys are part of a tougher competition for resources. Being among the selected and getting access to these resources has been found to be essential for young players' development [26], and provides obvious advantages for future development [3]. Coaches that focus on results and achievement among young players rely on a static perception of talent and utilize present performance levels and physical properties as the basis for identifying and selecting the best talent [24]. This could obviously affect the player's perception of his or her talent as a static condition. Coaches who are concerned about short-term results, in terms of winning football matches and giving playing time to the best players, will favor the best players at any given time.

4.2. Highly Specified or General Skills

In accordance with the literature of talent development [22], most talented players would agree to highlight training load as an essential factor in talent development. Even so, the importance of training quality and which skills one should develop is a more complicated question. One of the basic assumptions regarding talent focuses on talent as being domain-specific [2], indicating the importance of developing highly specified skills. When the players were asked whether they should develop highly specified skills or more general skills, there was dissensus. Similar to how players perceive talent and how to develop skills, the gender dimension was present with boys clearly prioritizing highly specified skills:

"I have always learned that if there is one thing I am good at I should focus on training more on that. To get even better at it" (B2).

"It is also important to have one very good skill" (B3).

"You can always get better at what you are good at. So it is important to work on it too" (B1).

A few of the boys were, however, somewhat more diffuse about whether they should pursue more specified skills or not.

"Mainly focus on what I do best and take what I'm worst at eventually" (B4).

"Both really. Develop what you are good at and what you are bad at actually" (B5).

As the quotes above show, all of the boys did not prioritize highly specified skills; rather, it seems like some of them prioritized both types of skills. The girls were even more concerned about finding the balance between general and specified skills, and some were quite clear that they prioritize general skills:

"I would have developed what I'm bad at. And continue to maintain what I am good at" (G5).

"I would have done both. But mostly what I'm bad at" (G4).

"It's important to practice what you might not be so good at. So you get good at it. But do not stop practicing what you are good at either. It's good that you have the advantage in something. And continue to work at it" (G2).

Overall, results show that boys prioritize highly specified skills rather than general skills. Girls in this sample seem to distribute equal value to general and highly specific skills. Asked to prioritize, several of the girls would give priority to developing general skills. Taken together, results in this study show a relationship between gender, perception of talent, and prioritization of highly specified or general skills. The girls have a more dynamic understanding of talent and prioritize general skills to a greater extent, confirming the perception of compensating for deficiencies in one area by strength in others [20]. One way of explaining these results is through combining what we know about coaches often utilizing present performance levels and physical properties as the basis for identifying and selecting the best talent [24], together with the tendency of selecting talented players by an early birth month, the relative age effect [15–17]. Since the relative age effect appears less pronounced for female players [14], we suggest that girls are part of a selection system that allows them to develop a more dynamic perception of talent compared with the boys.

Another potential explanation to why the boys focus on specific skills relates to Ericsson and his colleagues [18], understanding deliberate practice as a success factor in talent development. Highlighting the importance of deliberate practice could indicate specialization according to both playing position and developing specified skills, which girls in this study seem to deem less important compared to the boys. Even though the coaches' role in talent identification and development is obvious [23–25], the players' perception of their own talent and their tactics to overcome obstacles [5] is also important for their development. Earlier studies show that coaches have problems defining the criteria by which they identify talented players [7]. This is an obvious obstacle for the talented players if they are uncertain about which skills they should develop to heighten the possibility of becoming an elite-level player.

Accepting that boys have a more static perception of talent and are part of a selection system that relies more heavily on basic assumptions regarding talent development [8,11] has some interesting implications. First of all, coaches should be aware of the possible vulnerability following players' static perception of talent. Such players would typically explain a lack of success through lacking abilities and might not see the point of making an effort to improve their skills through training. Second, locking onto highly specified skills, instead of finding a balance between specified and general skills, might make for a less optimal preparation for the changing demands young players meet when moving through the different levels of play on their way to high-level football.

4.3. Limitations of the Study and Future Research

The relatively small number of participants is an obvious limitation of this study. Even if the recruited players were included based on the criteria of selection to a district, regional or age-specific national team during the latest 12 months, these players would mostly be representative of the regional football district. The limited number of topics in this study could also be seen as a limitation, since a broader span of topics could have given a better understanding of the players' perceived talent and abilities. The limitations of focus group interviews regarding the depth of information should also be mentioned [29]. It is, for instance, not exactly clear what the participants think are highly specified and general skills. It is reasonable to assume that the distinction would differ from player to player, and that semi-structured interviews would be beneficial in future research. Future research should also investigate how players from other districts perceive their own talent compared to the current study. Furthermore, it would also be of interest to investigate players with a lower skill level, not yet regarded as having talent, and how they perceive their talent and skill development. One could hypothesize a relationship between the players' perceived talent and selection, indicating that a selection could be seen as a confirmation of ability, thereby showing that these players perceive their abilities to be higher than those of non-selected talented players.

5. Conclusions

The objective of the article is to investigate how boys and girls perceive their talent and to discuss how various perceptions influence coaching practice in talent development. The first objective of this study was to investigate if players have a static or dynamic perception of their own talent. Results show that talented girl footballers experience a weak link between talent and heritage, and have a dynamic perception of the skill concept. Among talented boy footballers there exists a widespread perception of talent to be something innate. The boys in the sample connect talent to genes and something that players just *"have in them"*, and seem to have a more static perception of the skill concept, agreeing to many of the basic assumptions often associated with talent [2]. Even so, hard work is described as important. Players understand their own talent as having a kind of breaking point, being able to "surf" on their talent in younger years, but that their peers will catch up if they take a breather in developing as a player. This perception may be described as a dynamic perception of talent in accordance with Abbott and Collins [5]. The second objective was to investigate if the players consider specific or general skills most important in their skill development. Results show that the girls were more concerned about finding the balance between highly specified and general skills, and clearly give priority to general skills. The boys, however, were keen to develop highly specified skills, although some of the boys point out the importance of having both specified and general skills.

Author Contributions: Stig Arve Sæther conceived and designed the experiments; Stig Arve Sæther performed the experiments; Stig Arve Sæther and Ingar Mehus analyzed the data; Stig Arve Sæther and Ingar Mehus wrote the paper.

Conflicts of Interest: The authors declare no conflict of interest.

References

1. Simonton, J.L. Talent and its development: An emergenic and epigenetic model. *Psychol. Rev.* **1999**, *106*, 435–457. [CrossRef]
2. Durand-Bush, N.; Salmela, J.H. The development of talent in sport. In *Handbook of Sport Psychology*; Singer, R.N., Hausenblas, H.A., Janelle, C.M., Eds.; Wiley: New York, NY, USA, 2001.
3. Ashworth, J.; Heyndels, B. Selection bias and peer effects in team sports: The effect of age grouping on earnings of German soccer players. *J. Sports Econ.* **2007**, *8*, 355–377. [CrossRef]
4. Larsen, C.H.; Alfermann, D.; Henriksen, K.; Christensen, M.K. Successful talent development in soccer: The characteristics of the environment. *Sport Exerc. Perform. Psychol.* **2013**, *2*, 190–206. [CrossRef]
5. Abbott, A.; Collins, D. A theoretical and empirical analysis of a "state of the art"talent identification model. *High Abil. Stud.* **2002**, *13*, 157–178. [CrossRef]
6. Miller, P.K.; Cronin, C.; Baker, G. Nurture, nature and some very dubious social skills: An interpretative phenomenological analysis of talent identification practices in elite English youth soccer. *Qual. Res. Sport Exerc. Health.* **2015**, *7*. [CrossRef]
7. Sæther, S.A. Talent Identification in Soccer. What do Coaches Look for? Available online: http://idrottsforum.org/wp-content/uploads/2014/03/saether140319.pdf (accessed on 15 May 2015).
8. Helsen, W.F.; Hodges, N.J.; Winckel, J.V.; Starkes, J.L. The roles of talent, physical precocity and practice in the development of soccer expertise. *J. Sports Sci.* **2000**, *18*, 727–736. [CrossRef] [PubMed]
9. Reilly, T.; Williams, A.M.; Nevill, A.; Franks, A. A multidisciplinary approach to talent identification in soccer. *J. Sports Sci.* **2000**, *18*, 695–702. [CrossRef] [PubMed]
10. Williams, A.M.; Reilly, T. Talent identification and development in soccer. *J. Sports Sci.* **2000**, *18*, 657–667. [CrossRef] [PubMed]
11. Abbott, A.; Collins, D. Eliminating the dichotomy between theory and practice in talent identification and development: Considering the role of psychology. *J. Sport Sci.* **2004**, *22*, 395–408. [CrossRef] [PubMed]
12. Gledhill, A.; Harwood, C. A Systematic Review of Psychological Factors Associated with Talent Development in Soccer. In Proceedings of the 13th FEPSAC European Congress of Sport Psychology, Madeira, Portugal, 2–17 July 2011.
13. Van Yperen, N.W. Why some make it and others do not: Identifying psychological factors that predict career success in professional adult soccer. *Sport Psychol.* **2009**, *23*, 317–329.
14. Schorer, J.; Cobley, S.; Bilsch, D.; Brautigam, H.; Baker, J. Influences of competition level, gender, player nationality, career stage and playing position on relative age effects. *Scand. J. Med. Sci. Sports* **2009**, *19*, 720–730. [CrossRef] [PubMed]
15. Brewer, J.; Balsom, P.; Davis, J. Seasonal birth distribution amongst European soccer players. *Sports Exerc. Inj.* **1995**, *1*, 154–157.
16. Helsen, W.F.; Starkes, J.L.; Hodges, N.J. Team sports and the theory of deliberate practice. *J. Sports Exerc. Psychol.* **1998**, *20*, 13–35.
17. Simmons, C.; Paull, G.C. Season-of-birth in association football. *J. Sports Sci.* **2001**, *19*, 677–686. [CrossRef] [PubMed]
18. Ericsson, K.A.; Krampe, R.; Tesch-Römer, C. The role of deliberate practice in the acquisition of expert performance. *Psychol. Rev.* **1993**, *100*, 363–406. [CrossRef]
19. Cote, J.; Fraser-Thomas, J. Play, practice and athlete development. In *Developing Sport Expertise*; Farrow, D., Baker, J., MacMahon, C., Eds.; Routledge: London, UK, 2008; pp. 17–28.
20. Meylan, C.; Cronin, J.; Oliver, J.; Hughes, M. Reviews: Talent identification in soccer: The role of maturity status on physical, physiological and technical characteristics. *Int. J. Sports Sci. Coach.* **2010**, *5*, 571–592. [CrossRef]
21. Stølen, T.; Chamari, K.; Castagna, C.; Wisløff, U. Physiology of soccer: An update. *Sports Med.* **2005**, *35*, 501–536. [CrossRef] [PubMed]
22. Haugaasen, M.; Jordet, G. Developing football expertise: A football-specific research review. *Int. Rev. Sport Exerc. Psychol.* **2012**, *5*, 177–201. [CrossRef]
23. Carlson, R. *Vägen til landslaget. En retrospektiv Studie av Framgångsrika Ungdomar i sju Idrottar*; Høgskolen för lärarutbildning i Stockholm: Stockholm, Sweden, 1991.

24. Gagné, F. Understanding the complex choreography of talent development through DMGT-based analysis. In *International Handbook for Research on Giftedness and Talent*; Heller, K.A., Mönks, F.J., Sternberg, R.J., Subotnik, R., Eds.; Pergamon Press: Oxford, UK, 2000; pp. 67–79.
25. Martindale, R.J.J.; Collins, D.; Abraham, A. Effective talent development: The elite coach perspective in UK sport. *J. Appl. Sport Psychol.* **2007**, *19*, 187–206. [CrossRef]
26. Christensen, M.K.; Sørensen, J.K. Sport or school? Dreams and dilemmas for talented young Danish football players. *Eur. Phys. Educ. Rev.* **2009**, *15*, 115–133. [CrossRef]
27. Dowling, F.N. Naratives about Young Men and Masculinities in Organised Sport in Norway. *Sport Educ. Soc.* **2001**, *6*, 125–142.
28. Berg, B.L.; Lune, H. *Qualitative Research Methods for the Social Sciences*; Pearson: Boston, MA, USA, 2012.
29. Lune, H.; Enrique, P.; Koppel, R. *Perspectives in Social Research Methods and Analysis. A Reader for Sociology*; Sage Publications: Thousand Oaks, CA, USA, 2009.

7

The Effect of Recovery Duration on Technical Proficiency during Small Sided Games of Football

Scott McLean [1,*], Hugo Kerhervé [1], Mitchell Naughton [1], Geoff P. Lovell [2], Adam D. Gorman [1] and Colin Solomon [1]

1 School of Health and Sport Sciences, University of the Sunshine Coast, Sippy Downs, QLD 4556, Australia; hugokerherve@gmail.com (H.K.); mrn004@student.usc.edu.au (M.N.); agorman@usc.edu.au (A.D.G.); csolomon@usc.edu.au (C.S.)
2 School of Social Sciences, University of the Sunshine Coast, Sippy Downs, QLD 4556, Australia; glovell@usc.edu.au
* Correspondence: scott.mclean@research.usc.edu.au

Academic Editor: Filipe Manuel Clemente

Abstract: The aim of this study was to determine the effect of increasing the duration of the recovery periods separating serial bouts of small sided games (SSG) of football on technical skills (TS). Twelve semi-professional footballers (mean ± SD; age 21 ± 3 years; VO_{2peak} 64 ± 7 mL·min·kg^{-1}; playing experience 15 ± 3 years) completed two SSG sessions, consisting of 3 vs. 3 players and 6 bouts of 2 min, separated by either 30 s recovery (REC-30) or 120 s recovery (REC-120). Sixteen TS, including passing, possession, and defensive related variables, and exercise intensity (heart rate, rating of perceived exertion, time motion descriptors) during the bouts were measured. Repeated measures ANOVA were used to determine differences between-conditions, for TS. The number of successful tackles was significantly higher, and the average time each team maintained possession was significantly lower in REC-120 compared to REC-30. There were no significant differences for all other TS variables, or exercise intensity measures between REC-30 and REC-120. Overall, a four-fold increase in the duration of recovery separating SSG bouts did not alter the technical skill execution of players. The experience and skill level of the players, combined with an apparent regulation of effort through pacing, may have assisted in the maintenance of technical skill execution.

Keywords: small sided games; football; recovery; technical skill; pacing

---

1. Introduction

The execution of technical skills (TS) is the fundamental component of football [1,2]. Players must apply cognitive, perceptual, and motor skills in a process where decisions are made and executed in a rapidly changing environment [3–5]. Ultimately, the successful execution of TS, including passing, tackling, dribbling, and shooting, are likely to be primary determinants in the outcome of a match [2,3,6].

Successful execution of TS by football players could be decreased by the fatigue that occurs during a match [2,7]. Players experience temporary fatigue following phases of high intensity exercise during a match, and progressive fatigue across the duration of a match [8]. The mechanisms responsible for the accumulation of fatigue in players during match-play are varied, complex and not completely understood [9,10]. Depletion of energetic substrates (e.g., muscle glycogen, muscle creatine phosphate), increased metabolic by-products (e.g., lactate, potassium), increased pH, and dehydration, have all been proposed to contribute to the accumulation of fatigue during a football match [10]. Despite the lack of a definitive conclusion regarding the mechanisms of fatigue during a match, it is implied that a decline in TS in the later stages of a match is attributable to fatigue [9,11].

Investigations into the relationship between fatigue, TS, and decision making are often conducted using non-football match specific or laboratory-based football simulations [4,9,12,13]. Additionally, non-match specific simulations do not account for factors such as player interactions, field positioning, and match related stressors both physiological and psychological. Furthermore, the participants do not experience the same sensory state as in an actual match, therefore reducing arousal levels, which can influence playing performance [14]. Small sided games (SSG), although different to actual match-play, combine the physiological, technical, tactical, and decision making components of football [15–17], thereby providing a more representative test environment compared to non-match play and laboratory based studies. The SSG format is also an effective training method, using conditions that are representative of match demands [18]. Typically, SSG are used in an interval format, consisting of a series of bouts and recovery periods [19–22].

Progressive increases in heart rate (HR), rating of perceived exertion (RPE), blood lactate [La], and decreased high intensity running during SSG bouts have been associated with decreases in TS [19,20,23,24]. However, increasing the duration of recovery during repeated bouts of high intensity exercise increases physiological recovery and may allow physical performance to be maintained [25]. Mclean et al. (2016) have shown that increasing the duration of the recovery period from 30 s to 120 s separating serial SSG bouts, significantly increased physiological recovery, both systemically (HR), and locally (vastus lateralis muscle oxygenation, using near infrared spectroscopy) in experienced semi-professional players, [26].

Only one study has investigated the effect of the duration of the recovery period during SSG on TS, using recovery durations of 1, 2, 3, and 4 min separating the bouts [24]. The increased recovery duration produced an increased number of total and successful passes, tackles, and passes received, suggesting that the longer recovery duration may have decreased progressive fatigue and allowed the TS to be maintained during the SSG [24]. Increasing the duration of recovery periods separating serial bouts may reduce physiological and psychological stress in subsequent bouts, allowing players to maintain optimal arousal levels and the subsequent attentional levels required for successful TS execution [4,14]. Exercising at very high levels of intensity elevates arousal levels, and has a negative impact on attentional processes, resulting in players missing the important cues that are necessary for successful skill execution [4].

Despite only measuring five technical variables, Koklu et al. (2015) found that a shorter recovery duration decreased TS in youth participants [24]. To obtain a more comprehensive understanding of the effect of recovery duration separating SSG bouts on TS, it is necessary to assess additional TS variables, and use experienced players. Analyzing additional (to previously measured) technical variables, including first touch passing, the number of individual touches occurring during each possession, and time in possession for individuals and teams, will provide necessary information to establish whether TS execution is affected when the recovery periods separating SSG bouts are manipulated. First touch passing involves high technical difficulty and information processing to recognize the positioning of team members and defenders [20]. Determining the number of touches a player selects per possession, and the duration of time that each individual possesses the ball during SSG, will provide additional information on whether the technical components of football are influenced by fatigue.

Therefore, the aim of this study was to determine whether changing the recovery duration during the same 3 vs. 3 SSG format would have an effect on multiple, specific individual, and team TS variables. It was hypothesized that during serial bouts of SSG, a 120 s recovery period compared to a 30 s recovery period, would allow players to maintain their TS execution.

2. Materials and Methods

2.1. Participants

Twelve experienced male semi-professional football players (mean $\pm$ SD; age 21 $\pm$ 3 years; VO_{2peak} 64 $\pm$ 7 mL·min·kg^{-1}; playing experience 15 $\pm$ 3 years) [26], playing in the same team and competing in the second tier of football in Australia, participated in the study. Participants trained three times per week for an approximate weekly total of 240 min and competed in one match per week of 90 min duration. The study received institutional ethical approval and participants were informed of the study requirements and provided written informed consent.

2.2. Study Design

This study was conducted using a one-group, repeated measures design. The independent variables were the two different recovery durations, 30-s recovery (REC-30), and 120-s recovery (REC-120), and the number of bouts (1–6). The dependent variables were the individual and team technical skill variables. Participants completed the SSG sessions, and a peak aerobic capacity test (laboratory conditions). All testing and data collection was completed in an 11-week period during the participants' competitive season. The exercise intensity during the bouts of the SSG was monitored using heart rate (HR), rating of perceived exertion (RPE; Borg CR-10 scale), time motion descriptors (TMD) (speed and distance), as previously reported (see McLean et al., 2016, for the methods used for these measurements) [26]. In the current original sub-set of exercise intensity data there was a significant ($p < 0.05$) decrease for HR in REC-120 compared to REC-30 during the recovery periods. There were no significant ($p > 0.05$) differences for HR, RPE, or TMD between REC-30 and REC-120 during the bouts.

2.3. Small Sided Games

Each participant completed REC-30 and REC-120 under the same SSG format consisting of 3 vs. 3 players with 6 × 2 min bouts played on a 15 m × 20 m natural grass pitch [26]. Participants were tested in two separate sessions, separated by a minimum of 2 days and maximum of 5 days, and the order of conditions was counterbalanced. The SSG testing was completed in 8 sessions during a 5-week period. The SSG testing sessions were completed at the beginning of the participants' normal football training session and at the same time of day to avoid variations to circadian rhythm. The SSG teams were selected by the two experienced team coaches to ensure that similar levels of technical ability and physical capacity of players were evenly distributed across the two teams. The same team membership was used for all testing sessions. The objective of the SSG was to maintain possession as a team, with unlimited ball contacts per possession, with no goals or goalkeepers, and no coach encouragement. Additional balls were placed around the pitch to minimize time lost for balls out of play. Prior to testing, participants performed a standardized warm up. For the recovery periods, participants were instructed that they could walk within the playing area.

2.4. Technical Skills Analysis

The SSG were recorded using a high definition video recorder (Sony HDR-CX130) positioned on a tripod at approximately 3 m above the playing surface, at the center of the 20 m length of the playing area and approximately 10 m from the boundary of the playing area. Post hoc analysis of the video recordings was used to analyze the TS of participants. Technical actions were divided into 16 different categories (refer to Table 1 for definitions). Intra and inter-observer (2 observers) reliability were assessed by analysis of three randomly selected bouts. An observation by observation breakdown of the coding results was used for statistical analysis [19]. Intra- class correlations showed a high degree of intra-observer reliability (ICC > 0.801), as well as high inter-observer reliability using Cohen's Kappa ($k > 0.814$). The reliability results therefore indicated a very high level of agreement [19].

Table 1. Technical skill definitions.

Technical Action	Definition
Time (s) in possession (individual)	The amount of time (s) an individual player has possession.
Touches in possession (individual)	The number of occasions an individual player has contact with the ball (using the foot, thigh, head, or chest) per possession.
Time (s) in possession (team)	The amount of time (s) a team has possession.
Successful team passes	The number of passes each team completes for each possession.
Successful pass (%)	The percentage of successful passes completed during the bouts (both teams).
Intercept	A player from the non-possession team gains possession by intercepting a pass from the team in possession.
Deflection	A player is struck with the ball, without attempting to play at it resulting in a change/no change of team possession, or the ball goes out of play.
Unsuccessful pass	An incomplete attempted pass between players of same team.
Successful pass	The completion of an attempted pass between players of the same team.
Unsuccessful 1st touch pass	The incompletion of an attempted 1st touch pass between players of same team.
Successful 1st touch pass	The completion of an attempted 1st touch pass between players of the same team.
Successful tackle	A player from the non-possession team involved in a duel gains possession of the ball.
Unsuccessful tackle	A player in possession remains in possession after a duel.
Lost possession (miscontrol)	A player loses ball possession due to miscontrol
Total possessions per bout	The number of individual possessions, during the bouts (all players).
Technical actions per minute	The sum of successful and unsuccessful passes, successful and unsuccessful first touch passes, successful and unsuccessful tackles, and intercepts performed per minute of the bouts.
Time (s) ball is out of play	Time from when the ball leaves the playing area until a new ball is played back into the playing area.

Time in possession (individual) was recorded when a player first touched the ball until that player's final touch of the ball (from either a pass, lost possession, or tackle). Time in possession (team) was recorded from the first touch by the player in a passing sequence, to the final touch of the last player in the passing sequence. Deflections are described as an unintentional act, and are therefore not included in the technical actions per minute variable.

2.5. Statistical Analysis

Statistical power calculations (using G * Power) using the mean difference and standard deviation in the variable with the largest difference in mean values between conditions, average team possessions, was low (0.26). However, despite the low power we were able to detect a significant difference in two of the TS dependent variables, which indicates that the design and number of participants was satisfactory. Statistical analyses was performed using SPSS (version 22, IBM Corporation, Armonk, NY, USA). A two-way repeated-measures ANOVA was used for each dependant variable to assess the effect of condition (REC-120 and REC-30), bout (1-6), and condition $\times$ bout interactions for all dependent variables. Assumptions of sphericity using Mauchly's W test were used, with adjustments for significant results implemented using the Greenhouse-Geisser correction of degrees of freedom. Post hoc pairwise comparisons were used to investigate significant interactions, and were conducted using the least significant difference (LSD) method with no adjustments for multiple comparisons. A paired t-test was used to compare the total distances covered between REC-30 and REC-120, in the SSG sessions. Partial eta-squared (η_P^2), was used as an indicator of effect size, (range was small 0.01, medium 0.06, and large 0.14) [27], and statistical power were reported. Data are reported using mean $\pm$ SD, and the level of significance was set at $p < 0.05$.

3. Results

Technical Skill

For TS there was a significant main effect of condition with a large effect size for the number of successful tackles ($p = 0.023$; $\eta_p^2 = 0.071$; $\beta = 0.313$), with an increased number of tackles performed in REC-120. There was also a significant main effect and large effect size for the average time of team possessions ($p = 0.038$; $\eta_p^2 = 0.807$; $\beta = 0.660$), with possessions being lower in REC-120. There were no significant (all p values > 0.05) main effects for condition, or bout number, and no condition × bout interaction, for all other technical variables (Tables 2 and 3).

Table 2. Mean ± SD of technical actions.

Variable	Condition	B1	B2	B3	B4	B5	B6	SSG Session
Time in possession (s)	REC-30	2.2 ± 1.0	2.1 ± 0.9	2.1 ± 1.2	1.9 ± 0.8	2.2 ± 1.1	2.7 ± 3.2	2.2 ± 1.3
	REC-120	2.1 ± 1.1	1.9 ± 1.3	1.8 ± 0.8	1.9 ± 0.9	2.1 ± 0.9	2.3 ± 1.2	2.0 ± 1.0
Touches in possession	REC-30	3.3 ± 0.9	3.4 ± 0.9	3.3 ± 1.0	2.8 ± 0.5	3.4 ± 1.2	4.1 ± 2.3	3.4 ± 1.3
	REC-120	3.3 ± 1.4	3.1 ± 1.3	3.0 ± 0.8	3.2 ± 0.6	3.4 ± 1.1	3.6 ± 1.5	3.3 ± 1.1
* Average team possession (s)	REC-30	7.3 ± 3.4	9.3 ± 2.6	6.8 ± 1.9	7.9 ± 1.8	6.7 ± 2.0	9.8 ± 6.9	7.9 ± 3.4
	REC-120	5.9 ± 2.0	7.0 ± 2.7	6.5 ± 2.6	6.9 ± 4.5	6.5 ± 1.6	7.0 ± 1.9	6.6 ± 2.4
Pass/possession (team)	REC-30	1.8 ± 1.1	2.8 ± 0.3	1.9 ± 0.5	3.0 ± 2.0	1.6 ± 0.3	2.9 ± 2.7	3.2 ± 1.4
	REC-120	1.4 ± 0.5	1.9 ± 1.1	2.4 ± 1.2	3.5 ± 3.4	1.4 ± 0.3	1.7 ± 0.9	2.0 ± 1.6
Successful pass (%)	REC-30	79 ± 20	85 ± 12	84 ± 18	82 ± 15	82 ± 25	80 ± 15	80 ± 15
	REC-120	71 ± 29	81 ± 16	81 ± 18	77 ± 23	79 ± 23	76 ± 17	77 ± 21
Interceptions	REC-30	0.4 ± 0.7	0.4 ± 0.7	0.3 ± 0.7	0.4 ± 0.7	0.4 ± 0.5	0.2 ± 0.4	0.4 ± 0.6
	REC-120	0.8 ± 0.8	0.6 ± 0.7	0.3 ± 0.5	0.3 ± 0.5	0.7 ± 0.9	0.1 ± 0.3	0.5 ± 0.7
Deflections	REC-30	0.0 ± 0.0	0.2 ± 0.4	0.0 ± 0.0	0.2 ± 0.4	0.3 ± 0.7	0.3 ± 0.5	0.2 ± 0.4
	REC-120	0.5 ± 1.2	0.5 ± 0.5	0.4 ± 0.7	0.0 ± 0.0	0.3 ± 0.5	0.3 ± 0.6	0.3 ± 0.7
Unsuccessful pass	REC-30	0.9 ± 0.7	0.4 ± 0.5	0.4 ± 0.5	0.9 ± 0.8	0.6 ± 0.9	0.8 ± 1.0	0.7 ± 0.8
	REC-120	1.2 ± 1.1	0.7 ± 0.7	0.8 ± 0.9	1.3 ± 1.9	0.9 ± 1.0	0.8 ± 1.1	0.9 ± 1.1
Successful pass	REC-30	3.2 ± 2.3	4.0 ± 1.7	2.8 ± 1.5	3.2 ± 1.3	2.4 ± 1.6	3.1 ± 2.4	3.1 ± 1.8
	REC-120	2.4 ± 1.6	2.9 ± 1.8	3.1 ± 1.4	2.6 ± 1.0	2.8 ± 1.4	3.3 ± 1.5	2.8 ± 1.4
Unsuccessful 1st touch pass	REC-30	0.1 ± 0.3	0.5 ± 0.8	0.3 ± 0.5	0.3 ± 0.5	0.2 ± 0.4	0.4 ± 0.9	0.3 ± 0.6
	REC-120	0.4 ± 0.5	0.3 ± 0.5	0.3 ± 0.7	0.3 ± 0.7	0.3 ± 0.9	0.7 ± 0.5	0.4 ± 0.6
Successful 1st touch pass	REC-30	1.5 ± 1.3	1.7 ± 1.3	1.1 ± 0.9	1.9 ± 1.5	1.3 ± 0.8	2.0 ± 1.0	1.6 ± 1.2
	REC-120	1.5 ± 1.6	1.7 ± 1.3	1.3 ± 1.0	1.2 ± 1.0	1.2 ± 0.9	1.3 ± 0.8	1.4 ± 1.1
* Successful tackle	REC-30	0.5 ± 0.7	0.3 ± 0.5	0.9 ± 0.8	0.6 ± 0.7	0.8 ± 1.0	0.3 ± 0.8	0.6 ± 0.8
	REC-120	0.6 ± 0.7	1.1 ± 1.1	1.3 ± 1.2	0.9 ± 0.7	0.5 ± 0.7	0.7 ± 0.7	1.0 ± 0.9
Unsuccessful tackle	REC-30	0.8 ± 1.1	0.6 ± 0.7	0.9 ± 0.9	0.8 ± 0.7	0.8 ± 1.1	0.3 ± 0.5	0.7 ± 0.8
	REC-120	0.8 ± 0.8	0.9 ± 1.0	0.7 ± 1.0	0.8 ± 1.0	0.3 ± 0.5	0.4 ± 0.7	0.6 ± 0.8
Technical actions· min^{-1}	REC-30	3.7 ± 1.4	3.9 ± 1.2	3.4 ± 1.1	4.0 ± 1.3	3.3 ± 1.3	3.5 ± 1.4	3.6 ± 1.3
	REC-120	3.7 ± 1.6	4.1 ± 1.4	3.9 ± 1.6	3.7 ± 1.0	3.4 ± 1.1	3.6 ± 1.0	3.7 ± 1.3
Lost possession (miscontrol)	REC-30	0.5 ± 0.7	0.3 ± 0.5	0.4 ± 0.7	0.3 ± 0.5	0.7 ± 0.9	0.2 ± 0.4	0.4 ± 0.6
	REC-120	0.9 ± 12	0.5 ± 0.8	0.9 ± 1.1	0.3 ± 0.5	0.4 ± 0.9	0.5 ± 0.5	1.0 ± 0.9
Total possession per bout	REC-30	7.4 ± 3.0	7.5 ± 2.5	5.4 ± 1.6	7.5 ± 2.3	5.8 ± 1.9	7.1 ± 2.4	6.8 ± 2.4
	REC-120	6.9 ± 2.3	7.0 ± 2.7	6.8 ± 2.6	6.3 ± 1.9	6.7 ± 1.2	7.3 ± 2.5	6.8 ± 2.2

* Significant ($p < 0.05$) main effect of condition.

Table 3. Probability (p), F statistic (F), Observed power (β), Partial eta squared (effect size η_p^2) of technical variables for Condition, Bout, and Condition × Bout interaction.

Technical Variable	Condition				Bout				Interaction			
	p	F	β	η_p^2	p	F	β	η_p^2	p	F	β	η_p^2
Time in possession (s)	0.495	0.497	0.099	0.043	0.368	1.106	0.364	0.091	0.881	0.193	0.080	0.881
Touches in possession	0.672	0.189	0.068	0.017	0.099	1.961	0.617	0.151	0.586	0.617	0.154	0.053
Average team possession (s)	0.038 *	12.51	0.660	0.807	0.424	1.053	0.274	0.260	0.908	0.296	0.102	0.090
Pass/possession (team)	0.557	0.434	0.077	0.126	0.510	0.893	0.235	0.229	0.348	1.218	0.316	0.289
Successful pass (%)	0.305	1.157	0.166	0.095	0.710	0.586	0.199	0.051	0.992	0.099	0.070	0.009
Interceptions	0.223	1.669	0.219	0.132	0.089	2.028	0.634	0.156	0.602	0.732	0.244	0.062
Deflections	0.078	3.786	0.427	0.256	0.698	0.603	0.204	0.052	0.163	1.646	0.530	0.163
Unsuccessful pass	0.226	1.647	0.217	0.217	0.183	1.572	0.509	.125	0.996	0.071	0.064	0.006
Successful pass	0.523	0.435	0.093	0.038	0.330	1.181	0.388	0.097	0.246	1.465	0.327	0.118
Unsuccessful 1st touch pass	0.339	1.000	0.150	0.083	0.652	0.664	0.223	0.057	0.502	0.718	0.190	0.006
Successful 1st touch pass	0.128	2.708	0.324	0.198	0.514	0.859	0.284	0.072	0.310	1.224	0.401	0.100
Successful tackle	0.023 *	6.962	0.671	0.388	0.071	2.164	0.667	0.164	0.313	1.219	0.400	0.100
Technical action$\cdot$ min^{-1}	0.169	2.164	0.270	0.164	0.672	0.637	0.215	0.055	0.867	0.371	0.138	0.033
Unsuccessful tackle	0.652	0.214	0.071	0.019	0.323	1.196	0.392	0.098	0.780	0.493	0.172	0.043
Lost possession (miscontrol)	0.112	2.983	0.351	0.231	0.227	1.434	0.467	0.115	0.462	1.000	0.329	0.083
Total possession per bout	0.982	0.001	0.050	0.000	0.146	1.719	0.551	0.135	0.197	1.526	0.495	0.122

* Significant ($p < 0.05$) main effect of condition.

4. Discussion

This study was designed to determine the effect of increasing the recovery duration between serial bouts of SSG from 30 s to 120 s on a set of TS in experienced participants. Contrary to the hypothesis, the main result was that overall TS execution was not influenced by the increased recovery duration. From the TS that were analyzed in the current study, only two out of the sixteen variables were significantly different (and with large effect sizes): duration of team possessions (shorter), and the number of successful tackles (higher) in REC-120 compared to REC-30. The shorter duration of possessions measured in REC-120 may be due to the increased number of tackles performed in that condition. It is possible that the increased physiological recovery (HR) during REC-120 allowed the players to perform more tackles, subsequently reducing time in possession. The absence of any significant differences, between the conditions or across the bouts, for all other TS variables needs to be considered in the context of the low statistical power in the study design Nevertheless, the consistency of the means between the conditions and across the bouts indicates that practical differences were unlikely. The absence of an overall difference between conditions in TS occurred despite a significantly decreased HR, during the recovery periods in REC-120 compared to REC-30.

The current result is in contrast with those of the only other study that has investigated TS execution when using different recovery durations separating SSG bouts, in which there was an increase in total passes, successful passes, passes received, and tackles during bouts interspersed with recovery durations of 3 and 4 min, compared to the 1 min [24]. In the study of Koklu et al. [24], the HR in the 3 and 4 min recovery conditions were significantly lower than in 1 min recovery condition, indicating an increased physiological recovery, which may have affected performance of TS [24]. In the current study, TS was not affected with an increase in the duration of the recovery period. A possible explanation is that highly trained and skilled athletes are able to adapt to the demands to which they are exposed, including the maintenance of skill execution while experiencing fatigue [14]. In support of the current results, no declines were observed in the TS execution of professional midfield players during full-scale matches [11]. This was despite players experiencing end-game fatigue, as indicated by significant decreases in high speed running in the final 30 min of the game [11].

One of the critical attributes of skilled performers is their capability to continually adapt to the demands of the performance context [28–30]. Skilled athletes can compensate for changes in the performance environment to maintain consistent performance outcomes [14]. This is a potential explanation for the maintenance of TS between REC-30 and REC-120 in the current study. A further facilitator for the maintenance of TS, could be explained by the players regulating effort [26]. The exercise intensity measures in the current study were not different between the SSG conditions (REC-30, REC-120), indicating that the exercise intensity level and work performed during the SSG were similar for both of these conditions [26]. The ability to regulate effort to the appropriate level is increased when individuals are highly trained, have task-specific experience, and possess knowledge of the exercise endpoint [31–35]. The experience level (14.6 years), aerobic capacity (VO_{2peak} of 64 $mL \cdot min \cdot kg^{-1}$), experience in SSG (a regular component of training) of the participants, and known exercise endpoint, suggests that the current participants were well equipped to be able to regulate their effort to maintain their TS.

In addition to investigating individual TS variables, we measured the TS performed per minute, which allowed comparisons to the frequency of TS performed during matches. One study has reported that elite players were involved with the ball on approximately 45 occasions during a 90 min match, which equates to two ball related actions per minute [36]. In the current study, the TS performed per minute of the SSG was not significantly different between conditions, despite being almost double (REC-30 = 3.6, and REC-120 = 3.7) the TS performed per minute of a match [36].

Normalizing TS variables as a percentage of totals allows comparisons of specific TS variables across different SSG formats. Successful passing is a commonly used variable that is expressed as a percentage of total passes [20,37]. In the current study, successful passing was 80% (REC-30), and 77% (REC-120), and did not decline across the subsequent bouts. This is contrary to other 3 vs. 3 SSG formats with unlimited ball touches per possession [20], where the percentage of successful passes significantly decreased from bout 1 (76%) to the fourth and final bout (70%), and HR was significantly higher in the fourth bout compared to the first bout [20]. In the current study, the exercise intensity of participants (HR, RPE and TMD) was maintained across the bouts, which may have prevented declines in physical and cognitive performance, allowing TS execution to remain relatively constant across the multiple bouts.

In addition to previously measured TS variables, this study analyzed four TS variables not previously measured in SSG research. The findings of the current study that could assist with the planning of SSG training, are that players utilized three ball touches, with a possession duration of 2.2 s (REC-30), and 2.0 s (REC-120), when instructed to play with unlimited ball touches per individual possession. This is higher than the mean number of touches taken during regular professional matches (Defenders = 1.74, Attacking Midfielders = 2.26) [20], which could be explained by the increased number of passing options available during a normal game. For successful first touch passes there was no significant difference between the two conditions. However, successful first touch passes produced approximately 50% of total successful passes in both conditions. First touch passing tends to increase the pace of the game and requires high levels of information processing, both of which are characteristics of elite level football [20]. The high percentage of successful first touch passing in the current study indicates that SSG played with 3 vs. 3 could provide an appropriate stimulus to develop the information processing required for performance in the normal competitive environment.

Limitations of the current study include that a measure of pacing was not included in the current design, as a measure of pacing could have directly indicated if pacing was consciously used. It is suggested that future research could include objective and subjective measures of pacing to determine whether this strategy is a fundamental factor in maintaining TS while potentially experiencing fatigue. In addition, only one format of SSG was used, and so manipulation of variables such as modifying player numbers, pitch size, number of bouts and recovery periods, or including goals and goalkeepers may have provided further information of the effect of altering recovery duration on different SSG formats.

5. Conclusions

It is concluded that increasing the duration of the recovery period separating serial SSG bouts from 30 s to 120 s did not affect the TS execution of experienced and trained football players. It is likely that the trained football players were able to adapt to the increased physical demands of the shorter recovery duration to maintain TS. This is likely due to pacing, whereby players regulate their effort to maintain performance. During a 3 vs. 3 SSG format, experienced and trained football players prefer to take three touches of the ball while in possession, use a high number of first touch passing, and maintain possession for approximately 2 s. Future research in SSG could include the technical actions performed per minute, as in the current study, so that comparisons can be made between studies that utilize different SSG formats. Furthermore, future SSG research could determine the repeat sprint ability of participants as an additional exercise specific indicator of exercise capacity.

6. Practical implications

Planning SSG training with 30 s recovery periods separating bouts may provide a more time efficient training session, without compromising the technical skill execution of players. Further, coaches should consider playing experience, and training status of players when designing SSG training sessions, as these will influence the SSG training outcomes. In addition, coaches often impose restrictions on players' touches in training to encourage playing with fewer touches. In the current SSG format, players chose to take three touches, and to spend approximately 2 s in possession.

Acknowledgments: The authors gratefully acknowledge the participation of the players and coaches from the Sunshine Coast Football Club for participating in the current study.

Author Contributions: Conceived and designed the study: S.M., C.S., H.K., A.D.G.; Performed the experiment: S.M., H.K., M.N.; Analyzed the data: S.M., H.K., C.S., G.P.L., A.D.G., M.N.; Wrote the paper: S.M., C.S., H.K., A.D.G., G.P.L.

Conflicts of Interest: The authors declare no conflicts of interest.

References

1. Stolen, T.; Chamari, K.; Castagna, C.; Wisloff, U. Physiology of soccer: An update. *Sports Med. (Auckl. N. Z.).* **2005**, *35*, 501–536. [CrossRef]
2. Stone, K.J.; Oliver, J.L. The effect of 45 minutes of soccer-specific exercise on the performance of soccer skills. *Int. J. Sports Physiol. Perform.* **2009**, *4*, 163–175. [PubMed]
3. Ali, A. Measuring soccer skill performance: A review. *Scand. J. Med. Sci. Sports* **2011**, *21*, 170–183. [CrossRef] [PubMed]
4. McMorris, T.; Graydon, J. The effect of exercise on the decision-making performance of experienced and inexperienced soccer players. *Res. Q. Exerc. Sport* **1996**, *67*, 109–114. [CrossRef] [PubMed]
5. Abernethy, B. Training the visual-perceptual skills of athletes: Insights from the study of motor expertise. *Am. J. Sports Med.* **1996**, *24*, S89–S92. [PubMed]
6. Mohr, M.; Krustrup, P.; Bangsbo, J. Match performance of high-standard soccer players with special reference to development of fatigue. *J. Sports Sci.* **2003**, *21*, 519–528. [CrossRef] [PubMed]

7. Russell, M.; Benton, D.; Kingsley, M. The effects of fatigue on soccer skills performed during a soccer match. *Int. J. Sports Physiol. Perform.* **2011**, *6*, 221–233. [PubMed]
8. Mohr, M.; Krustrup, P.; Bangsbo, J. Fatigue in soccer: A brief review. *J. Sports Sci.* **2005**, *23*, 593–599. [CrossRef] [PubMed]
9. Rampinini, E.; Impellizzeri, F.M.; Castagna, C.; Azzalin, A.; Ferrari Bravo, D.; Wisloff, U. Effect of match-related fatigue on short-passing ability in young soccer players. *Med. Sci. Sports Exerc.* **2008**, *40*, 934–942. [CrossRef] [PubMed]
10. Bangsbo, J.; Marcello Iaia, F.; Krustrup, P. Metabolic Response and Fatigue in Soccer. *Int. J. Sports Physiol. Perform.* **2007**, *2*, 111–127. [PubMed]
11. Carling, C.; Dupont, G. Are declines in physical performance associated with a reduction in skill-related performance during professional soccer match-play? *J. Sports Sci.* **2011**, *29*, 63–71. [CrossRef] [PubMed]
12. Bullock, W.; Panchuk, D.; Broatch, J.; Christian, R.; Stepto, N. An intergrative test of agility, speed and skill in soccer: Effects of exercise. *J. Sci. Med. Sport* **2012**, *15*, 431–436. [CrossRef] [PubMed]
13. Marriott, J.; Reilly, T.; Miles, A.; Reilly, T.; Clarys, J.; Stibbe, A. The effect of physiological stress on cognitive performance in a simulation of soccer. In *Science and Football II*; Taylor & Francis: Abingdon, UK, 1993; pp. 261–264.
14. Royal, K.A.; Farrow, D.; Mujika, I.; Halson, S.L.; Pyne, D.; Abernethy, B. The effects of fatigue on decision making and shooting skill performance in water polo players. *J. Sports Sci.* **2006**, *24*, 807–815. [CrossRef] [PubMed]
15. Casamichana, D.; Castellano, J. Time-motion, heart rate, perceptual and motor behaviour demands in small-sides soccer games: Effects of pitch size. *J. Sports Sci.* **2010**, *28*, 1615–1623. [CrossRef] [PubMed]
16. Dellal, A.; Hill-Haas, S.; Lago-Penas, C.; Chamari, K. Small-sided games in soccer: Amateur vs. professional players' physiological responses, physical, and technical activities. *J. Strength Cond. Res./Natl. Strength Cond. Assoc.* **2011**, *25*, 2371–2381. [CrossRef] [PubMed]
17. Hill-Haas, S.V.; Dawson, B.; Impellizzeri, F.M.; Coutts, A.J. Physiology of small-sided games training in football: A systematic review. *Sports Med. (Auckl. NZ).* **2011**, *41*, 199–220. [CrossRef] [PubMed]
18. Gabbett, T.J.; Jenkins, D.G.; Abernethy, B. Game-Based Taining for Improving Skill and Physical Fitness in Team Sports. *Int. J. Sports Sci. Coach.* **2009**, *4*, 273–283. [CrossRef]
19. Kelly, D.M.; Drust, B. The effect of pitch dimensions on heart rate responses and technical demands of small-sided soccer games in elite players. *J. Sci. Med. Sport/Sports Med. Aus.* **2009**, *12*, 475–479. [CrossRef] [PubMed]
20. Dellal, A.; Lago-Penas, C.; Wong Del, P.; Chamari, K. Effect of the number of ball contacts within bouts of 4 vs. 4 small-sided soccer games. *Int. J. Sports Physiol. Perform.* **2011**, *6*, 322–333. [PubMed]
21. Rampinini, E.; Impellizzeri, F.M.; Castagna, C.; Abt, G.; Chamari, K.; Sassi, A.; Marcora, S.M. Factors influencing physiological responses to small-sided soccer games. *J. Sports Sci.* **2007**, *25*, 659–666. [CrossRef] [PubMed]
22. Katis, A.; Kellis, E. Effects of small-sided games on physical conditioning and performance in young soccer players. *J. Sports Sci. Med.* **2009**, *8*, 374–380. [PubMed]
23. Dellal, A.; Drust, B.; Lago-Penas, C. Variation of activity demands in small-sided soccer games. *Int. J. Sports Med.* **2012**, *33*, 370–375. [CrossRef] [PubMed]
24. Koklu, Y.; Alemdaroglu, U.; Dellal, A.; Wong, D.P. Effect of different recovery durations between bouts in 3-a-side games on youth soccer players' physiological responses and technical activities. *J. Sports Med. Phys. Fit.* **2015**, *55*, 430–438.
25. Balsom, P.D.; Seger, J.Y.; Sjodin, B.; Ekblom, B. Maximal-intensity intermittent exercise: Effect of recovery duration. *Int. J. Sports Med.* **1992**, *13*, 528–533. [CrossRef] [PubMed]
26. McLean, S.; Kerhervé, H.; Lovell, G.P.; Gorman, A.D.; Solomon, C. The Effect of Recovery Duration on Vastus Lateralis Oxygenation, Heart Rate, Perceived Exertion and Time Motion Descriptors during Small Sided Football Games. *PLoS ONE* **2016**, *11*, e0150201. [CrossRef] [PubMed]
27. Cohen, J. *Statistical Power Analysis for the Behavioural Sciences*; Lawrence Earlbaum Associates: Hillside, NJ, USA, 1988.
28. Bartlett, R.; Wheat, J.; Robins, M. Is movement variability important for sports biomechanists? *Sports Biomech.* **2007**, *6*, 224–243. [CrossRef] [PubMed]

29. Davids, K.; Glazier, P.; Araújo, D.; Bartlett, R. Movement systems as dynamical systems. *Sports Med.* **2003**, *33*, 245–260. [CrossRef] [PubMed]
30. Davids, K.W.; Button, C.; Bennett, S.J. *Dynamics of skill acquisition: A constraints-led approach*; Human Kinetics: Champaign, IL, USA, 2008.
31. Waldron, M.; Highton, J. Fatigue and Pacing in High-Intensity Intermittent Team Sport: An Update. *Sports Med.* **2014**, *44*, 1645–1658. [CrossRef] [PubMed]
32. Tucker, R.; Noakes, T.D. The physiological regulation of pacing strategy during exercise: A critical review. *Br. J. Sports Med.* **2009**, *43*, e1. [CrossRef] [PubMed]
33. St Clair Gibson, A.; Lambert, E.V.; Rauch, L.H.; Tucker, R.; Baden, D.A.; Foster, C.; Noakes, T.D. The role of information processing between the brain and peripheral physiological systems in pacing and perception of effort. *Sports Med. (Auckl. N. Z.)* **2006**, *36*, 705–722. [CrossRef]
34. Gabbett, T.; Walker, B.; Walker, S. Influence of prior knowledge of exercise duration on pacing strategies during game-based activities. *Int. J. Sports Physiol. Perform.* **2015**, *10*, 298–304. [CrossRef] [PubMed]
35. Johnston, R.D.; Gabbett, T.J.; Jenkins, D.G. The Influence of Physical Fitness and Playing Standard on Pacing Strategies during a Team-Sport Tournament. *Int. J. Sports Physiol. Perform.* **2015**, *1*, 18.
36. Rampinini, E.; Impellizzeri, F.M.; Castagna, C.; Coutts, A.J.; Wisloff, U. Technical performance during soccer matches of the Italian Serie A league: Effect of fatigue and competitive level. *J. Sci. Med. Sport/Sports Med. Aus.* **2009**, *12*, 227–233. [CrossRef] [PubMed]
37. Dellal, A.; Owen, A.; Wong, D.P.; Krustrup, P.; van Exsel, M.; Mallo, J. Technical and physical demands of small vs. large sided games in relation to playing position in elite soccer. *Hum. Mov. Sci.* **2012**, *31*, 957–969. [CrossRef] [PubMed]

8

Can Fundamental Movement Skill Mastery Be Increased via a Six Week Physical Activity Intervention to Have Positive Effects on Physical Activity and Physical Self-Perception?

Elizabeth S. Bryant [1,*], Michael J. Duncan [2,†], Samantha L. Birch [2,†] and Rob S. James [2,†]

1 London Sports Institute, Middlesex University, The Burroughs, London NW4 4BT, UK
2 Research Centre for Applied Biological and Exercise Sciences, Coventry University, Priory Street, Covenrty CV1 5FB, UK; aa8396@coventry.ac.uk (M.J.D.); aa0052@coventry.ac.uk (S.L.B.); apx214@coventry.ac.uk (R.S.J.)
* Correspondence: L.Bryant@mdx.ac.uk
† These authors contributed equally to this work.

Academic Editor: Eling de Bruin

Abstract: Background: Previous research has suggested a positive relationship between fundamental movement skills (FMS) mastery and physical activity (PA) level. Research conducted on interventions to improve FMS mastery is equivocal and further research is needed. Methods: An intervention group of 82 children (35 boys and 47 girls) and a control group of 83 children (42 boys and 41 girls) were recruited from Years 4 and 5 (mean age ± SD = 8.3 ± 0.4 years) of two schools in Central England. The intervention included a combination of circuits and dancing to music. Pre and post intervention tests were conducted. Tests included: subjective assessment of eight FMS; objective measurement of two FMS; four day pedometer step count recording; height and mass for Body Mass Index (BMI); and the completion of Harter *et al.*'s (1982) self-perception questionnaire. Results: Following a two (pre to post) by two (intervention and control group) mixed-model ANOVA it was highlighted that the intervention group improved mastery in all eight FMS, and increased both daily steps and physical self-perception. Conclusions: It can be concluded that focussing one Physical Education (PE) lesson per week on the development of FMS has had a positive benefit on FMS, PA level and physical self-perception for the children in this study.

Keywords: fundamental movement skills; children; physical activity; obesity; intervention

1. Introduction

The mastery of Fundamental Movement Skills (FMS) in children has been assessed in an attempt to identify any mechanisms underlying physical activity (PA) levels and weight status [1–4]. Research has recently identified that previous mastery in FMS can predict future PA levels in children [3–5]. These findings demonstrate the importance of FMS competency in childhood for maintenance of PA levels and in turn a healthy weight status. This has particular relevance for school Physical Education (PE) as the development of physical literacy and FMS is a key component of the National Curriculum for PE (NCPE) at key stages 1 and 2 in England [6].

Given this focus for school PE and the recent findings of Bryant *et al.*, (2014) [4], a key further step would be to determine whether it is possible to intervene and create an ecologically valid intervention to increase a child's FMS competency to acquire the benefit of sustained PA participation. Primary school children in the United Kingdom currently have two hours of statutory PE per week [7]. This PE time needs to provide children with the skills and tools to be able to lead a physically active lifestyle [8].

An additional target for PE lessons proposed by the National Association for Sport and Physical Education [9] is that 50% of each lesson should be comprised of time in moderate-vigorous PA (MVPA) to contribute to the Department for Health's "Start Active, Stay Active" daily target of at least 60 min of MVPA [10]. Consequently schools provide PE lessons to meet this target, often via team games [11,12]. However, this may be short-sighted, as engaging children in team games (to meet this target [9,13–16]) when they do not have mastery of FMS may be detrimental to future PA participation [17].

PE lessons that are less active but promote the teaching of skill-related fitness [16] may be more important in the long term to provide children with the skills to be physically active in later life [4]; which is the main goal in the NCPE [9]. According to Stodden *et al.*, (2008) [18] PA participation level and weight status are mediated by a combination of actual and perceived motor competence (PMC). Stodden *et al.*, (2008) [17] explains that when children reach middle to-late childhood (7–10 years old) their cognitive ability has developed to a stage where they can compare themselves to their peers [18]. Furthermore, children who obtain a higher PMC due to a higher actual motor competence (AMC) will perceive tasks as being easier and are more likely to engage in them. This engagement in PA will allow a child to practice and develop their AMC, sustain their PA level and maintain a healthy weight status [17]. Previous research has identified significant relationships between PMC, PA levels and weight status [19–21]. Although this significant relationship has been identified it needs to be distinguished as to whether PMC can be changed through an intervention to gain the benefit of an increased PA level. It is important to note that there are many factors that affect lifestyle behaviours, such as PA and weight status, and that motor development is just one such factor that contributes to this.

To date, no studies appear to have examined whether a short-term intervention, focusing on FMS during one out of two statutory school PE session, might result in greater benefit than engaging in two sessions of statutory PE per week. The current study sought to address this issue by: running an exploratory six week trial that replaced one out of two statutory PE lessons per week focused on the teaching of FMS; and determining the efficacy of such an intervention on PA, weight status and physical self-perception.

2. Method

2.1. Sample

Three primary schools in Central England were invited to take part in the study, of which two schools accepted. The schools were chosen from the same bracket of electoral wards (50%–59%) for deprivation and socio-economic status [22] as a means to ensure that extremes of affluence and deprivation did not confound the results of the study. When the schools were chosen, it was ensured that they were not currently, or had not previously been, part of any specialist PE programmes/interventions. Following informed consent from parents/guardians, 165 Years 4 and 5 children, mean ($\pm$SD) age of 8.3 $\pm$ 0.4 years, were recruited to take part in the study. Each school had two classes per year group. From the two classes per year group, one class was selected by a teacher to complete the intervention, whilst the other class was the control group. The intervention group consisted of 82 children (35 boys and 47 girls) and the control group consisted of 83 children (42 boys and 41 girls).

2.2. Study Design

The intervention group and control group were both tested to determine baseline values for FMS, daily steps, physical self-perception and weight status. The intervention group in each school underwent the 6 week intervention programme as detailed in Table 1. Only one PE lesson was replaced in an attempt to have little disturbance in the school's curriculum, and to create a design that could be realistically repeated by class teachers in schools. The control group continued their normal physical education (PE) lessons. Immediately post completion of the intervention the control and intervention groups were both retested for FMS, daily steps, physical self-perception and weight status. Both schools involved in the intervention had two classes per year group; one class acted as the intervention group and one as the control group. Further details on all methods are given below.

Table 1. The Content of the Six Week Intervention (30 s rest between each activity).

Weeks 1–3	Aim	Content	Equipment (for 30 Children)
Warm up (5 min)	To steadily increase the children's heart rate. Prepare the body for similar movements that they are about to undertake.	Dancing to a song (cha cha slide, DJ Casper). This song is popular for the age group completing the research and includes instructions that the children have to follow, for example, hopping, jumping and sliding.	CD player
Instruction time (8 min)	To identify key coaching points of each skill to the children.	Coaching points from the POC [23] were explained and demonstrated to the children.	N/A
Circuits 1. Running (3 min)	The use of the hurdles will encourage children to lift their knees higher to increase efficiency of the sprint [24].	Running over hurdles. Hurdles would start on the lowest level (10 cm) and increase in height each week (17.5 and 25 cm). Children were instructed to stay on the balls of their feet and drive their arms.	Five agility hurdles
2. Balance (3 min)	For children to control a balance board by engaging core muscles to improve balance.	Standing on balance boards. They were instructed to not let the board touch the floor. If they found this too easy then they were told to close their eyes. They were instructed to tense their stomach muscles.	Eight wobble boards
3. Throwing and catching (3 min)	For children to learn the correct technique to throw and catch a ball.	Children were in pairs standing five metres apart and practiced throwing and catching to each other with a tennis ball. They were given instructions for: the throw-start standing side on and step forward with the opposite leg; and the catch-meet the ball with your hands and bring it in to your body.	Eight tennis balls and 16 cones
4. Kicking (3 min)	For the children to learn the correct technique of the kick.	Children stood five metres from each other in pairs and kicked a ball back to each other. Children were instructed to take a step and swing back the leg, and keep their eye on the ball.	Eight small soft round playground footballs
		Songs	
1. Jumping (Kriss Kross, Jump)	For children to learn the technique of the jump through a song that they will engage with.	Children were demonstrated the correct technique of a counter movement jump and were asked to complete this jump every time they heard the word jump in the song.	CD player
2. Hopping (One Direction, One way or another)	For children to learn the technique of hopping through a song that they will engage with.	Children were split into four teams. The children were demonstrated the correct technique of the hop with coaching points such as "stay on your toes". Children then completed hopping relays in their teams.	CD player, cones
3. Gallop (PSY, Gangnam style)	For children to learn the technique of galloping through a song that they will engage with.	Children were demonstrated the correct technique of the gallop and given coaching points such as, "make sure your hips and shoulders stay straight and do not twist". Children would gallop in a circle around the room and when the chorus came on they would all come to the middle of the hall and perform the "gangnam style" dance to the music.	CD player
Cool down-song (Harlum shake)	To progressively cool the body down with lighter exercise to decrease the children's heart rate and to recap the movements learnt in the session.	Children had to pick a skill that they had performed in the session and mime it to the speed of the music. This was repeated three times with them choosing a different skill each time.	CD player

Table 1. *Cont.*

Weeks 3–6	Aim	Content	Equipment (for 30 Children)
Warm up (7 min)	To steadily increase the children's heart rate. Prepare the body for similar movements that they are about to undertake.	Pirate ship game. Commands were shouted out to the children to which they had to perform a response. These were: Starboard: side gallop to the right hand side of the hall. Port side: hop to the left hand side of the hall. Climb the riggings: pretend to climb up a ladder getting their knees high and parallel to the ground. Scrub the deck: the children had to get onn the floor on their hands and knees pretending to wash the floor. Invasion: children had to pretend to throw bombs at other pirates. Spying: children had to pretend to throw bombs at invading pirates. Walk the plank: children had to stand on one leg as if they were on the end of a plank.	N/A
Instruction time (8 min)	To identify key coaching points of each skill to the children.	Coaching points from the POC[23] were explained and demonstrated to the children.	N/A
Circuits 1. Hopping (3 min)	To be able to hop over all the hurdles without the use of the other leg.	Hurdles were set at the lowest level and children were asked to hop on one leg over each hurdle. Legs were then alternated between goes.	Five agility hurdles
2. Kicking (3 min)	To put the technique of the kick that the children have learnt into practise via competition.	Yellow stars were stuck on the wall and children had to kick and aim at the star. If they hit a star they scored one point. Children would compete against their partner.	Six cardboard stars and four small soft playground footballs
3. Throwing (3 min)	To put the technique of the throw that the children have learnt into practice via competition.	Multi coloured cut outs of hands were stuck onto a wall and children had to throw a tennis ball, aiming at the hands. If they hit a hand then they would score one point. Each child competed against their partner.	Six cardboard hands and four tennis balls
4. Jumping (3 min)	To complete the jump on a trampet to help increase height and encourage children to control the jump.	Children would do three consecutive jumps on a trampet, with the final jump landing on a mat in front.	Trampet
5. Balance (3 min)	To successfully walk along the benches without falling off.	Balance. Children would walk along three upside down gym benches with a cone on their head.	Three gymnasium benches
Relays (6 min)	To successfully complete the gallop and the run in a competitive situation.	Children remained in their five teams and completed running and galloping relay races. Children were demonstrated the correct technique and given coaching points.	10 cones
Cool down-game (7 min)	To play a more static game to decrease heart rate and to successfully catch the ball in a competitive situation.	Children were split into two teams. Within each team children had to stand in two lines with a partner in front of them. Children had to throw the ball back and forth, from person to person, and work it up the line so that everyone had to touch the ball. If someone dropped that ball then that team had to start again from the beginning. The first team to get the ball to the other end without dropping it were the winners. To begin with, children had to have their hands behind their backs before catching that ball. This was to prove that it is much harder to catch a ball if you don't have your hands prepared to catch. It then would progress to having your hands waiting in a cupped position with a stable stance and as a consequence each team would complete the challenge quicker, therefore reinforcing the importance of being prepared.	Two tennis balls

2.2.1. Instrumentation

Anthropometric Measurements

Anthropometric measurements were carried out individually in a sports hall prior to the performance of the fundamental movement skills (FMS). Children wore shorts and a t-shirt, but shoes were removed. Height (cm) and body mass (kg) were recorded to the nearest cm and 0.1 kg respectively using a stadiometer and electronic weighing scales (SECA Instruments Ltd., Hamburg, Germany), respectively. Body Mass Index (BMI) was calculated as Kg/m^2. Children were classed as overweight if they were in the 85th centile and obese if in the 95th centile [25]. Using these criteria, 64% of children were classified as "normal weight" and 36% as "overweight/obese".

2.2.2. Fundamental Movement Skill Assessment

Subjective Measurement

FMS was assessed using the Process Orient Checklist (POC) [23]. Children were demonstrated each skill once with no coaching points. Children were asked to perform each skill three times. This checklist is comprised of eight different FMS; Sprint Run, Side Gallop, Hop, Kick, Catch, Overarm Throw, Vertical Jump and Static Balance. Each Skill is broken down into five or six components; depending on how many components the child demonstrated a percentage of mastery was calculated. The average percentage of mastery for the three trials was used for further analysis. In addition to the percentage of mastery being calculated, if a child demonstrated all components of the skill then they were rated as having "mastery"; if they demonstrated all but one of the components of the skill then "near mastery" and if more than one component were deemed to be missing then the participant was said to have no mastery of the skill [23].

Each FMS was video recorded (Sony video camera, Sony, Surrey, UK) and subsequently edited into single film clips of single skills on a computer using Quintic biomechanics analysis software (Quintic Consultancy Ltd., Sutton Coldfield, UK). Each video clip was given a unique identification code and did not indicate if the clip was from the intervention group or pre or post assessment. The clips were coded by a researcher who was not involved in analysis of the videos. This allowed researchers to be blinded to which group each participant was in and which stage of the research the participants were at to limit subjective and unconscious preferable scoring. The skills were also analysed using this software, enabling the videos to be slowed down, magnified and replayed. Prior to analysis inter- and intra-rater reliability analysis was performed for all the FMS between each researcher and the lead researcher. Inter-rater reliability was 91% and intra-rater reliability was 92%, demonstrating good reliability [20].

Objective Measurement

A 10 m sprint run was timed (s) using Smartspeed® gates (Smartspeed, Fusion Sport, Coopers Plains, Queensland, Australia). Two laser gates were set up ten meters apart. The children were asked to sprint through the two gates. The height (cm) of the vertical jump was measured using a Myotest jump monitor (Myotest, Sion, Switzerland), as recommended by Bubanj *et al.*, (2010) [24]. The children had three attempts at each test and the best score was taken for analysis.

2.2.3. Physical Activity Assessment

Habitual physical activity (PA) was measured using a sealed pedometer (Yamax Digi-Walker; SW 700, Yamax, TX, USA) worn over four days (two weekdays and two weekend days) [26]. Average daily steps were recorded for analysis. If children failed to collect data on any of the four days and/or values of <1000 steps or >40,000 steps per day were recorded on any day then all data for that child was excluded from the analysis in accordance with recommendations for the treatment of pedometer derived PA [27]. Children kept a diary of the step count that they completed each day. This diary was signed off by their parents to ensure that the legitimate pedometer data was recorded and used for analysis.

2.2.4. Children's Self-Perception of Skill Ability Assessment

A modified version of The Perceived Physical Competence Subscale for Children questionnaire (PPCSC) was used [18]. The questionnaire was reduced to 10 questions to represent popular activities which have been shown to have good discrimination between self-efficacy levels. The modifications made to the PPCSC replicated those made in other publications that have also utilized the PPCSC [28–30]. The questionnaire was completed in a classroom in the presence of the project coordinator and a class teacher.

2.3. Data Analysis

No children missed more than one session out of the six weeks, therefore data from all participants was retained and analysed.

Firstly, the Q-Q plot and the kurtosis and skewness values for each variable were assessed to identify whether each variable was normally distributed. The values for skewness and kurtosis were all between <1 and >−1 and therefore normally distributed [31], allowing the use of parametric testing.

Independent t test were conducted on baseline characteristics between the intervention group and the control group to ensure that they were comparable prior to intervention. The independent *t* tests highlighted no significant difference ($p > 0.05$) between the intervention (I) and control (C) group for gender (I: 46.6% boys and 53.4% girls and C: 50% boys and 50% girls), age (I: 8.35 ± 0.47 years and C: 8.34 ± 0.47 years), BMI (I: 18.01 ± 2.9 kg/m^2 and C: 18.33 ± 3.3 kg/m^2), average daily steps (I: 9682 ± 6109 steps and C: 10,036 ± 8527 steps) and overall motor competency percentage (I: 45.16% ± 15.02% and C: 47.34% ± 11.71%).

Children who had full mastery of a particular FMS at baseline, and therefore could no longer improve, were removed from the analysis of that FMS. *i.e.*, their data was only removed for the tasks that they showed full mastery for, not for all the FMS. This resulted in a number of children being removed from the FMS analysis as follows: Intervention boys: run 1; hop 0; gallop 9; catch 2; throw 2; kick 1; jump 0; balance 10. Intervention girls: run 0; hop 0; gallop 8; catch 8; throw 0; kick 0; jump 1; balance 15. Control boys: run 0; hop 0; gallop 11 catch 3; throw 3; kick 1; jump 0; balance 13. Control girls: run 0; hop 0; gallop 5; catch 6; throw 0; kick 0; jump 0; balance 14.

A two (pre to post) by two (intervention and control group) mixed model ANOVA was conducted to analyse any main effects and pre to post by group interactions for FMS mastery, daily steps, BMI, and physical self-perception scores. Levene's test was used to determine whether variances were equal between each group. Where variances were unequal we have taken a more conservative approach and used $p < 0.001$ as the critical p value. Where significant interactions were highlighted, paired samples *t* test was conducted on the variable to identify if the intervention or control group significantly increased. Significance was set at $p < 0.05$.

3. Results

3.1. FMS Changes

3.1.1. Subjective Measure

Boys

Following the two (pre/post) by two (intervention/control) mixed model ANOVA there was an overall main effect from pre to post for all eight fundamental movement skills (FMS) (All eight FMS $p < 0.001$ in each case).

A pre to post significant interaction between intervention and control group was highlighted for seven out of the eight FMS (Hop and gallop $p < 0.05$; catch, throw, kick, balance and jump $p < 0.001$).

Paired t tests highlighted that for the seven skills with a significant interaction there was a significant increase in skill mastery level between pre and post for the intervention group. (Intervention group, Hop, gallop, throw, kick, balance and jump $p < 0.001$; catch $p < 0.5$). For the same seven skills the paired samples t tests highlighted that five skills also significantly increased in mastery level for the control group (Hop, gallop, throw and jump $p < 0.001$). Although the control group also significantly improved from pre to post in five measures of FMS, the intervention group improved by a greater magnitude compared to the control group (Figure 1).

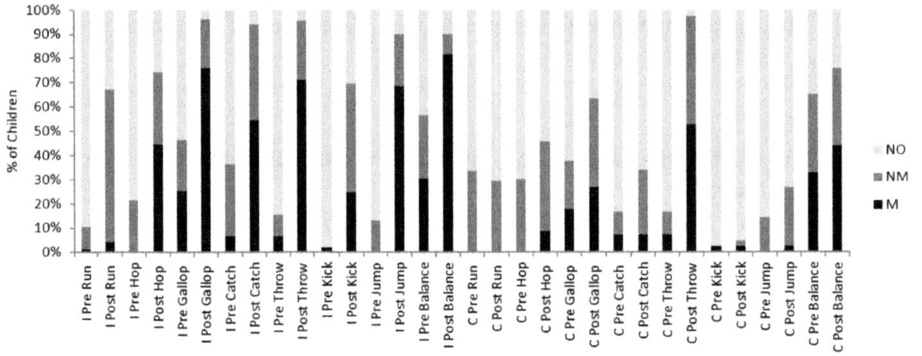

Figure 1. Percentage of Boys Classed as M (Mastery), NM (Near Mastery) and NO (No Mastery) for all eight fundamental movement skills (FMS) Pre and Immediately Post the Six Week Intervention (N = 35) and Control Group (N = 42). I = Intervention Group; C = Control Group.

Girls

Following the two (pre/post) by two (intervention/control) mixed model ANOVA there was an overall main effect from pre to post for all eight FMS (All eight FMS $p < 0.001$).

A pre to post between intervention and control group significant interaction was highlighted for seven out of the eight FMS (Hop and gallop $p < 0.05$; catch, throw, kick balance and jump $p < 0.001$). Paired t tests highlighted that for the seven skills with a significant interaction there was a significant increase in skill mastery level between pre and post for the intervention group. (Intervention group, Hop, gallop, throw, kick, balance and jump $p < 0.001$; catch $p < 0.05$). For the same seven skills the paired samples t tests highlighted that five skills also significantly increased in mastery level in the control group (Hop, gallop, throw balance and jump $p < 0.001$) Although the control group also significantly improved from pre to post in five measures of FMS, the intervention group improved by a greater magnitude compared to the control group (Figure 2).

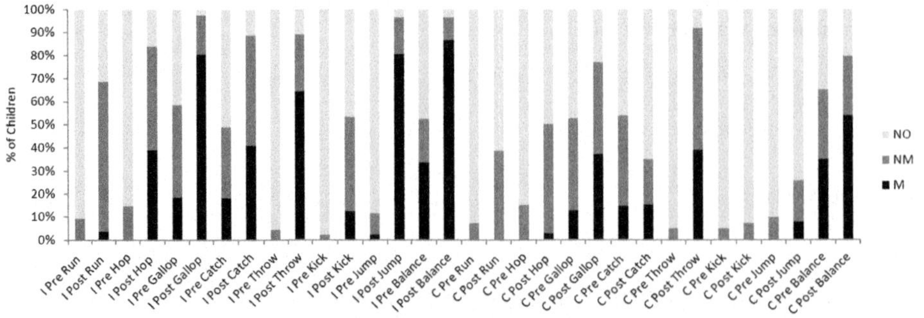

Figure 2. Percentage of Girls Classed as M (Mastery), NM (Near Mastery) and NO (No Mastery) for all eight fundamental movement skills (FMS) Pre and Immediately Post the Six Week Intervention (N = 47) and Control Group (N = 41). I = Intervention Group; C = Control Group.

3.1.2. Objective

Boys

There was a significant main effect for pre to post jump height for the intervention and control group (ANOVA $F(1) = 10.3$, $p < 0.05$). There was no significant interaction between the intervention and control group. There was no significant main effect for pre to post sprint speed for the intervention and control group ($f(1) = 3.3$, $p > 0.05$).

Girls

There was a significant main effect for pre to post jump height for the intervention and control group (ANOVA $F(1) = 23.6$, $p < 0.05$). There was no significant interaction between the intervention and control group for jump height. There was no significant main effect for pre to post sprint speed for the intervention and control group ($f(1) = 1.58$, $p > 0.05$). However, there was a significant interaction between the intervention and control group, pre to post assessments ($f(1) = 4.46$, $p < 0.05$). There was no significant difference from pre to post measurement of the sprint run for the intervention group (paired t test, $t(46)$ 0.66, $p > 0.05$). However, there was a significant difference between pre to post measurement for the control group ($t(40)$ −2.17, $p < 0.05$). The mean (±SD) for the sprint speed and jump height, pre and post intervention, for the intervention and the control groups are displayed in Table 2.

Table 2. Mean ± SD for objectively measured fundamental movement skills (FMS) pre and post intervention, for intervention (N = 35 boys and 47 girls) and control groups (N = 42 boys and 41 girls).

Gender	Intervention		Control	
Boys	Pre	Post	Pre	Post
Jump height (cm)	21.6 ± 4.9	25.3 ± 1.65	19.4 ± 6.4	21.3 ± 4.2 *
Sprint speed (sec)	2.09 ± 0.69	1.96 ± 0.86 *	2.18 ± 0.75	2.36 ± 0.45
Girls	Pre	Post	Pre	Post
Jump height (cm)	21.2 ± 4.0	23.2 ± 4.5 *	19.4 ± 6.4	21.3 ± 4.2 *
Sprint speed (sec)	2.41 ± 0.68	2.34 ± 0.85	2.18 ± 0.75	2.36 ± 0.45

Note: * Significantly different from pre intervention or control ($p < 0.05$).

3.1.3. Body Mass Index

There was no significant change in body mass index (BMI) in the intervention or control group from pre to post measurements (ANOVA $p > 0.05$) for both boys and girls.

3.2. Physical Activity Changes

Boys

There was a significant main effect for the intervention and control group (ANOVA $F(1) = 8.3$, $p < 0.05$). However, there was no significant interaction between pre/post and the intervention and control group ($f(1) = 0.71$, $p < 0.05$).

Girls

There was a significant main effect for the intervention and control group (ANOVA $F(1) = 21$, $p < 0.001$). There was also a significant interaction between the intervention and control group from pre to post intervention ($f(1) = 13.7$, $p < 0.001$). There was a significant increase in daily steps from pre to post (paired t test, $t(20)$ −4.55, $p < 0.001$). However, there was no significant difference in daily steps from pre to post control group ($t(18)$ 01.68), $p > 0.05$). Mean (±SD) average daily steps for pre and post intervention and control are displayed in Figure 3.

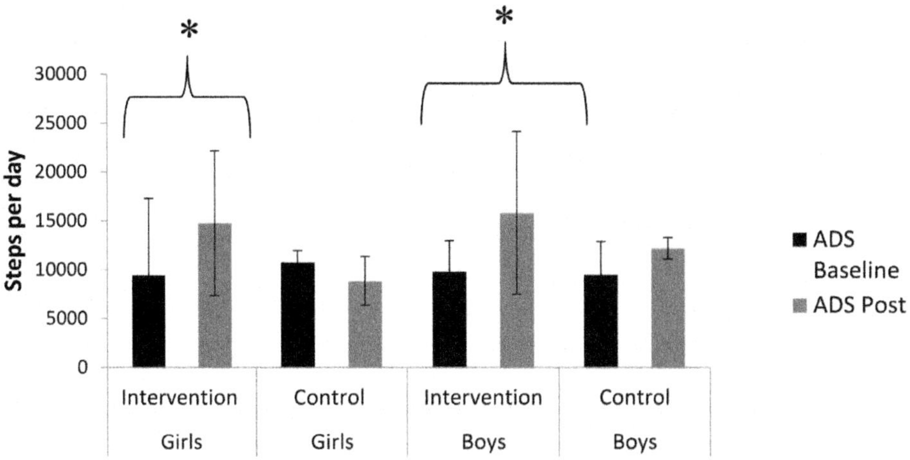

Figure 3. Mean (±SD) of Pedometer Step Counts for Girls and Boys For Intervention Group at Baseline, Post Six Weeks and for the Control Group at Baseline and Post Six Week Control. * Significant increase from baseline to post intervention ($p < 0.05$). (ADS: Average Daily Steps).

3.3. Physical Self-Perception

Boys

There was a significant main effect for the intervention and control group ($f(1) = 4.75$, $p < 0.05$) for physical self-perception scores. There was no significant interaction between the intervention and control group from pre to post measurement ($f(1) = 0.016$, $p > 0.05$).

Girls

There was a significant main effect for the intervention and control group ($f(1) = 11.8$, $p < 0.001$) for physical self-perception scores. There was no significant interaction between the intervention and control group from pre to post measurement ($f(1) = 0.13$, $p > 0.05$). The mean (±SD) PPSCS score for pre and post intervention and control are displayed in Table 3.

Table 3. The mean (±SD) for self-perception according to the Phyisical Percieved Competency Scale for Children (PPCSC) for pre and post intervention and control.

Gender	Intervention		Control	
Boys	Pre	Post	Pre	Post
PPCSC Score	28.94 ± 6	31.06 ± 4.6	27.18 ± 6.5	29.49 ± 6.1
Girls	Pre	Post	Pre	Post
PPCSC Score	26.14 ± 5.6	28.8 ± 6.5	27.24 ± 5.4	30.25 ± 5.47

4. Discussion

This current study has identified that the children who completed this intervention increased significantly more than the control group mastery of fundamental movement skills (FMS), pedometer step counts and physical self-perception.

The study is novel as it presents an ecologically valid FMS intervention (the materials and methods could realistically be repeated in a school by class teachers) which positively influences FMS, physical activity (PA) and physical self-perception. Stodden *et al.*, (2008) [17] identified that a combination of actual motor competence (AMC) and perceived motor competence (PMC) will influence PA and then weight status. To the author's knowledge, no other study has identified whether all three of these variables will be influenced from an increase in AMC through an intervention. This study is also novel in that it sought to modify one school PE lesson per week rather than add additional PA sessions (such as work by Cliff *et al.*, (2007) [32]; Graf *et al.*, (2008) [33]) or to completely change the physical education (PE) curriculum [34]. Thus, not only is the intervention efficacious effective, it is also ecologically valid and feasible for primary schools to implement.

4.1. Overall Changes in FMS

The number of children who were classed as having mastery for all eight subjectively measured skills increased post intervention. This is consistent with the findings of Mitchell *et al.*, (2011) who reported a significant increase in the number of children who were classed as having mastery for all 12 FMS that were assessed after a minimum of a six week intervention. Mitchell *et al.*'s (2011) [35] intervention was conducted on children aged 5–12 years old which provided teachers with a FMS manual to use through PE lessons and fitness classes. At baseline, the children in Mitchell *et al.*'s (2011) [35] study had a higher amount of children classed as having mastery levels (21.4%–84.6%) compared to the children at baseline in this study (0%–25.3%). Post intervention, the percentage of children classed as having mastery of the skills in Mitchell *et al.*'s (2011) [35] study ranged from 49.8% to 98.3%, compared to 3.6%–81.2% in the present study. Although Mitchells *et al.*'s (2011) [35] study reports a larger amount of children as having mastery of the skills, the Test of Gross Motor Development 2 (TGMD-2) was used to assess the FMS. Although it is still a process orient based method, it only has 3–4 components for each skill and therefore it is much easier for children to gain mastery of the skills. This is similar for Hardy *et al.*, (2010) [36] who also used the TGMD-2 to assess FMS and reported that 20.5%–76% of children had mastery of the same FMS. In this current study the POC, which was used to assess FMS, has 5–6 components for each skill, therefore making it much harder to gain full mastery of them. Okely *et al.*, (2004) [2] also used the POC and also reported lower numbers of children classed as having mastery 0%–35%. Although two different scales have been used between this intervention and Mitchell *et al.*'s (2011) [35] intervention, the two skills with the lowest and highest percentage of children classed as having mastery, were also the lowest and highest skills post intervention. This finding suggests that if all skills are focused on throughout an intervention then they will develop at similar rates with the extremes still remaining the extremes.

Out of the two skills that were measured objectively, jump height significantly improved post intervention, but sprint speed did not. Research has identified that locomotor skills such as the sprint run are harder to master [37,38]. This is reflected in the subjective result of the sprint run, as it was the skill that the least amount of children could master. This suggests that the new/correct technique that the children have learnt is not yet autonomous and that the children still have to concentrate when performing the skill which inhibits their objective performance outcome of the sprint run. Further research is needed to identify how long it takes for each skill to become autonomous to influence the amount of time needed to be spent on each skill in PE lessons in primary school. When children learn a new skill for the first time, they will get to the autonomous stage of learning quicker compared to when having to re learn a new skill [39]. The objective measure of the sprint run was measured over 10 m, therefore assessing acceleration rather than sprint speed. The technique that the children would have learnt is appropriate for sprinting at speed, not the acceleration phase of the sprint. This might also help to explain why the children improved in the subjective measure, but not the objective measure. In future children should be allowed a flying start when having their technique of the sprint run assessed.

An, explanation as to why there are differing numbers for the amount of girls and boys gaining mastery of FMS could be gender bias in activities. Research has highlighted that boys favour activities that require locomotor skills such as running and girls favour creative activities such as dance and gymnastics [39]. This difference in gender and FMS performance is consistent with previous research [2,40–42]. The intervention group significantly gained mastery in all eight FMS and the control group significantly gained mastery in six out of the eight FMS. Initially, when the control group improved alongside the intervention group it suggested that the change was not down to the intervention. Although the control groups were in a different class they were in the same year group at the same school. Some of the children in the intervention group had friends in the control group and when they met them in the playground they taught them the skills they had learnt; this was reported to the lead researcher by the children who participated in the intervention sessions. This highlights the importance of using separate schools as control groups to control for this limitation. Although, the control groups did significantly improve, the significant interactions highlighted that the intervention group improved significantly more than the control group.

The findings from this study indicate that an intervention in one group of children has wider benefits by significantly increasing FMS mastery in another group of children. From the perspective of the children this is a positive consequence. As previously stated the number of children who are classed as having mastery of the FMS increases for both the intervention group and the control group. This is inconsistent with previous research that had control groups at different schools to the intervention groups [39]. However, the significant interactions highlighted that the intervention group improved significantly more than the control group. If the control group from this study was at a different school, improvements in the control group may have differed from these results.

4.2. Physical Activity Changes

Children who completed the intervention were associated with having higher daily steps compared to the children who did not complete the intervention. Daily steps significantly increased in post intervention compared to baseline for the intervention group. Van Beurden *et al.*, (2003) [43] also found a significant increase, by 7.8%, in time spent in MVPA post intervention. On the contrary, Cliff *et al.*, (2007) [32] reported an overall decrease of 18% of time spent in MVPA. It was explained that this decrease was due to a ceiling effect and that baseline measures were 20% higher than the average for children that age in the area [32]. There are limited studies that have reported PA data alongside an intervention for FMS, however when they have, it has been MVPA that has been reported. Conversely, Westerterp and Plasqui (2004) [44] highlighted that it is activities of low and high intensity that are the main contributors to a child's PA level. Therefore, by measuring their habitual PA level, like in the current study, it includes all levels of intensity that will contribute to a child's PA status. This allows for the results to provide a better indication of the overall effect that an increase in FMS will have on habitual PA, which has been highlighted to be important to health [41]. However, with the limitations that pedometers hold, as discussed in the limitations section below, this statement about the results must be taken with caution.

4.3. Changes in Self Perception Scores

Perceived Physical Competence Scales for Children (PPCSC) scores significantly increased from baseline to post intervention. Previous research has suggested that children who have a higher self-perception are more likely to have better FMS competency [19–21]. Ekeland *et al.*, (2004) [45] completed a systematic review on exercise/PA and self-esteem in children and concluded that exercise has positive short term effects on self-esteem. Whilst these studies have identified this relationship between the two variables, the cause and effect relationship has still remained unanswered. It could be that if children perceive themselves as being more competent, in turn perceiving tasks as being easier, then they spend more time participating in PA, resulting in an increase in ACM [46,47]. Or on the other hand, it could be argued that children who spend more time in PA allow themselves to develop these skills, thus increasing their PMC due to a higher AMC.

Due to no follow up assessment being conducted it is unknown whether the PPCSC scores revert back to their original levels. However, once children have mastery of a skill they are highly unlikely to lose it and according to Stodden *et al.*, (2008) [17] the age of the children in this study should be able to accurately perceive their AMC. Therefore, with the number of children who have gained mastery of the FMS it seems unlikely that the PPCSC score would revert back to its original score [17].

4.4. Limitations

Six weeks after the intervention had finished follow up assessments were conducted on the intervention group. Unfortunately it was not possible to conduct the follow up assessments on the control group; therefore this is why this data was not included in the analysis in this paper. Six weeks after the cessation of the intervention, children increased in mastery in six out of the eight skills (not the throw and kick) compared to immediately post intervention. For daily steps, children remained significantly higher compared to baseline, however they had significantly decreased from immediately post intervention, therefore highlighting the possibility that PA levels could revert back to original levels. Further research is needed with longer follow up assessments that are conducted on both the intervention and control group.

An additional key limitation of the present study was the use of the control group from the same year group and school as the intervention group. It was speculated that the reason for the increase in the percentage of children, in the control group, classed as having mastery was due to the children in the intervention group teaching the control group in the playground. Another limitation was the use of pedometers as it did not give the measurement of intensity of physical activity. Although the aim of the study was to assess habitual PA, if intensity had been measured it would have given information as to whether this intervention could have also contributed to the NICE PE target of 50% of their lesson at MVPA [10]. Furthermore, the intervention content involved diverse movements and types of activities that would not necessarily be identified by a step counter and therefore the intervention effect may have been underestimated. The generalisability of the results of this study is limited due to only two schools being used from the same area in central England. Therefore, it is unknown whether the same results would be seen in culturally different children.

5. Conclusions

It can be concluded that by focussing one PE lesson on the development of FMS (one hour per week for six weeks) it will have a positive benefit on PA level and physical self-perception. This study highlights a unique and efficacious way in which children could be taught the FMS. Teachers should take this information and use it to aid in the teaching of FMS. Using circuits as way of getting children to repeat the skill, but allowing them to move on quickly will enable children to stay engaged in the session whilst practising the skills. By interspersing the circuits with dancing to songs, it again keeps the children engaged and practising the techniques of skills. Although this intervention was in a six week block that was based on one school term in the UK, it can be adapted to suit any school structure by using the successful mechanisms elucidated in this intervention.

Acknowledgments: Thanks to Hollyfast Primary School and Eastern Green Junior School in Coventry, Central England for participation in this intervention.

Author Contributions: Elizabeth S. Bryant was the lead researcher, designing, collecting, analyzing the data and writing the paper. Michael J. Duncan was involved with the study design, analysis of the data and writing of the paper. Samantha L. Birch was involved with the study design, analysis of the data and writing of the paper. Rob S. James was involved with the study design, analysis of the data and writing of the paper.

Conflicts of Interest: The authors declare no conflict of interest.

References

1. McKenzie, T.L.; Sallis, J.F.; Broyles, S.L.; Zive, M.M.; Nader, P.R.; Berry, C.C.; Brennan, J.J. Childhood movement skills: Predictors of physical activity in anglo american and mexican american adolescents? *Res. Q. Exerc. Sport* **2002**, *73*, 238–244. [CrossRef] [PubMed]
2. Okely, A.D.; Booth, M.L.; Chey, T. Relationships between body composition and fundamental movement skills among children and adolescents. *Res. Q. Exerc. Sport* **2004**, *75*, 238–247. [CrossRef] [PubMed]
3. Barnett, L.M.; Morgan, P.J.; van Beurden, E.; Beard, J.R. Perceived sports competence mediates the relationship between childhood motor skill proficiency and adolescent physical activity and fitness: A longitudinal assessment. *Int. J. Behav. Nutr. Phys. Act.* **2008**, *5*, 1–12. [CrossRef] [PubMed]

4. Bryant, E.S.; James, R.; Birch, S.; Duncan, M. Does prior or current FMS predict future habitual physical activity (PA) levels and weight status? *J. Sports Sci.* **2014**, *32*, 1775–1782. [CrossRef] [PubMed]
5. Okely, A.D.; Booth, M.L.; Patterson, J.W. Relationship of physical activity to fundamental movement skills among adolescents. *Med. Sci. Sports Exerc.* **2001**, *33*, 1899–1904. [CrossRef] [PubMed]
6. Physical Education Programmes of Study: Key Stages 1 and 2. 2013. Available online: https://www.gov.uk/government/uploads/system/uploads/attachment_data/file/239040/PRIMARY_national_curriculum_-_Physical_education.pdf (accessed on 8 October 2015).
7. Bardens, J.B.; Long, R.; Gillie, C. *School Report*; House of Commons Report; The Stationery Office Limited: London, UK, 2012.
8. Green, K. *Understanding Physical Education*; SAGE: London, UK, 2008.
9. Qualifications and Curriculum Authority (QCA). *Physical Education: Programme of Study for Key Stage 3 and Attainment Target*; QCA: London, UK, 2007.
10. Department of Helath. Physical Activity Guidelines for Children and Young People. 2011. Available online: https://www.gov.uk/government/uploads/system/uploads/attachment_data/file/213739/dh_128144 (accessed on 8 October 2015).
11. Fairclough, S.J. Physical activity levels during key stage 3 physical education 34. *Br. J. Teach. Phys. Educ.* **2003**, *34*, 40–45.
12. Warburton, P.; Woods, J. Observation of children's physical activity levels during primary school physical education lessons. *Eur. J. Phys. Educ.* **1996**, *1*, 56–65. [CrossRef]
13. Hodges-Kulinna, P.; Martin, J.; Lai, Q.; Kliber, A.; Reed, B. Student physical activity patterns: Grade, gender and activity influences. *Br. J. Teach. Phys. Educ.* **2003**, *22*, 298–310.
14. McNamee, G.D. The One Who Gathers Children: The work of vivian gussin paley and current debates about how we educate young children. *J. Early Child. Teach. Educ.* **2005**, *25*, 275–296. [CrossRef]
15. Trudeau, F.; Shephard, R.J. Contribution of school programmes to physical activity levels and attitudes in children and adults. *Sports Med.* **2005**, *35*, 89–105. [CrossRef] [PubMed]
16. Stratton, G.; Fairclough, S.J.; Ridgers, N.D. Physical Activity Levels during the School Day. In *Youth Physical Activity and Sedentary Behaviour: Challenges and Solutions*; Smith, A.L., Biddle, S.J.H., Eds.; Human Kinetics: Champaign, IL, USA, 2008; pp. 321–350.
17. Stodden, D.F.; Goodway, J.D.; Langendorfer, S.J.; Roberton, M.A.; Rudisill, M.E.; Garcia, C. A developmental perspective on the role of motor skill competence in physical activity: An emergent relationship. *Quest* **2008**, *60*, 290–306. [CrossRef]
18. Harter, S. The perceived competence scale for children. *Child Dev.* **1982**, *53*, 87–97. [CrossRef]
19. Hands, B. Changes in motor skill and fitness measures among children with high and low motor competence: A five-year longitudinal study. *J. Sci. Med. Sport* **2008**, *11*, 155–162. [CrossRef] [PubMed]
20. Jones, R.A.; Okely, A.D.; Caputi, P.; Cliff, D.P. Perceived and actual competence among overweight and non-overweight children. *J. Sci. Med. Sport* **2010**, *13*, 589–596. [CrossRef] [PubMed]
21. Southall, J.E.; Okely, A.D.; Steele, J.R. Actual and perceived physical competence in overweight and non-overweight children. *Pediatr. Exerc. Sci.* **2004**, *16*, 15–24.
22. Coventry City Council. Key Statistics. 2004. Available online: http://www.coventry.gov.uk/info/200088/information_and_statistics/749/key_statistics (accessed on 23 September 2013).
23. New South Wales Department of Health. *Move It, Groove It—Physical Activity in Primary Schools Summary Report*; Northern NSW Health Promotion: Lismore, NSW, Australia, 2003.
24. Bubanj, S.; Stankovic, R.; Bubanj, R.; Bojiv, I.; Dindic, B.; Dimic, A. Reliability of myotest test by a countermovement jump. *Acta Kinesiol.* **2010**, *2*, 46–48.
25. Cole, T.J.; Freeman, J.V.; Preece, M.A. Body mass index reference curves for the UK. *Arch. Dis. Child.* **1990**, *73*, 25–29. [CrossRef]
26. Trost, S.G.; Pate, R.R.; Freedson, P.S.; Sallis, J.F.; Taylor, W.C. Using objective physical activity measures with youth: How many days of monitoring are needed? *Med. Sci. Sports Exerc.* **2000**, *32*, 426–431. [CrossRef] [PubMed]
27. Rowe, D.A.; Mahar, M.T.; Raedeke, T.D.; Lore, J. Measuring physical activity in children with pedometers: Reliability, reactivity, and replacement of missing data. *Pediatr. Exerc. Sci.* **2004**, *16*, 1–12.
28. Horn, T.; Hasbrook, C. Psychological Characteristics and the Criteria Children use for Self-Evaluation. *J. Sport Psychol.* **1987**, *9*, 208–221.

29. Duncan, T.E.; Duncan, S.C. A latent growth curve approach to investigating developmental dynamics and correlates of change in children's perceptions of physical competence. *Res. Q. Exerc. Sport* **1991**, *62*, 390–398. [CrossRef] [PubMed]
30. Kimiecik, J.; Horn, T.; Shurin, C. Relationship among children's beliefs, perceptions of their parent's beliefs, and their moderate to vigorous physical activity. *Res. Q. Exerc. Sport* **1996**, *67*, 324–336. [CrossRef] [PubMed]
31. Kline, R.B. *Principles and Practice of Structural Equation Modelling*; The Guilford Press: New York, NY, USA, 2005.
32. Cliff, D.P.; Wilson, A.; Okely, A.D.; Mickle, K.J.; Steele, J.R. Feasibility of SHARK: A physical activity skill-development program for overweight and obese children. *J. Sci. Med. Sport* **2007**, *10*, 263–267. [CrossRef] [PubMed]
33. Graf, C.; Koch, B.; Falkowski, G.; Jouck, S.; Christ, H.; Staudenmaier, K.; Tokarski, W.; Gerber, A.; Predel, H.; Dordel, S. School-based prevention: Effects on obesity and physical performance after 4 years. *J. Sports Sci.* **2008**, *26*, 987–994. [CrossRef] [PubMed]
34. Jones, R.A.; Riethmuller, A. Promoting fundamental movement skill development and physical activity in early childhood settings: A cluster randomized controlled trial. *Pediatr. Exerc. Sci.* **2011**, *23*, 600–615. [PubMed]
35. Mitchell, B.; McLennan, S.; Latimer, K.; Graham, D.; Gilmore, J.; Rush, E. Improvement of fundamental movement skills through support and mentorship of class room teachers. *Obes. Res. Clin. Pract.* **2011**, *7*, 230–234. [CrossRef] [PubMed]
36. Hardy, L.L.; King, L.; Espinel, P.; Okely, A.D.; Bauman, A. Methods of the NSW schools physical activity and nutrition survey 2010 (SPANS 2010). *J. Sci. Med. Sport* **2011**, *14*, 390–396. [CrossRef] [PubMed]
37. Schmidt, R.A. A Schema theory of discrete motor skill learning. *Psychol. Rev.* **1975**, *82*, 225–260. [CrossRef]
38. Westendorp, M.; Houwen, S.; Hartman, E.; Visscher, C. Are gross motor skills and sports participation related in children with intellectual disabilities? *Res. Dev. Disabil.* **2011**, *32*, 1147–1153. [CrossRef] [PubMed]
39. Fitts, P.M.; Posner, M.I. *Human Performance*; Brooks/Cole: Belmont, CA, USA, 1967.
40. Blatchford, P.; Baines, E.; Pellegrini, A. The social context of school playground games: Sex and ethnic differences, and changes over time after entry to junior school. *Br. J. Dev. Psychol.* **2003**, *21*, 481–505. [CrossRef]
41. Vandaele, B.; Cools, W.; de Decker, S.; de Martelaer, K. Mastery of fundamental movement skills among 6-year-old flemish pre-school children. *Eur. Phys. Educ. Rev.* **2011**, *17*, 3–17. [CrossRef]
42. Bryant, E.S.; Duncan, M.J.; Birch, S.L. Fundamental movement skills and weight status in british primary school children. *Eur. J. Sports Sci.* **2014**, *14*, 730–736. [CrossRef] [PubMed]
43. Beurden, E.V.; Barnett, L.M.; Zask, A.; Dietrich, U.C.; Brooks, L.O.; Beard, J. Can we skill and activate children through primary school physical education lessons? move it groove it—A collaborative health promotion intervention. *Prev. Med.* **2003**, *36*, 493–501. [CrossRef]
44. Westerterp, K.R.; Plasqui, G. Physical activity and human energy expenditure. *Curr. Opin. Clin. Nutr. Metab. Care* **2004**, *7*, 607–613. [CrossRef] [PubMed]
45. Ekeland, E.; Heian, F.; Hagan, K.B.; Abbott, J.M.; Nordheim, L. Exercise to improve self-esteem in children and young people. *Cochrane Database Syst. Rev.* **2004**, *1*, 1–37.
46. Goodway, J.D.; Rudisill, M.E. Perceived physical competence and actual motor competence of african american preschool children. *Adapt. Phys. Act. Q.* **1997**, *14*, 314–326.
47. Weiss, M.R.; Amorose, A.J. Children's self-perception, in the physical domain: Between- and within-age variability in level, accuracy, and sources of perceived competence. *J. Sport Exerc. Psychol.* **2005**, *27*, 226–244.

9

How Confident Can We Be in Modelling Female Swimming Performance in Adolescence?

Shilo J. Dormehl [1], Samuel J. Robertson [2,†] and Craig A. Williams [1,*,†]

[1] University of Exeter, Children's Health and Exercise Research Centre, College of Life and Environmental Sciences, St Luke's Campus, Heavitree Road, Exeter EX1 2LU, UK; sjd223@exeter.ac.uk
[2] Victoria University, Institute of Sport, Exercise & Active Living, Melbourne 3011, Australia; Sam.Robertson@vu.edu.au
* Correspondence: C.A.Williams@exeter.ac.uk

† These authors contributed equally to this work.

Academic Editor: Eling Douwe de Bruin

Abstract: The purpose of this research was to determine the expected progression of adolescent female swimming performances using a longitudinal approach. The performances of 514 female swimmers (12–19 year olds) who participated in one or more FINA-regulated annual international schools' swimming championships over an eight-year period were analysed. Quadratic functions for each of the seven individual events (50, 100, 200 m freestyle, 100 m backstroke, breaststroke, butterfly, 200 m individual medley) were determined using mixed linear models. The predicted threshold of peak performance ranged from 16.8 ± 0.2 (200 m individual medley) to 20.6 ± 0.1 (100 m butterfly) years of age, preceded by gradual rates of improvement (mean rate of 1.6% per year). However, following cross validation, only three events (100 m backstroke, 200 m individual medley and 200 m freestyle) produced reliable models. Identifying the factors that contribute to the progression of female performance in this transitory period of life remains challenging, not least since the onset of puberty is likely to have occurred prior to reaching 12 years of age, the minimum competition age for this championship.

Keywords: puberty; tracking; talent-development; sub-elite; competition

---

1. Introduction

Based on the increasing pressure for nations to develop talented athletes and win medals at the highest level, many sporting bodies have directed strategies and resources to increasing performance levels in all sports; swimming is no exception [1–3]. Trying to separate the performance gains that are made by athletes due to training as opposed to natural growth and development has been one of the most important challenges to overcome. Malina [4] highlighted the need for longitudinal studies to better understand how and when athletes' performances progressed. There have been a number of approaches to predictive modelling in a variety of different sports, including physiological, mathematical or probability strategies [5]. However, these authors suggest that until all factors such as biomechanical, physiological and psychological parameters that influence human performance are fully understood and accounted for, modelling will continue to lack sufficient accuracy to meaningfully predict future performance. Nevertheless, numerous studies have considered how changes in physical, physiological and biomechanical parameters affect performance during adolescence [6,7].

To date, research exploring the development of youth swimmers during adolescence has focussed mainly on male subjects [8–11] with comparatively fewer targeting solely young females [7,12]. In one of the few studies on young female swimmers, Lätt, Jürimäe, Haljaste, Cicchella, Purge and Jürimäe [7]

found that development of biomechanical factors such as velocity, stroke length, stroke rate and in particular stroke index, rather than bioenergetics, contributed more to improved performance times in the 400 m freestyle event.

The performance gap between adult males and females in swimming has reportedly been stable at 8.9% since 1979 [13]. Despite the negligible differences in swimming performance between the sexes before puberty, from age 12 years onwards the performance gap appears to increase [14]. Indeed, it is the greater stroke-specific power of males compared with females that is purported to be a key contributing factor to this difference [15,16]. However, it has been proposed that since females mature physically earlier than males, they are better equipped to compete equitably with older females after reaching the age of 15 years [14]. From a physical standpoint, males can only start competing with an equal chance of success against mature males from the age of 17 years [14].

Baxter-Jones [17] questioned the age at which athletes should formally start competing and this debate remains as relevant today. In contradiction to competition entry requirements, the Amateur Swimming Association's (ASA) "The Swimmer Pathway" [18] advocated that only 15 year old female swimmers should consider racing at the "training to compete" stage of the Long Term Athlete Development model [19]. However, Grange and Gordon [20] indicated that the youngest competition age was 9 years and the distances over which these younger swimmers competed continued to change, with no distinction being made between sexes [21]. Furthermore, the latest version of the ASA handbook does not make any reference to race distances for these younger swimmers [22]. Despite this, Light, Harvey and Memmert [3] found that, given the appropriate setting, club swimmers drawn from France, Germany and Australia (mean age of 10.39 ± 1.07 years), were in fact demonstrating early specialisation and were not averse to competing at an early age. The findings of Barynina and Vaitsekhovskii [23] suggested that young swimmers would benefit from later specialisation within the sport (after the age of 12 years) and less training before reaching the age of 11 years. These findings add support to the sampling approach to sport advocated by the Development Model of Sports Participation [24]. However, Erlandson, Sherar, Mirwald, Maffulli and Baxter-Jones [12] found the development process of young female elite athletes did not appear to be adversely affected by intensive participation in sports, including swimming. The multitude of conflicting ideas regarding the minimum age for specialisation and/or competition suggested by various research groups, sporting bodies and development models confirms that, as yet, there is no definitive conclusion to this debate.

Longitudinal studies have the potential to help coaches gain perspective on the success of young athletes and enables them to give sound career advice [8]. A longitudinal study by Sokolovas [25] was one of the first to draw attention to the value of tracking elite swimmers retrospectively through their careers. With recent improvements in statistical methods, Allen *et al.* [26] and Dormehl *et al.* [27] have extended this concept by creating mixed linear models of elite-level, and sub-elite adolescent male swimmers respectively.

Since there are many challenges associated with constructing accurate models of human performance, besides the performance of young female sub-elite swimmers, it is unsurprising that no quantifiable baseline model currently exists. While it is tempting to create an all-encompassing model of swimming as a single sport, it is of more value to coaches and swimmers to acknowledge the individual specialisms within this multi-disciplinary sport. The aim of the present study was therefore to create the first models of the performance progression of sub-elite adolescent female swimmers for common strokes and distances. Identifying the threshold ages of peak performance in adolescent female swimmers could provide coaches and sporting associations with some potentially useful benchmarking tools to identify talent, and possibly provide evidence to determine realistic qualifying times as well as a justifiable minimum competition age for females.

2. Methods

Performance times for all female entrants (n = 514, aged between 12–19 years) who competed in one of seven individual events (Table 1) were extracted from the official results of an annual schools' swimming championships from 2006 to 2013. The 13 competing schools were American, British and International schools, predominantly located in Western Europe. Team sizes were limited and the competition rules limited swimmers to a maximum of three individual events per championship. The data were in the public domain and downloaded from the relevant tournament websites. All swimmers were assigned individual identity codes to ensure anonymity. The study was approved by the institutional ethics committee and conformed to the recommendations of the Declaration of Helsinki. The single best performances in each of the seven events entered (in either the heats or the finals) over the 8-year analysis period are described in Table 1. The swimmers' ages at the time of each competition were also obtained.

Table 1. Cumulative number of performances over the 8-year analysis period (between 2006 and 2013) for female swimmers between the ages of 12 and 19 years in each event.

Number of Performances (Years)	50 m Freestyle	100 m Freestyle	200 m Freestyle	100 m Backstroke	100 m Breaststroke	100 m Butterfly	200 m Individual Medley
1*	414	310	233	223	217	135	163
2	167	109	92	83	84	48	64
3	69	42	28	34	33	22	23
4	22	17	10	14	12	8	8
5	7	3	5	5	3	6	2
6	2	0	2	0	1	2	0

Note: The drop in the number of repeat performances was likely to have been caused by a change in event choice, team selection, the transitory nature of scholars at international schools, injury or dropout. * This row of data denotes the total number of swimmers competing in each event, since this table sums the consecutive number of years swum. *i.e.*, the total number of entrants in the 50 m freestyle event was 414, 167 of whom competed for two or more years with 2 of whom went on to swim in this event for 6 consecutive years (the maximum number of years over which any swimmer could compete between age 12 and 19 years).

2.1. Statistical Analysis

The raw datasets for all performances in each of the seven events were tested for normality using the Shapiro–Francia test [28] in STATA ver. 13 (StataCorp. 2013. *Stata Statistical Software: Release 13.* College Station, TX, USA: StataCorp LP). The trajectories of the curves showing the progression in performance during maturation were analysed using mixed or multi-level modelling (MLM) in STATA. Time was zero centred at 12 years of age, using an unstructured covariance approach. The fit of the models in fixed and random effects were compared with maximum likelihoods, using a hierarchical method. The final models were quadratic functions for fixed effects (y = ax^2 + bx + c). The fixed effects of time represented polynomial changes of the population with age and the random effects reflected individual deviations from the sample mean trajectory. Inter-class correlation coefficients were calculated and R^2 values determined in order to measure the difference between and within person variability and effect size respectively.

2.2. Evaluation of Models

The datasets for certain events had non-normal distributions. As a result, to validate the proposed models, cross-validations were performed whereby the datasets were randomly split into 1/3 and 2/3 sub-groups. Cross-validation of models is highly recommended under such circumstances in order to determine the generalisability of the findings [29].

The percentage rate of improvement was determined through differentiation of the quadratic functions for each event separately, as $y = \left(\frac{2a}{c} \times 100\right) x + \left(\frac{b}{c} \times 100\right)$, where y = percent change in performance time and $x + 12$ = age, in years. The threshold age of peak performance was calculated as the axis of symmetry of the quadratic function *i.e.*, $\frac{-b}{2a}$.

3. Results

Many of the probability values for the coefficients of the functions were greater than 0.05 (Table 2), resulting in reduced confidence in those models. This included the full model of the fixed quadratic for the 100 m butterfly and at least one of the cross-validation models for the 50 and 100 m freestyle in addition to the 100 m backstroke and breaststroke. Cross validation confirmed that the full models for the 200 m freestyle and the 100 m backstroke events fit the data well in comparison to those for the other events. In the remaining five events however, at least one coefficient of the cross-validation models fell just outside of the standard error (SE) of the full model, but all fell within the 95% confidence interval (C.I.) of the full model. Of all the models, the 100 m freestyle event had the poorest fit.

The models indicate that female swimmers are likely to reach their threshold of peak performance earliest in the 200 m individual medley (16.8 years) and latest in the 100 m butterfly, the latter of which was predicted to occur beyond the age range of the dataset (Figure 1 and Table 3). The slowest rate of improvement between the ages of 12 and 16.8 years was observed in 100 m butterfly swimmers, whereas the greatest rate of improvement (over the same age range) was predicted to occur in the 200 m freestyle event. For the modelled improvement rates from 12 years through to the threshold age, 200 m freestyle swimmers remain the fastest improving, while breaststroke swimmers replace butterfly swimmers as the slowest to improve (Table 3).

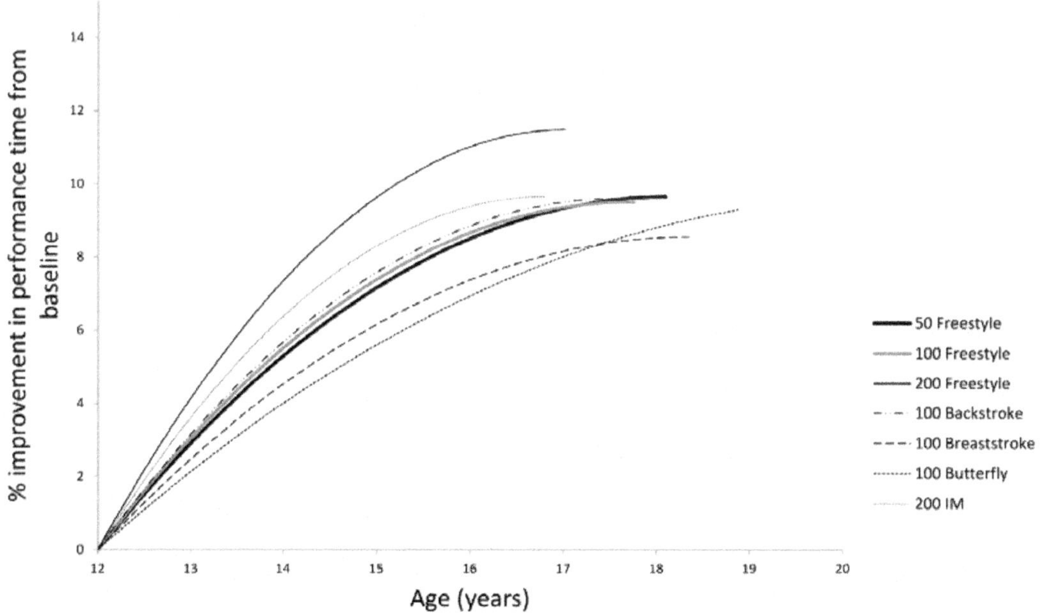

Figure 1. Quadratic functions of the progression in performance for each of the seven events modelled for females from the baseline age of 12 years to the threshold age of peak performance.

Table 2. Summary of models for all events with cross validation for each of the fixed effects of the quadratic functions.

Predictor	50 m Freestyle		100 m Freestyle		200 m Freestyle		100 m Backstroke		100 m Breaststroke		100 m Fly		200 m Individual Medley	
	Mean	*p*	Mean	*p*	Mean	*p*	Mean	*p*	Mean	*p*	Mean	*p*	Mean	*p*
Fixed Quadratic (a)	0.095	<0.001	0.24	<0.001	0.83	<0.001	0.29	<0.001	0.217	0.012	0.12	0.333	0.83	<0.001
(SE)	(0.02)		(0.06)		(0.13)		(0.07)		(0.09)		(0.12)		(0.19)	
95% C.I.	0.05		0.11		0.25		0.13		0.17		0.24		0.37	
Cross val. 2/3 diff.	−0.03	<0.001	0.10	0.072	0.071	<0.001	−0.05	<0.001	−0.001	0.054	0.048	0.637	0.035	0.001
Cross val. 1/3 diff.	0.03	0.089	−0.11	<0.001	0.045	0.001	0.01	<0.077	−0.03	0.128	−0.09	0.299	−0.26	0.001
Fixed Linear (b)	−1.16	<0.001	−2.73	<0.001	−8.31	<0.001	−3.22	<0.001	−2.77	<0.001	−2.05	0.031	−7.96	<0.001
(SE)	(0.17)		(0.45)		(0.97)		(0.52)		(0.63)		(0.95)		(1.40)	
95% C.I.	0.34		0.87		1.90		1.02		1.24		1.86		2.73	
Cross val. 2/3 diff.	0.22	<0.001	−0.73	<0.001	−0.53	<0.001	0.19	<0.001	0.22	<0.001	−0.54	0.196	−0.202	<0.001
Cross val. 1/3 diff.	−0.15	<0.001	0.72	<0.001	−0.30	<0.001	−0.51	0.001	−0.67	0.027	1.13	0.045	1.26	0.002
Fixed Intercept in seconds (c)	36.69	<0.001	81.66	<0.001	181.21	<0.001	93.06	<0.001	103.25	<0.001	90.59	<0.001	197.62	<0.001
(SE)	(0.32)		(0.92)		(2.1)		(1.10)		(1.19)		(1.79)		(2.86)	
95% C.I.	0.62		1.81		4.11		2.15		2.33		3.51		5.60	
Cross val. 2/3 diff.	−0.27	<0.001	1.29	<0.001	1.03	<0.001	0.59	<0.001	−0.42	<0.001	1.37	<0.001	1.36	<0.001
Cross val. 1/3 diff	−0.12	<0.001	−1.27	<0.001	−0.03	<0.001	−0.68	<0.001	1.30	<0.001	−2.89	<0.001	−2.44	<0.001
ICC	0.90		0.96		0.97		0.97		0.95		0.90		0.97	
χ^2 df	133.12 [df = 5]		70.41 [df = 7]		93.31 [df = 7]		60.32 [df = 7]		46.47 [df = 7]		26.4 [df = 5]		45.41 [df = 7]	
Total R^2	0.03		0.05		0.08		0.04		0.02		0.04		0.17	
n	414		310		233		223		217		135		163	

Notes: Cross val. diff. is the difference between the cross validation split and the whole sample mean; SE = standard error; C.I. = confidence interval; df = degrees of freedom.

Table 3. Descriptors determined for the full models of the seven events.

Predictor	50 m Freestyle	100 m Freestyle	200 m Freestyle	100 m Backstroke	100 m Breaststroke	100 m Fly	200 m Individual Medley
% Rate of improvement (12 year—threshold age)	9.65	9.50	11.48	9.60	8.56	9.66	9.66
% Rate of improvement (from 12 to 16.8 year)	9.21	9.28	11.46	9.43	8.04	7.81	9.66
Threshold age at peak performance (year)	18.1 (0.02)	17.8 (0.06)	17.0 (0.13)	17.6 (0.07)	18.4 (0.09)	20.6 (0.12)	16.8 (0.19)
Performance time (s) at threshold age	33.15 (0.14)	73.81 (0.14)	160.42 (4.87)	84.04 (0.36)	94.42 (0.32)	81.85 (0.11)	178.50 (6.70)

4. Discussion

The aim of the study was to model the performance of female swimmers in all strokes between the ages of 12 and 19 years. However, only the 200 m freestyle, the 100 m backstroke and, to a lesser extent, the 200 m individual medley events produced functions that can be interpreted with any confidence (Table 2).

Although Kojima, Jamison and Stager [14] did not aim to determine a peak age—they predicted that females could already start competing equally with older females from as young as 15 years of age. In contrast, the quadratic functions of this study indicated thresholds of peak performance occurred later, i.e. from the age of 16.8 years (Table 3). A possible reason for this apparent discrepancy is that our dataset only included females from the age of 12 years (Figure 1), as this was the minimum entry age for the particular competition studied, while in the Kojima study there were swimmers as young as 7 years of age [14]. The unexpectedly late age of predicted peak performance for swimmers competing in the 100 m butterfly (20.6 years), was largely due to the shallow gradients (approx. 1.1% per year) of modelled improvement for this event. According to Malina, *et al.* [30], puberty begins at approximately 8 to 10 years of age for females and the mean age of menarche has been reported as 12.9 years [31]. It is therefore possible that the majority of females in this study may already have experienced meaningful gains in performance due to maturational development prior to competing in these events.

The threshold age of peak performance for the sub-elite female swimmers in this study were on average only 0.7 years younger than their male counterparts at the same championships [27], even though females are expected to mature approximately 2 years earlier [30]. This finding supports the authors' concerns about combining data on all strokes and distances into one single model, as the relatively late predicted age of peak performance in the butterfly will undoubtedly have contributed to the higher mean threshold age calculated for the females in this study. However, the relative rate of improvement for adolescent female swimmers is confounded by numerous additional factors. Since females mature earlier than males, their improvement between the ages 12 and 19 years is likely to be affected less by biological processes and potentially more by external factors, including biomechanical development, psychological and social pressures [32]. While the growth and maturational process to adulthood starts prior to the age of 12 years for females, it has been questioned whether they have sufficient cognitive development to deal with the rigours of high level competition and the concomitant pressures [33], or whether they should be specialising at such a young age [34].

The expected plateau in performance as biological maturation nears its peak, experienced earlier in females than males, is a factor possibly leading to waning interest and commitment to training and potentially higher dropout rates in females [12]. In accordance with the findings of Cornett and Stager [35], who examined the effect of the number of entrants in a 50 yard freestyle event on the level of performance, it is also possible that the lower number of entrants in the older age groups (data not shown) may also have contributed to reduced competitiveness in these groups. Nevertheless, these sub-elite females were predicted to attain their threshold of peak performance 5.1 years earlier than the peak performance age reported for elite-level swimmers in the same events analysed by Allen, Vandenbogaerde and Hopkins [26]. The difference is likely due in part to their study exclusively containing a narrower sample of elite swimmers and, importantly, included performance data that progressed beyond their teenage years.

While the predicted models in this study provide poor fit for many of the events, there is value in examining the comparisons between events. Females reach their threshold of peak performance in longer distance events such as the 200 m individual medley and the 200 m freestyle at a younger age than shorter distance events (Table 3), confirming a phenomenon reported on by Arellano, *et al.* [36] and Allen, Vandenbogaerde and Hopkins [26]. Swimmers competing in the 200 m freestyle event also demonstrated the highest rate of improvement between the ages of 12 and 16.8 years (Figure 1). It is possible that females improve most in the longer distance events due to changes in body composition as a result of puberty. Post-pubertal females are known to have greater buoyancy, which has been suggested to give them an energy efficiency advantage over males [37] and is most noticeable in longer distance events [13,38].

Practical Applications

Rather than being limited to mere mathematical comparisons of combined threshold times of numerous specialisms within swimming, the value of the individual models developed in this study promotes many potential applications for coaches, swimmers and governing bodies. Swimmers can set realistic targets for the following season and coaches can measure the performance of their adolescent female swimmers against the average expected progressions for each of the events modelled. Furthermore, swimmers who consistently exceed the modelled rates of progression might be considered for talent development or alternatively may be identified as early or late maturers. With further refinements of the models, they could one day also assist governing bodies in the setting of justifiable qualifying times for national and international competitions.

5. Conclusions

Despite the poor fit of some of the models generated, the novel analysis of individual events allows for some interesting comparisons to be made. The authors feel that this approach is of more value than a one size fits all model for the sport. The models suggest that females achieve thresholds of peak performance earlier in longer distance events. Use of this particular international schools' swimming competition provided a consistent minimum age over many consecutive years and consequently ensured high validity of the dataset. However, the slow rate of progression seen in the quadratic functions generated in comparison to those found for the male adolescents by Dormehl, Robertson and Williams [27] indicates that the process of maturation had likely already begun for many of the females in this study. Compared with data for male swimmers [27], confidently identifying the contribution of maturation to performance improvement in females through adolescence remains an elusive goal. Future research should therefore consider collecting longitudinal data on very young swimmers in competition, as these could generate more robust models and higher levels of confidence. Finding a suitable sub-elite competition setting for this may however prove difficult until such time as a consensus is reached on a suitable minimum age of competition, and whether this age should be the same for both males and females. Overcoming these issues could lead to the development of useful benchmarking tools for potential talent identification of sub-elite athletes or the setting of realistic development goals.

Author Contributions: S.J.D. and C.A.W designed the study, S.J.D collected the data, S.J.R. & S.J.D. statistically analysed the data, S.J.D. wrote the first draft, C.A.W. supervised the study. All authors critically reviewed, contributed to and approved the final manuscript.

Conflicts of Interest: The authors declare no conflict of interest.

References

1. Barreiros, A.; Côté, J.; Fonseca, A.M. From early to adult sport success: Analysing athletes' progression in national squads. *Eur. J. Sport Sci.* **2014**, *14*, S178–S182. [CrossRef] [PubMed]
2. Bergeron, M.F.; Mountjoy, M.; Armstrong, N.; Chia, M.; Côté, J.; Emery, C.A.; Faigenbaum, A.; Hall, G.; Kriemler, S.; Léglise, M.; *et al.* International Olympic committee consensus statement on youth athletic development. *Br. J. Sports Med.* **2015**, *49*, 843–851. [CrossRef] [PubMed]
3. Light, R.L.; Harvey, S.; Memmert, D. Why children join and stay in sports clubs: Case studies in Australian, French and German swimming clubs. *Sport Educ. Soc.* **2013**, *18*, 550–566. [CrossRef]
4. Malina, R.M. Physical-activity and training: Effects on stature and the adolescent growth spurt. *Med. Sci. Sports Exerc.* **1994**, *26*, 759–766. [CrossRef] [PubMed]
5. Liu, Y.; Paul, S.; Fu, F.H. Accomplishments and compromises in prediction research for world records and best performances in track and field and swimming. *Meas. Phys. Educ. Exerc. Sci.* **2012**, *16*, 167–182. [CrossRef]

6. Baxter-Jones, A.D.G.; Goldstein, H.; Helms, P. The development of aerobic power in young athletes. *J. Appl. Physiol.* **1993**, *75*, 1160–1167. [PubMed]
7. Lätt, E.; Jürimäe, J.; Haljaste, K.; Cicchella, A.; Purge, P.; Jürimäe, T. Physical development and swimming performance during biological maturation in young female swimmers. *Coll. Antropol.* **2009**, *33*, 117–122. [PubMed]
8. Costa, M.J.; Marinho, D.A.; Bragada, J.A.; Silva, A.J.; Barbosa, T.M. Stability of elite freestyle performance from childhood to adulthood. *J. Sports Sci.* **2011**, *29*, 1183–1189. [CrossRef] [PubMed]
9. De Mello Vitor, F.; Böhme, M.T.S. Performance of young male swimmers in the 100-meters front crawl. *Pediatr. Exerc. Sci.* **2010**, *22*, 278–287.
10. Barbosa, T.M.; Costa, M.; Marinho, D.A.; Coelho, J.; Moreira, M.; Silva, A.J. Modeling the links between young swimmers' performance: Energetic and biomechanic profiles. *Pediatr. Exerc. Sci.* **2010**, *22*, 379–391. [PubMed]
11. Baxter-Jones, A.D.G.; Helms, P.; Maffulli, N.; Bainespreece, J.C.; Preece, M. Growth and development of male gymnasts, swimmers, soccer and tennis players: A longitudinal study. *Ann. Hum. Biol.* **1995**, *22*, 381–394. [CrossRef] [PubMed]
12. Erlandson, M.C.; Sherar, L.B.; Mirwald, R.L.; Maffulli, N.; Baxter-Jones, A.D.G. Growth and maturation of adolescent female gymnasts, swimmers, and tennis players. *Med. Sci. Sports Exerc.* **2008**, *40*, 34–42. [CrossRef] [PubMed]
13. Thibault, V.; Guillaume, M.; Berthelot, G.; El Helou, N.; Schaal, K.; Quinquis, L.; Nassif, H.; Tafflet, M.; Escolano, S.; Hermine, O.; *et al.* Women and men in sport performance: The gender gap has not evolved since 1983. *J. Sports Sci. Med.* **2010**, *9*, 214–223. [PubMed]
14. Kojima, K.; Jamison, P.L.; Stager, J.M. Multi-age-grouping paradigm for young swimmers. *J. Sports Sci.* **2012**, *30*, 313–320. [CrossRef] [PubMed]
15. Toussaint, H.M.; Hollander, A.P.; Berg, C.; Vorontsov, A. Biomechanics of swimming. In *Exercise and Sport Science*; Garrett, W.E., Kirkendall, D.T., Eds.; Lippincott, Williams & Wilkins: Philadelphia, PA, USA, 2000; pp. 639–660.
16. Wells, G.D.; Schneiderman-Walker, J.; Plyley, M. Normal physiological characteristics of elite swimmers. *Pediatr. Exerc. Sci.* **2006**, *18*, 30–52.
17. Baxter-Jones, A.D.G. Growth and development of young athletes: Should competition levels be age related? *Sports Med.* **1995**, *20*, 59–64. [CrossRef] [PubMed]
18. Amateur Swimming Association. *The Swimmer Pathway: Long Term Athlete Development*; ASA: Loughborough, UK, 2003.
19. Balyi, I.; Hamilton, A. *Long-Term Athlete Development: Trainability in Childhood and Adolescence—Windows of Opportunity, Optimal Trainability*; National Coaching Institute British Columbia and Advanced Training and Performance Ltd.: Victoria, BC, Canada, 2004.
20. Grange, J.; Gordon, R. *Success is Long Term: Long Term Athlete Development Related to the Journey through Swimming*; Amateur Swimming Association: Loughborough, UK, 2004; pp. 1–12.
21. Amateur Swimming Association. *Success is Long Term: Long-Term Athlete Development Related to the Journey through Swimming*; Amateur Swimming Association: Loughborough, UK, 2010.
22. Amateur Swimming Association. *The ASA handbook 2014*; Amateur Swimming Association: Loughborough, UK, 2014.
23. Barynina, I.I.; Vaitsekhovskii, S.M. The aftermath of early sports specialization for highly qualified swimmers. *Fitness Sports Rev. Int.* **1992**, *27*, 132–133.
24. Côté, J.; Fraser-Thomas, J. Youth involvement in sport. In *Sport Psychology: A Canadian Perspective*; Crocker, P., Ed.; Pearson: Toronto, AB, USA, 2007; pp. 270–298.
25. Sokolovas, G. Analysis of USA swimming's all-time top 100 times. In Proceedings of the Xth International Symposium on Biomechanics and Medicine in Swimming; Vilas Boas, J.P., Alves, F., Marques, A., Eds.; University of Porto: Porto, Portugal, 2006; pp. 315–317.
26. Allen, S.V.; Vandenbogaerde, T.J.; Hopkins, W.G. Career performance trajectories of Olympic swimmers: Benchmarks for talent development. *Eur. J. Sport Sci.* **2014**, *14*, 643–651. [CrossRef] [PubMed]
27. Dormehl, S.J.; Robertson, S.J.; Williams, C.A. Modelling the progression of male swimmers' performances through adolescence. *Sports* **2016**, *4*, 2. [CrossRef]

28. Mbah, A.K.; Paothong, A. Shapiro-Francia test compared to other normality test using expected p-value. *J. Stat. Comput. Sim.* **2015**, *85*, 3002–3016. [CrossRef]
29. Witten, I.H.; Frank, E. *Data Mining: Practical Machine Learning Tools and Techniques*, 2nd ed.; Morgan Kaufmann Publishers Inc.: San Francisco, CA, USA, 2005.
30. Malina, R.M.; Bouchard, C.; Bar-Or, O. *Growth, Maturation and Physical Activity*, 2nd ed.; Human Kinetics: Champaign, IL, USA, 2004.
31. Whincup, P.H.; Gilg, J.A.; Odoki, K.; Taylor, S.J.C.; Cook, D.G. Age of menarche in contemporary British teenagers: Survey of girls born between 1982 and 1986. *Br. Med. J.* **2001**, *322*, 1095–1096. [CrossRef]
32. Saavedra, J.M.; Escalante, Y.; Rodriguez, F.A. A multivariate analysis of performance in young swimmers. *Pediatr. Exerc. Sci.* **2010**, *22*, 135–151. [PubMed]
33. Wiersma, L.D. Risks and benefits of youth sport specialization: Perspectives and recommendations. *Pediatr. Exerc. Sci.* **2000**, *12*, 13–22.
34. Côté, J.; Lidor, R.; Hackfort, D. ISSP position stand: To sample or to specialize? Seven postulates about youth sport activities that lead to continued participation and elite performance. *Int. J. Sport Exerc. Psychol.* **2009**, *7*, 7–17. [CrossRef]
35. Cornett, A.C.; Stager, J.M. Large n: A strategy for improving regional sport performance. *Int. J. Sports Physiol. Perform.* **2015**, *10*, 626–629. [CrossRef] [PubMed]
36. Arellano, R.; Brown, P.; Cappaert, J.; Nelson, R.C. Analysis of 50-, 100-, and 200-m freestyle swimmers at the 1992 Olympic games. *J. Appl. Biomech.* **1994**, *10*, 189–199.
37. Ratel, S.; Duche, P.; Williams, C.A. Muscle fatigue during high-intensity exercise in children. *Sports Med.* **2006**, *36*, 1031–1065. [CrossRef] [PubMed]
38. Chatterjee, S.; Laudato, M. An analysis of world record times of men and women in running, skating, and swimming. *J. Strength Cond. Res.* **1996**, *10*, 274–278.

10

Martial Arts and Metabolic Diseases

Hidetaka Hamasaki [1,2]

1 Department of Internal Medicine, National Center for Global Health and Medicine Kohnodai Hospital, 1-7-1 Kohnodai, Chiba 272-8516, Japan; hhamasaki78@gmail.com
2 Hamasaki Clinic, 2-21-4 Nishida, Kagoshima 890-0046, Japan

Academic Editor: Eling de Bruin

Abstract: Different forms of martial arts are practiced worldwide, each with various intensities of physical activity. These disciplines are potentially an effective exercise therapy for metabolic diseases. Tai chi is the most well-studied style of martial arts and has shown evidence of its effect on metabolic diseases; however, little evidence is available regarding the association between other styles of martial arts and metabolic health. To summarize and evaluate the effects of martial arts on metabolic diseases, eligible articles were searched by using Pubmed. To date, systematic reviews provide no definite conclusion on the effectiveness of tai chi for treating metabolic diseases because of a small numbers of subjects, short durations of clinical trials, and some biases involved in testing. However, there are several clinical studies on subjects with metabolic diseases, which show that tai chi improves obesity, glycemic control, blood pressure control, and lipid profiles. Currently, some limited evidence suggests that other martial arts, such as kung fu and karate, may be beneficial for body composition, glycemic control, and arterial stiffness. To clarify the effectiveness of martial arts for treating metabolic diseases, well-designed prospective studies, preferably with a larger number of subjects and of longer duration, are warranted.

Keywords: martial arts; tai chi; metabolic disease; diabetes

1. Introduction

Many studies evaluating the benefits of physical activity on health generally recommend 30–60 min/day of moderate to vigorous intensity of physical activity for at least five days/week [1]. Such physical activity intensity is classified using metabolic equivalents (METs), *i.e.*, 3.0–5.9 METs, including various sports activities (Table 1) [1,2]. Conversely, physical inactivity is one of the leading causes of mortality, and in fact, 31% of people cannot achieve the recommended level of physical activity [3].

Table 1. Excerpt of various sports activities with moderate intensity.

Sports	METs
Gymnastics, general	3.8
Golf, general	4.8
Tennis, doubles	4.5
Volleyball, non-competitive, general	3.0
Softball, practice	4.0
Bowling	3.8
Basketball, shooting practice	4.5
Martial arts, practice, slow pace	5.3

Each activity is quoted from Ainsworth *et al.* 2011 Compendium Physical Activities [2]. METs = metabolic equivalents.

Judo, karate, aikido, kung fu, and tai chi are examples of some of the various styles of martial arts. In addition, the intensity of physical activity involved in martial arts varies according to its style. Performing tai chi is equal to 1.5–3.0 METs (light to moderate intensity), practicing various martial arts at a slow pace is equal to 5.3 METs (moderate intensity), and practicing combat martial arts, such as judo, karate, and kick boxing, at a moderate pace is equal to 10.3 METs (vigorous intensity) [2]. In terms of physical activity for health, martial arts have proven to provide beneficial effects on the human body. It has been reported that tai chi has beneficial effects on blood pressure, muscle strength, and the subject's ability to maintain balance [4]. Recent studies have shown that tai chi also improves glycemic control [5], health-related quality of life (HR-QOL) [6], and peripheral nerve conduction velocity [7] as well as reducing oxidative stress [8] and improving immunity in patients with type 2 diabetes [9]. Tai chi is the most well-studied style of martial arts, and there is sufficient evidence for its effect on metabolic diseases; however, little evidence is available regarding the association between other styles of martial arts and metabolic health.

This review is aimed at summarizing and evaluating the effects of tai chi and other martial arts on metabolic diseases, providing clinicians and patients with new insights into the strategy of using martial arts as an exercise therapy for metabolic diseases.

2. Methods

I searched literature written in English on martial arts and metabolic diseases by using Pubmed from its inception to March 2016. I used the following combined Medical Subject Headings (MeSH) terms. Search terms were "martial arts", "tai ji [MeSH] or tai chi", "metabolic disease", "diabetes mellitus", "hypertension", and "dyslipidemias". I aimed primarily at reviewing controlled trials, but also included reviews and other types of clinical studies such as before-after studies, case-control studies, and cross-sectional studies. I found 61 published articles, and the titles and abstracts of identified articles were reviewed to determine their relevance. Twenty-seven articles were eligible. Clinical studies which did not have study participants with metabolic diseases or outcomes related to metabolic diseases were excluded.

3. Tai Chi

Tai chi is an ancient Chinese martial art, which is characterized by slow, smooth, and fluid movements. The level of physical activity intensity of tai chi depends on its style, form, and duration. The most popular is the classical Yang style, which is a moderate intensity exercise [10]. The efficacy and safety of tai chi have been investigated in several clinical studies, as well as in the publication of several systematic reviews. Hartley *et al.* evaluated the effectiveness of tai chi in the prevention of cardiovascular disease (CVD) by researching previous randomized controlled trials (RCTs) of tai chi in healthy subjects and individuals at a high risk for CVD, without language restrictions. Although some trials showed that tai chi lowered blood pressure and ameliorated lipid profiles, none showed consistent beneficial effects of tai chi on CVD risk factors. The authors pointed out some of the potential problems with the study, including small numbers of subjects, short durations of the trials, and some risk of bias [11]. On the other hand, another systematic review to investigate the effectiveness of tai chi for the primary prevention of stroke in middle-aged and elderly individuals revealed that tai chi intervention significantly reduced the incidence of nonfatal stroke (relative risk = 0.11, 95% CI; 0.01–0.85) and cardio-cerebrovascular disease (relative risk = 0.33, 95% CI; 0.11–0.96). This study also demonstrated that tai chi exercise was associated with the improvement of metabolic diseases such as obesity, hypertension, dyslipidemia, and diabetes [12]. Lee *et al.* [13] independently evaluated the systematic reviews of tai chi because the previous RCTs had different characteristics of the study population, and their conclusions were contradictory. Although the evidence for fall prevention, improving psychological health, and health benefits for the elderly was relatively clear, the evidence for improving metabolic diseases was not definitive [13]. Recently, Yang *et al.* [14] evaluated a total of 507 clinical studies, including systematic reviews, RCTs, observational studies, case series, and case reports, to summarize the evidence of the effect of tai chi on health. Among the 507 studies, 317 were conducted in China (62.5%) with various tai chi styles for interventions (Yang style, 72.84%; Chen style, 3.88%; Sun style, 4.53%; Wu style, 1.9%; and others, 23.71%), and the duration of the tai chi interventions varied from five days to three years. These wide variations in style, intensity, duration, and practicing methods of the interventions may demonstrate the limitations of the previous studies. They concluded that further well-designed studies would be required to confirm the effects of tai chi for diseases.

A few systematic reviews evaluated the effectiveness of tai chi for type 2 diabetes. Lee *et al.* investigated whether tai chi reduced fasting blood glucose levels and glycosylated hemoglobin A1c (HbA1c) in RCTs and controlled clinical trials. The meta-analysis failed to show beneficial effects of tai chi on glycemic control; therefore, it may be concluded that tai chi is not an effective therapy for type 2 diabetes [15,16]. In systematic reviews, evidence that tai chi is effective for improving metabolic diseases, such as hypertension, dyslipidemia, and type 2 diabetes, is controversial. However, the heterogeneity of the study population, variety of the intensity, and duration of the tai chi interventions could affect the results [14].

Further, this review focuses on clinical studies investigating the effects of tai chi on metabolic diseases (Table 2).

Table 2. Clinical trials investigating the effects of tai chi on health in patients with metabolic diseases.

Authors, Year	Study Design	Subjects	Tai Chi Exercise (Style, Frequency, and Duration)	Results
Tsang *et al.*, 2007 [16]	RCT	38 patients with type 2 diabetes, ⩾50 years of age	12 movements from Yang and Sun styles 1 h, 2 sessions/week, 16 weeks	No improvements in balance, physical performance, muscle performance and HR-QOL
Zhang and Fu, 2008 [18]	RCT	20 women with type 2 diabetes	24-style 1 h, 5 days/week, 14 weeks	Fasting plasma glucose↓, glycated serum proteins↓, triglycerides↓, and fasting plasma insulin↑. No significant group effects
Sun and Buys., 2015 [19]	RCT	266 subjects with hypertension	No descriptions of style 3 h/week in group and 2h/week at home, 12 months	Blood pressure↓, BMI↓, eGFR→, HR-QOL↑
Liu *et al.*, 2013 [6]	RCT	41 subjects with elevated blood glucose or diabetes	KaiMai tai chi/qiong style 1.5 h, 3 times/week,12 weeks	Physical QOL↑
Chen *et al.*, 2010 [8]	RCT	104 obese patients with type 2 diabetes	Chen style, 99-form 1 h, 3 times/week, 12 weeks	BMI↓, triglycerides↓, HDL-cholesterol↑ C-reactive proteins↓, malondialdehyde↓
Hung *et al.*, 2009 [7]	Before-after study	28 patients with type 2 diabetes and 32 healthy adult controls	Cheng style 40 min, 3 sessions/week, 12 weeks	Improvement of nerve conduction velocities in patients with type 2 diabetes
Yeh *et al.*, 2007, 2009 [9,24]	Before-after study	32 patients with type 2 diabetes 30 pairs of type 2 diabetic patients and controls	Cheng style, 37-form 40 min, 3 days/week, 12 weeks	Improvement of immunity

RCT = randomized controlled trial; HR-QOL = health related quality of life; BMI = body mass index; eGFR = estimated glomerular filtration rate; HDL = high density lipoprotein.

Tsang *et al.* [16] conducted a single-blind, randomized controlled trial among 38 sedentary older patients with type 2 diabetes. Study participants completed supervised one-hour tai chi practices twice a week, for 16 weeks. The tai chi exercise consisted of 12 movements from the Yang and Sun styles. Static and dynamic balance abilities, maximal gait speeds, and habitual physical activity levels significantly increased in the tai chi group; however, there were no group effects found in the control group. Unfortunately, this study did not evaluate metabolic risk factors, such as blood glucose levels, lipid profiles, and blood pressure. The tai chi intervention for diabetes was not sufficient for the improvement of balance, physical performance, muscle performance, or HR-QOL in older patients with type 2 diabetes [17]. Zhang and Fu investigated the effects of the 24-style of tai chi on metabolic control in female patients with type 2 diabetes. Twenty subjects were randomly assigned to tai chi training and control groups. Subjects in the training group performed supervised tai chi exercises for 1 h/day, five days/week, for 14 weeks. After 14 weeks of tai chi exercises, fasting plasma glucose, glycated serum proteins, and triglycerides were reduced, whereas fasting plasma insulin levels increased. However, group effects between the tai chi training and control groups were not significant [18]. A recent study examined the long-term effects of tai chi on weight, blood pressure, lipid profiles, renal function, and quality of life. A total of 266 subjects with hypertension were randomly assigned to tai chi intervention and control groups. Subjects in the intervention group attended a tai chi exercise program for 12 months. Systolic blood pressure, diastolic blood pressure, and body mass index (BMI) significantly decreased after the tai chi intervention. Renal function, represented by estimated glomerular filtration rate (eGFR), was maintained, and HR-QOL improved; however, dyslipidemia and hyperglycemia did not improve. Additionally, there were significant between-group differences in terms of blood pressure, eGFR, and BMI. It appears that long-term tai chi exercise may be effective in the management of risk factors associated with hypertension. This is the first RCT to show the long-term effects of tai chi on metabolic diseases; however, details of the intervention, such as style, intensity, and duration of tai chi, were not described in the paper [19]. Liu *et al.* assessed the effects of tai chi on HR-QOL in individuals with impaired glucose tolerance and diabetes, using the Medical Outcomes Study 36-Item Short-Form Health Survey (SF-36), although metabolic parameters were not measured. Forty-one participants were randomly allocated to tai chi intervention and usual medical care control groups. Tai chi intervention was a supervised group program with 1.5 h of practice, three times/week, for 12 weeks. The exercise was KaiMai tai chi/qiong style. They noted that because of differences in individual health and fitness levels, the intensity of the exercise varied among the participants. There were significant between-group differences for the tai chi intervention group in physical functioning, role-physical, bodily pain, and vitality [6]. They previously reported that the tai chi exercise improved BMI, waist circumference, blood pressure, HbA1c, insulin resistance, stress, depressive symptoms, and the SF-36 score. However, this was a small, non-controlled study, and a single group before-after study [20]. Thus, it appears that tai chi improves physical QOL, but its beneficial effects on metabolic diseases are uncertain. Chen *et al.* conducted a RCT in a single center among 104 obese patients with type 2 diabetes. Fifty-six patients were allocated to the tai chi intervention group, and 48 patients were allocated to the conventional exercise group. The tai chi exercise session consisted of 30 min of Chen-style tai chi chuan 99-form, lasting up to 1 h, three times/week, for 12 weeks. Although no significant improvement in BMI, lipid profiles, or oxidative stress profiles was observed in the conventional exercise group, serum triglycerides, C-reactive protein, and malondialdehyde decreased, and high-density lipoprotein cholesterol increased in the tai chi intervention group. HbA1c values did not significantly decrease. The intensity of the exercise was monitored by the heart and respiration rates of the subjects during exercise, and both groups performed at a similar intensity (moderate intensity); however, there were between-group differences in changes of metabolic parameters. The authors stated that the key benefits of tai chi exercise do not depend on energy expenditure but on the efficacy of cardiopulmonary function, antioxidative action, and improved metabolism [8]. Although RCTs are the gold standard study design to reveal the efficacy of tai chi for metabolic diseases, there was considerable heterogeneity between the studies. Specifically, we should assess the methodological quality of each article to discuss the evidence of whether tai chi is really effective for improving metabolic diseases. Table 3 shows the methodological differences among the above-mentioned clinical studies.

Table 3. Comparison of methodologies in RCTs investigating the effects of tai chi on health in patients with metabolic diseases.

Authors, Year	Inclusion Criteria	Exclusion Criteria	Subjects	Controls	Statistical Method
Tsang *et al.*, 2007 [16]	Type 2 diabetes ⩾50 years of age ⩽2 exercise sessions/week	Cognitive impairment (MMSE ⩽ 24) Changes in medication Hip or knee arthritis Current tai chi participation Residence in a nursing home Amputation of a limb Severe visual impairment	Age: 65 ± 8 years Sex: 8 men, 30 women Ethnicity: 89.5% of subjects were Caucasian BMI: 32.2 ± 6.3 kg/m^2 Dropout: One subject	Sham exercise (calisthenics and gentle stretching)	Described in detail
Zhang and Fu, 2008 [18]	Type 2 diabetes	Insulin therapy Exercise ⩾2 times/week Resistance training participation Changes in medication Serum creatinine levels ⩾200 M Proteinuria >1 g/day Blood pressure >160/95 mmHg	Age: 57.4 ± 6.2 years Sex: 20 women Ethnicity: Asian BMI: Not described Dropout: None	Free activity program	Not described in detail (e.g., How to randomize and calculate sample size)
Sun and Buys., 2015 [19]	Hypertension ⩾45 years of age Residence in Changshu city	Not described in detail	Age: 66.5% of subjects aged 45–64 years, 33.5% of subjects aged over 65 years Sex: 48 men, 218 women Ethnicity: Asian BMI: 23.4 ± 3.1 kg/m^2 Dropout: 30 subjects, 34 subjects were also excluded from analysis	Non-exercise-related activities such as reading and computing	Described in detail
Liu *et al.*, 2013 [6]	Type 2 diabetes or IFG and IGT No medication	Type 1 diabetes Diabetic medication BMI >45 kg/m^2 Aged <30 years, >71 years Serious injury No time Residence not in Brisbane Blood glucose level unknown	Age: 59 ± 8 years Sex: 16 men, 25 women Ethnicity: Not described BMI: Not described Dropout: One subject	Usual medical care	Described in detail
Chen *et al.*, 2010 [8]	Type 2 diabetes (HbA1c > 7%) ⩾40 years of age BMI ⩾ 30–35	Serious operation Myocardial infarction Stroke Severe liver or kidney disease Gait disturbance Regular exercise ⩾ 3 times/week	Age: 59.1 ± 6.2 years (tai chi group), 57.4 ± 5.8 years (control group) Sex: 45 men, 59 women Ethnicity: Asian BMI: 33.5 ± 4.7 kg/m^2 (tai chi group), 33.2 ± 4.1 kg/m^2 (control group) Dropout: 13 subjects	Conventional exercise (aerobic dance)	Described in detail

RCT = randomized controlled trial; MMSE = mini mental state examination; BMI = body mass index; IFG = impaired fasting glucose; IGT = impaired glucose tolerance.

There are interesting but non-randomized and non-controlled clinical studies that investigated the effects of tai chi on nerve function and immunity in patients with type 2 diabetes. Hung *et al.* evaluated changes in peripheral nerve modulation in 28 patients with type 2 diabetes and 32 healthy adult controls. All participants performed Cheng-style tai chi exercise for 40 min/session, three sessions/week, for 12 weeks. The relative intensity of the exercise was light to moderate, according to heart rate– and Borg rate–perceived exertion. After the 12-week tai chi exercise course, fasting blood glucose levels decreased in diabetic patients, as compared with healthy controls. No significant change in nerve conduction velocity, distal latency, or proximal and distal amplitude was found in the control group. However, the nerve conduction velocity of the tibial and median nerves, as well as the distal sensory latency of the ulnar nerves, in patients with type 2 diabetes improved after the 12-week tai chi exercise program [7]. This study suggests that tai chi may improve diabetic neuropathy as a result of microangiopathy. Nitric oxide may play an important role in the pathogeneisis of diabetic neuropathy [21] as shown in previous studies, where regular tai chi exercise was associated with the dilation of microvasculature mediated by nitric oxide [22,23]. Yeh *et al.* investigated the association between tai chi exercise and immunity in patients with type 2 diabetes. A before-after study among 32 patients with type 2 diabetes showed that the percentages of CD4 and CD8 lymphocyte subpopulations decreased, both proportional and absolute counts of CD4CD25 regulatory T-lymphocytes increased, and the proportional count of CD8CD28 cytotoxic lymphocytes decreased, along with the decrement of HbA1c levels, after a 12-week tai chi exercise regimen. Subjects performed Cheng-style tai chi 37-form, supervised by an expert, for 40 min/practice, three days/week, for 12 weeks. The study demonstrated that tai chi exercise could improve glucose metabolism, leading to a beneficial effect on immune regulatory functions in type 2 diabetic patients [24]. They also investigated the effect of a 12-week tai chi exercise regimen on helper T cell reactions in patients with type 2 diabetes. Thirty pairs of type 2 diabetic patients and age-matched controls participated in the study. After 12 weeks of tai chi exercise, the interleukin (IL)-12 levels increased and IL-4 levels decreased in the diabetic patients, but not in the controls. One of the Th1 transcription factors, T-bet m-RNA levels, also increased in type 2 diabetic patients. From this we may conclude that tai chi exercise may improve immunity as well as glucose metabolism [9].

4. Other Martial Arts

To the best of my knowledge, there are no systematic reviews or meta-analysis concerning the effects of other types of martial arts, such as judo, karate, tae kwon do, kung fu, or kick boxing, on metabolic diseases. A narrative review assessed the effect of such hard/external martial arts on physical fitness, including balance, flexibility, strength, cardiorespiratory fitness, and mental functions in people >40 years of age, but it failed to show sufficient evidence of the effect of martial arts on health because of the methodological shortcomings of previous clinical studies [25]. However, several clinical studies have shown significant associations between martial arts and metabolic diseases.

Tsang and her colleagues investigated whether kung fu, a Chinese martial art, was effective for improving body composition in overweight/obese adolescents, with a randomized placebo-controlled trial. A total of 20 subjects, aged six to 12 years, overweight/obese and sedentary, were investigated. Subjects were randomly assigned to kung fu or tai chi (control) groups, and they practiced each exercise three times, in 1 h sessions each week, for over six months. The kung fu training was based on the Choy Lee Fut Hung Sing Gwoon style. The resulting total body fat and abdominal fat mass, measured using dual-energy X-ray absorptiometry, physical fitness, muscle strength, and metabolic parameters, including HbA1c and serum lipid profiles, were assessed. Due to natural growth, their height, weight, bone mineral density, and lean mass increased during the study. However, total mass and abdominal fat mass were significantly reduced in both groups without a significant group effect. This study suggests that not only tai chi but also kung fu may be effective for the improvement of obesity in adolescents [26]. Kung fu training also resulted in greater improvements in submaximal cardiovascular fitness, lower muscle endurance, and upper body muscle velocity compared with those observed by tai chi training. The kung fu exercise improved physical fitness in overweight/obese adolescents with low physical fitness [27]. Moreover, although there were no between-group differences, HbA1c tended to decrease over time. Significant associations of increased lean body mass, with reductions in HbA1c, insulin resistance, triglycerides, and total cholesterol, suggest that the increase of lean mass by kung fu training may have favorable effects on metabolic health, independent of changes in fat mass [28]. Benbenek-Klupa *et al.* examined glycemic control in patients with type 1 diabetes who were engaged in combat sports. Three out of the five study participants were mixed martial arts competitors, and two were kick boxers. Each patient received multiple daily insulin injection therapy or continuous subcutaneous insulin infusion therapy, and glycemic control without hypoglycemia and hyperglycemia, pre- and post-combat sports, was expected to be very difficult. A detailed protocol for glycemic management was made in case of the occurrence of hypoglycemia and hyperglycemia related to performing combat sports, during the study period. In comparison with physically inactive control subjects, whose age, sex, and initial HbA1c were matched, the self-monitoring of blood glucose was more frequent. Glycemic control in all patients was improved or maintained, without diabetic ketoacidosis and severe hypoglycemia, during the follow-up. Type 1 diabetic patients who regularly engage in hard-contact martial arts can achieve or maintain satisfactory glycemic control without the increased risk of severe hyperglycemia and hypoglycemia if they have the access to expertise in physical activity and diabetes management. However, this is only a very small retrospective study, and a further prospective study will be needed for confirmation [29]. Benedini *et al.* reported metabolic and hormonal responses to a session of karate. Ten subjects practicing karate, with a mean training period of 10–12 h/week, were recruited. All subjects participated in two experimental exercises (3 min for kata and kumite) in a randomized crossover design. The kata session is a simulation of combat, combinations of punches and kicks, and a sequence of a pattern of fighting. The kumite session is fighting with punches and kicks against an opponent. Plasma glucose levels increased after the karate exercise, and after the kumite session, plasma glucose levels were significantly higher than those after the kata session. Epinephrine and norepinephrine also increased after the karate exercise. There were no significant changes in plasma insulin or cortisol levels; however, testosterone increased after the karate exercise. These results should not be applied to patients with metabolic diseases because the study subjects were healthy, elite karate athletes. The kumite exercise is not a favorable exercise for patients with diabetes, particularly with progressed diabetic complications, because an acute glycemic response to kumite could cause severe hyperglycemia in patients with diabetes [30]. A cross-sectional study investigated the association between martial arts and arterial stiffness. Douris *et al.* recruited 20 middle-aged subjects who were divided into martial arts and sedentary control groups. The martial artists practiced Soo Bahk Do, a traditional Korean martial art similar to karate, for approximately 20 years. The paper described that a typical Soo Bahk Do class lasted 1 h, but the intensity and frequency of the exercises were not described in detail. The martial artists had lower pulse wave velocity than did the sedentary control group. Trunks and hamstrings in the martial artists were also more flexible than in the controls, suggesting that martial arts training, with an emphasis on flexibility, is associated with less arterial stiffness [31]. Douris and his colleagues previously showed that Soo Bahk Do practitioners had higher levels of glutathione than the age-matched sedentary controls. This may demonstrate that martial arts could have a protective effect against oxidative stress [32]. Table 4 shows a summary of the above-mentioned clinical studies.

Table 4. Clinical studies investigating the associations of martial arts with metabolic parameters.

Authors, Year	Study Design	Subjects	Martial Arts (Style, Frequency and Duration)	Results
Tsang *et al.*, 2009 , 2010 [26,27]	Randomized placebo-controlled trial	20 overweight/obese subjects, aged 6 to 12 years	Kung fu 1 h, 3 times/week, over 6 months	Total and abdominal fat mass↓(without group effect) Submaximal cardiovascular fitness↑, lower muscle endurance↑, upper body muscle velocity↑ Lean body mass↑, HbA1c↓, insulin resistance↓, triglycerides↓, total cholesterol↓
Benbenek-Klupa *et al.*, 2015 [29]	Case-control study	5 patients with type 1 diabetes, aged 18 to 34 years	Mixed martial arts and kick boxing	Improvement or maintenance of glycemic control without diabetic ketoacidosis and severe hypoglycemia during at least a 2-year follow-up
Benedini *et al.*, 2012 [30]	Randomized crossover study	10 healthy subjects, university students	Karate (*kata* and *kumite* sessions)	Plasma glucose levels↑ Epinephrine↑, norepinephrine↑, testosterone↑
Douris *et al.*, 2009 [32]	Cross-sectional study	10 martial artists and 10 sedentary subjects, middle-aged	Soo Bahk Do	Lower pulse wave velocity in martial artists
Douris *et al.*, 2013 [31]	Matched-pair design	9 martial artists and 9 sedentary subjects, middle-aged	Soo Bahk Do	Higher levels of glutathione and lower levels of glutathione disulfide in martial artists

HbA1c = hemoglobin A1c.

5. Adverse Effects of Martial Arts

The incidence of injuries and accidents associated with martial arts should also be discussed. Most of the tai chi styles are soft/internal styles, and the incidence rate of injuries tends to be small. Although tai chi seems to have no serious adverse effects, a systematic review have shown that it is associated with minor musculoskeletal pain (e.g., knee and back pain) [33]. Martial arts practiced as a full-contact style seems to have a high incidence rate of injuries. Several systematic reviews have shown that an average injury risk is approximately 11%–12% in judo [34], 2%–14% in taekwondo [35], and 23% in mixed martial arts [36] in young elite athletes. However, when martial arts are performed in a light or no-contact style, the incidence rate of injuries is low [37]. Zetaruk *et al.* conducted a retrospective cohort study, involving 263 martial arts practitioners, to analyze and compare five styles of martial arts with respect to injury incidents. The incidence rate of injuries was 59% for tae kwon do, 51% for aikido, 38% for kung fu, 30% for karate, and 14% for tai chi. No sex differences were found. Subjects >18 years of age (odds ratio = 3.95; 95% CI, 1.48–8.52) had >three years of experience (odds ratio = 2.46; 95% CI, 1.51–4.02), practiced for >3 h/week (odds ratio = 1.85; 95% CI, 1.13–3.05), and were associated with an increased risk of injury. Although the types of injuries varied depending on the styles of martial arts, martial arts seem to be safe for young individuals and beginners [38]. Considering that patients with metabolic diseases are relatively old, fragile, and inactive, the practice of a hard-contact style of martial arts should be avoided. However, no-contact and/or solo-practice martial arts, such as tai chi and kata of karate, can be performed without serious injuries. Such soft/internal styles of martial arts may be recommended as exercise for patients with metabolic diseases. Moreover, vigorous exercise may increase the risk of acute coronary events and sudden cardiac arrest in susceptible individuals who do not engage in regular exercise [39,40], and we should be careful when older patients with metabolic diseases perform martial arts. Umeda *et al.* [41,42] reported that energy restriction combined with intense exercise might have impaired muscle and immune function in judo athletes. We should also note whether individuals have adequate energy intake in martial arts participation. Combat sports usually have weight categories, and most elite athletes take drastic measures (e.g., starvation, restriction of fluid intake, and sweating) to achieve target body weight [43]. Indeed, the prevalence of rapid weight loss (typically 2%–10% weight reduction) in combat sports is as high as 50% [44], and it must be harmful for athletes' health.

6. Conclusions

Systematic reviews of RCTs investigating the effectiveness of tai chi for metabolic diseases, including hypertension, dyslipidemia, and type 2 diabetes, showed that no sufficient evidence exists. However, when non-controlled studies, observational studies, and case series were included in this analysis, tai chi was found to be effective for reducing the risk of stroke and improving metabolic diseases. Other styles of martial arts, such as kung fu and karate, may be beneficial for body composition, glycemic control, and arterial stiffness; however, evidence is currently limited. The strength of this review is first to summarize the current literature in the effects of various styles of martial arts, not limited to tai chi, on metabolic diseases. Most previous studies evaluating the effects of martial arts on health were limited by a small numbers of subjects and short study durations. Previous RCTs also have methodological heterogeneity which makes it difficult to evaluate the efficacy of martial arts on metabolic diseases. Some confounding factors such as dietary intake may also affect the study results. For standardized evaluation of the quality and validity of clinical studies, clinicians should note how studies are conducted, including inclusion/exclusion criteria, sample size, randomization, and details of intervention and control group. Well-designed prospective studies, preferably RCTs with larger numbers of subjects, are warranted to clarify the effectiveness of martial arts for treating metabolic diseases. Another problem with past studies is a biased distribution of the ages of the subjects. There were few intervention studies investigating the effects of tai chi in children/adolescents or hard/external style martial arts in the elderly. Elderly patients with metabolic diseases should not perform a hard-contact style of martial arts against a real opponent because the incidence rate of injuries and accidents would be very high. However, they can practice a solo style of hard/external martial arts, under the supervision of experts in physical activity and metabolic diseases. In addition, the influence of a soft/internal style of martial arts, such as tai chi, on the growth of children provides an interesting perspective. Finally, traditional martial arts include unique forms of training, such as breathing techniques and manipulating bones and muscles. Investigating the clinical effects of such training on health, beyond the intensity and frequency of the exercise, may constitute a promising future study.

Conflicts of Interest: The authors declare no conflict of interest.

Abbreviations

The following abbreviations are used in this manuscript:

METs	metabolic equivalents
HR-QOL	health-related quality of life
CVD	cardiovascular disease
RCT	randomized controlled trial
CI	confidence intervals
eGFR	estimated glomerular filtration rate

References

1. Physical Activity Guidelines Advisory Committee Report, 2008. To the Secretary of Health and Human Services. Part A: Executive Summary. *Nutr. Rev.* **2009**, *67*, 114–120.
2. Ainsworth, B.E.; Haskell, W.L.; Herrmann, S.D.; Meckes, N.; Bassett, D.R., Jr.; Tudor-Locke, C.; Greer, J.L.; Vezina, J.; Whitt-Glover, M.C.; Leon, A.S. 2011 Compendium of Physical Activities: A second update of codes and MET values. *Med. Sci. Sports Exerc.* **2011**, *43*, 1575–1581. [CrossRef] [PubMed]
3. Kohl, H.W., 3rd; Craig, C.L.; Lambert, E.V.; Inoue, S.; Alkandari, J.R.; Leetongin, G.; Kahlmeier, S.; Lancet Physical Activity Series Working Group. The pandemic of physical inactivity: Global action for public health. *Lancet* **2012**, *380*, 294–305. [CrossRef]
4. Jahnke, R.; Larkey, L.; Rogers, C.; Etnier, J.; Lin, F. A comprehensive review of health benefits of Qigong and Tai Chi. *Am. J. Health Promot.* **2010**, *24*, e1–e25. [CrossRef] [PubMed]
5. Song, R.; Ahn, S.; Roberts, B.L.; Lee, E.O.; Ahn, Y.H. Adhering to a Tai Chi program to improve glucose control and quality of life for individuals with type 2 diabetes. *J. Altern. Complement. Med.* **2009**, *15*, 627–632. [CrossRef] [PubMed]
6. Liu, X.; Miller, Y.D.; Burton, N.W.; Chang, J.H.; Brown, W.J. The effect of Tai Chi on health-related quality of life in people with elevated blood glucose or diabetes: A randomized controlled trial. *Qual. Life Res.* **2013**, *22*, 1783–1786. [CrossRef] [PubMed]
7. Hung, J.W.; Liou, C.W.; Wang, P.W.; Yeh, S.H.; Lin, L.W.; Lo, S.K.; Tsai, F.M. Effect of 12-week Tai Chi Chuan exercise on peripheral nerve modulation in patients with type 2 diabetes mellitus. *J. Rehabil. Med.* **2009**, *41*, 924–929. [CrossRef] [PubMed]
8. Chen, S.C.; Ueng, K.C.; Lee, S.H.; Sun, K.T.; Lee, M.C. Effect of Wai Chi exercise on biochemical profiles and oxidative stress indicators in obese patients with type 2 diabetes. *J. Altern. Complement. Med.* **2010**, *16*, 1153–1159. [CrossRef] [PubMed]
9. Yeh, S.H.; Chuang, H.; Lin, L.W.; Hsiao, C.Y.; Wang, P.W.; Liu, R.T.; Yang, K.D. Regular Tai Chi Chuan exercise improves T cell helper function of patients with type 2 diabetes mellitus with an increase in T-bet transcription factor and IL-12 production. *Br. J. Sports Med.* **2009**, *43*, 845–850. [CrossRef] [PubMed]
10. Lan, C; Chen, S.Y.; Lai, J.S. The exercise intensity of Tai Chi Chuan. *Med. Sports Sci.* **2008**, *52*, 12–19.
11. Hartley, L.; Flowers, N.; Lee, M.S.; Ernst, E.; Rees, K. Tai Chi for primary prevention of cardiovascular disease. *Cochrane Database Syst. Rev.* **2014**, *4*. [CrossRef]
12. Zheng, G.; Huang, M.; Liu, F.; Li, S.; Tao, J.; Chen, L. Tai Chi Chuan for the primary prevention of stroke in middle-aged and elderly adults: A systematic review. *Evid. Based Complement. Altern. Med.* **2015**, *2015*. [CrossRef] [PubMed]
13. Lee, M.S.; Ernst, E. Systematic reviews of T'ai Chi: An overview. *Br. J. Sports Med.* **2012**, *46*, 713–718. [CrossRef] [PubMed]
14. Yang, G.Y.; Wang, L.Q.; Ren, J.; Zhang, Y.; Li, M.L.; Zhu, Y.T.; Luo, J.; Cheng, Y.J.; Li, W.Y.; Wayne, P.M.; *et al.* Evidence base of clinical studies on Tai Chi: A bibliometric analysis. *PLoS ONE* **2015**, *10*. [CrossRef] [PubMed]
15. Lee, M.S.; Pittler, M.H.; Kim, M.S.; Ernst, E. Tai Chi for Type 2 diabetes: A systematic review. *Diabet. Med.* **2008**, *25*, 240–241. [CrossRef] [PubMed]
16. Tsang, T.; Orr, R.; Lam, P.; Comino, E.J.; Singh, M.F. Health benefits of Tai Chi for older patients with type 2 diabetes: The "Move It For Diabetes study"—A randomized controlled trial. *Clin. Interv. Aging* **2007**, *2*, 429–439. [PubMed]
17. Lee, M.S.; Choi, T.Y.; Lim, H.J.; Ernst, E. Tai Chi for management of type 2 diabetes mellitus: A systematic review. *Chin. J. Integr. Med.* **2011**, *17*, 789–793. [CrossRef] [PubMed]
18. Zhang, Y.; Fu, F.H. Effects of 14-week Tai Ji Quan exercise on metabolic control in women with type 2 diabetes. *Am. J. Chin. Med.* **2008**, *36*, 647–654. [CrossRef] [PubMed]
19. Sun, J.; Buys, N. Community-Based Mind-Body Meditative Tai Chi Program and Its Effects on Improvement of Blood Pressure, Weight, Renal Function, Serum Lipoprotein, and Quality of Life in Chinese Adults With Hypertension. *Am. J. Cardiol.* **2015**, *116*, 1076–1081. [CrossRef] [PubMed]
20. Liu, X.; Miller, Y.D.; Burton, N.W.; Brown, W.J. A preliminary study of the effects of Tai Chi and Qigong medical exercise on indicators of metabolic syndrome, glycaemic control, health-related quality of life, and psychological health in adults with elevated blood glucose. *Br. J. Sports Med.* **2010**, *44*, 704–709. [CrossRef] [PubMed]

21. Kilo, S.; Berghoff, M.; Hilz, M.; Freeman, R. Neural and endothelial control of the microcirculation in diabetic peripheral neuropathy. *Neurology* **2000**, *54*, 1246–1252. [CrossRef] [PubMed]
22. Wang, J.S.; Lan, C.; Wong, M.K. Tai Chi Chuan training to enhance microcirculatory function in healthy elderly men. *Arch. Phys. Med. Rehabil.* **2001**, *82*, 1176–1180. [CrossRef] [PubMed]
23. Wang, J.S.; Lan, C.; Chen, S.Y.; Wong, M.K. Tai Chi Chuan training is associated with enhanced endothelium-dependent dilation in skin vasculature of healthy older men. *J. Am. Geriatr. Soc.* **2002**, *50*, 1024–1030. [CrossRef] [PubMed]
24. Yeh, S.H.; Chuang, H.; Lin, L.W.; Hsiao, C.Y.; Wang, P.W.; Yang, K.D. Tai Chi Chuan exercise decreases A1C levels along with increase of regulatory T-cells and decrease of cytotoxic T-cell population in type 2 diabetic patients. *Diabetes Care* **2007**, *30*, 716–718. [CrossRef] [PubMed]
25. Van Dijk, G.P.; Leffers, P.; Lodder, J. The Effectiveness of Hard Martial Arts in People over Forty: An Attempted Systematic Review. *Societies* **2014**, *4*, 161–179. [CrossRef]
26. Tsang, T.W.; Kohn, M.; Chow, C.M.; Singh, M.F. A randomised placebo-exercise controlled trial of Kung Fu training for improvements in body composition in overweight/obese adolescents: The "Martial Fitness" study. *J. Sports Sci. Med.* **2009**, *8*, 97–106. [PubMed]
27. Tsang, T.W.; Kohn, M.R.; Chow, C.M.; Fiatarone Singh, M.A. Kung Fu training improves physical fitness measures in overweight/obese adolescents: The "martial fitness" study. *J. Obes.* **2010**, *2010*. [CrossRef] [PubMed]
28. Tsang, T.W.; Kohn, M.; Chow, C.M.; Singh, M.F. A randomized controlled trial of Kung Fu training for metabolic health in overweight/obese adolescents: The "martial fitness" study. *J. Pediatr. Endocrinol. MeTable* **2009**, *22*, 595–607. [CrossRef]
29. Benbenek-Klupa, T.; Matejko, B.; Klupa, T. Metabolic control in type 1 diabetes patients practicing combat sports: At least two-year follow-up study. *Springerplus* **2015**, *4*, 133. [CrossRef] [PubMed]
30. Benedini, S.; Longo, S.; Caumo, A.; Luzi, L.; Invernizzi, P.L. Metabolic and hormonal responses to a single session of kumite (free non-contact fight) and kata (highly ritualized fight) in karate athletes. *Sport Sci. Health* **2012**, *8*, 81–85. [CrossRef] [PubMed]
31. Douris, P.C.; Ingenito, T.; Piccirillo, B.; Herbst, M.; Petrizzo, J.; Cherian, V.; McCutchan, C.; Burke, C.; Stamatinos, G.; Jung, M.K. Martial arts training attenuates arterial stiffness in middle aged adults. *Asian J. Sports Med.* **2013**, *4*, 201–207. [CrossRef] [PubMed]
32. Douris, P.C.; Elokda, A.S.; Handrakis, J.P.; Principal, S.; Rondo, E.; Bovell, J.; Coughlin, W.P.; Mastroianni, C.N.; Wong, M.J.; Zimmerman, T. Martial art training enhances the glutathione antioxidant system in middle-aged adults. *J. Strength Cond. Res.* **2009**, *23*, 1518–1523. [CrossRef] [PubMed]
33. Wayne, P.M.; Berkowitz, D.L.; Litrownik, D.E.; Buring, J.E.; Yeh, G.Y. What do we really know about the safety of tai chi? A systematic review of adverse event reports in randomized trials. *Arch. Phys. Med. Rehabil.* **2014**, *95*, 2470–2783. [CrossRef] [PubMed]
34. Pocecco, E.; Ruedl, G.; Stankovic, N.; Sterkowicz, S.; Del Vecchio, F.B.; Gutiérrez-García, C.; Rousseau, R.; Wolf, M.; Kopp, M.; Miarka, B.; *et al.* Injuries in judo: A systematic literature review including suggestions for prevention. *Br. J. Sports Med.* **2013**, *47*, 1139–1143. [CrossRef] [PubMed]
35. Pieter, W.; Fife, G.P.; O'Sullivan, D.M. Competition injuries in taekwondo: A literature review and suggestions for prevention and surveillance. *Br. J. Sports Med.* **2012**, *46*, 485–491. [CrossRef] [PubMed]
36. Lystad, R.P.; Gregory, K.; Wilson, J. The Epidemiology of Injuries in Mixed Martial Arts: A Systematic Review and Meta-analysis. *Orthop. J. Sports Med.* **2014**, *2*. [CrossRef] [PubMed]
37. Burke, D.T.; Al-Adawi, S.; Lee, Y.T.; Audette, J. Martial arts as sport and therapy. *J. Sports Med. Phys. Fit.* **2007**, *47*, 96–102.
38. Zetaruk, M.N.; Violán, M.A.; Zurakowski, D.; Micheli, L.J. Injuries in martial arts: A comparison of five styles. *Br. J. Sports Med.* **2005**, *39*, 29–33. [CrossRef] [PubMed]
39. Maron, B.J. The paradox of exercise. *N. Engl. J. Med.* **2000**, *343*, 1409–1411. [CrossRef] [PubMed]
40. Siscovick, D.S.; Weiss, N.S.; Fletcher, R.H.; Lasky, T. The incidence of primary cardiac arrest during vigorous exercise. *N. Engl. J. Med.* **1984**, *311*, 874–877. [CrossRef] [PubMed]
41. Umeda, T.; Nakaji, S.; Shimoyama, T.; Kojima, A.; Yamamoto, Y.; Sugawara, K. Adverse effects of energy restriction on changes in immunoglobulins and complements during weight reduction in judoists. *J. Sports Med. Phys. Fit.* **2004**, *44*, 328–334.

42. Umeda, T.; Nakaji, S.; Shimoyama, T.; Yamamoto, Y.; Totsuka, M.; Sugawara, K. Adverse effects of energy restriction on myogenic enzymes in judoists. *J. Sports Sci.* **2004**, *22*, 329–338. [CrossRef] [PubMed]
43. Artioli, G.G.; Saunders, B.; Iglesias, R.T.; Franchini, E. It is Time to Ban Rapid Weight Loss from Combat Sports. *Sports Med.* **2016**, in press. [CrossRef] [PubMed]
44. Franchini, E.; Brito, C.J.; Artioli, G.G. Weight loss in combat sports: Physiological, psychological and performance effects. *J. Int. Soc. Sports Nutr.* **2012**, *9*. [CrossRef] [PubMed]

11

Modelling the Progression of Male Swimmers' Performances through Adolescence

Shilo J. Dormehl [1], Samuel J. Robertson [2,†] and Craig A. Williams [1,†,*]

Academic Editor: Eling Douwe de Bruin

1 University of Exeter, Children's Health and Exercise Research Centre, College of Life and Environmental Sciences, St Luke's Campus, Heavitree Road, Exeter EX1 2LU, UK; sjd223@exeter.ac.uk
2 Victoria University, Institute of Sport, Exercise & Active Living, Melbourne 3011, Australia; Sam.Robertson@vu.edu.au
* Correspondence: C.A.Williams@exeter.ac.uk

† These authors contributed equally to this work.

Abstract: Insufficient data on adolescent athletes is contributing to the challenges facing youth athletic development and accurate talent identification. The purpose of this study was to model the progression of male sub-elite swimmers' performances during adolescence. The performances of 446 males (12–19 year olds) competing in seven individual events (50, 100, 200 m freestyle, 100 m backstroke, breaststroke, butterfly, 200 m individual medley) over an eight-year period at an annual international schools swimming championship, run under FINA regulations were collected. Quadratic functions for each event were determined using mixed linear models. Thresholds of peak performance were achieved between the ages of 18.5 $\pm$ 0.1 (50 m freestyle and 200 m individual medley) and 19.8 $\pm$ 0.1 (100 m butterfly) years. The slowest rate of improvement was observed in the 200 m individual medley (20.7%) and the highest in the 100 m butterfly (26.2%). Butterfly does however appear to be one of the last strokes in which males specialise. The models may be useful as talent identification tools, as they predict the age at which an average sub-elite swimmer could potentially peak. The expected rate of improvement could serve as a tool in which to monitor and evaluate benchmarks.

Keywords: adolescent; specialisation; quadratic functions; talent-identification; sub-elite

---

1. Introduction

Elite-level athletes have been well characterised compared with sub-elite adolescents. Retrospective studies such as those conducted by Sokolovas [1], Costa *et al.* [2] and Allen *et al.* [3] have enabled the performance of individual top-ranked swimmers to be tracked as they progressed through their careers, in the anticipation that the process may map the path to potential elite performance. The majority of longitudinal studies in swimming have also focused on adult athletes who had already reached elite status. These studies aimed to characterise both the consistency and rate of development of individual performances [2–5] *inter alia* and claimed to enable practitioners the ability to predict potential medallists and/or determine realistic individual performance goals [6,7].

Talent identification (TI) has been defined as the process whereby current performers are recognised as having the potential to become future elite athletes and talent development (TD) as the provision of a suitable, opportunity-rich, learning environment [8]. As improved TI and TD programmes become more widely implemented, former and current elite athletes are unlikely to reflect the pathway of future champions because they were products of an era of rudimentary TI practices. Furthermore it is likely that there would be a decrease in the mean age to reach elite-level standard and the start of the "peak-performance window", a term coined by Allen, Vandenbogaerde and Hopkins [3]. Therefore current "atypically-young" elite athletes could become the future norm.

To date, the prediction of future talent in young children has seldom shown to be accurate [9,10]. The majority of TI programmes continue to be based on cross-sectional studies [9] despite it being evident that many of the physical components being assessed may change or may not be as important at the elite adult level [11]. If future talent is to be successfully identified in adolescents, sporting organisations should aim to avoid summative discrete measurements and rather focus on creating environments conducive to longitudinal formative assessments [12]. This is pertinent because skill acquisition is non-linear and athletes and their training environments should thus be considered as complex dynamic systems [13].

However, since there is a dearth of longitudinal research on athletes of this age, there is a need to better understand the broad pool from which future talent is likely to arise, *viz.* the sub-elite athlete. Sub-elite athletes have been defined as those athletes who are yet to represent their country at international level [14]. Despite the challenges of categorising such an unstable, developing group of athletes, it is important to prioritise this often overlooked category of swimmer if the use of valid performance measures in TI is to progress.

The consequences of poor TI processes result in many late-developing athletes with potential being de-selected, frequently leading to dropout and often result in exclusivity rather than inclusivity [15]. Another outcome of many dated TI processes is that they inevitably lead to athletes choosing to specialise early in a sport in which they are believed to show potential. This practice may be due to the fact that immediate successful performance is prioritised over unrealised potential in the long term [10].

A further limitation that potentially explains the lack of success of many TI approaches relates to the types of assessments used. Specifically, many TI assessments fail to accurately represent the competition setting, often relying on generic physical evaluations or closed skill tests that do not correlate well with the demands that athletes will face in competition [16]. The rationale for undertaking this longitudinal study of male adolescent swimmers, in the competitive setting, was to: (a) model performance progression through adolescence; and (b) predict the ages at which performance plateaued. Advancements in statistical modelling have recently provided researchers with a more refined and rigorous method of interpreting longitudinal data [17,18], but until now, sub-elite athletes have been underrepresented. Additionally, swimming has commonly been considered as a single sport [3,19], rather than a sport with multiple specialisms in the form of different stroke techniques and distances. Where the individual strokes have been characterised, it is still rare to find simultaneous analyses of all strokes together. The aim of this study was to create a tool that will enable the progression and variability of performances throughout puberty to be tracked in relation to a modelled mean and as such, assist coaches with the setting of realistic goals when devising individually-tailored training programmes. Finally, the models produced in this study could potentially be used as instruments for identifying talented young male swimmers.

2. Methods

Performance times for all male entrants ($n = 446$, aged between 12 and 19 years) who competed in one of seven individual events (Table 1) were extracted from the official results of an annual international schools swimming championships from 2006 to 2013. The data was in the public domain and downloaded from the relevant tournament websites. All swimmers from the 13 competing schools were assigned individual identity codes to ensure anonimity. The study was approved by the institutional ethics committee and conformed to the recommendations of the Declaration of Helsinki. The number of observations in each of the seven events entered over the 8 year analysis period are described in Table 1. The swimmers' ages at the time of each competition were also obtained.

Table 1. Cumulative number of performances (between 2006 and 2013) for male swimmers between the ages of 12 and 19 years in each event.

Number of Performances (years)	50 m Freestyle	100 m Freestyle	200 m Freestyle	100 m Backstroke	100 m Breaststroke	100 m Butterfly	200 m Individual Medley
1	376	280	190	178	196	132	139
2	151	103	87	74	69	55	65
3	69	49	37	34	37	26	38
4	25	17	16	14	21	14	18
5	9	3	6	1	9	4	6
6	2	1	1	0	3	2	1

2.1. Statisical Analysis

The raw datasets for all performances in each of the seven events were tested for normality using the Shapiro-Francia test in STATA ver. 13. The datasets for all events had non-normal distributions. The trajectories of the curves showing the progression in performance during adolescence were analysed using mixed or multi-level modelling (MLM) in STATA. Time was zero centred at the first point of observation (12 years of age), using an unstructured covariance approach. The fit of the models for fixed and random effects were compared by obtaining maximum likelihoods using a hierarchical method. The final models were quadratic functions for fixed effects ($y = \mathrm{a}x^2 + \mathrm{b}x + \mathrm{c}$). The fixed effects of time represented polynomial changes of the population with age and the random effects reflected individual deviations from the sample mean trajectory. Inter-class correlations were calculated and R^2 values determined in order to measure the difference between and within person variability and effect size respectively.

2.2. Evaluation of Models

Cross-validation of models is highly recommended to ensure the generalizability of the findings [20]. Cross-validation was therefore performed for each of the seven models separately, whereby the datasets were randomly split into training (66%) and test (33%) sets. Performance of each test set was determined through obtaining the mean difference in model performance.

The percentage rate of improvement was determined through differentiation of the quadratic functions for each event separately, as $y = \left(\frac{2a}{c} \times 100\right) x + \left(\frac{b}{c} \times 100\right)$, where y = % change in performance time and $x + 12$ = age, in years. The age at peak performance was calculated as the axis of symmetry of the quadratic function *i.e.*, $\frac{-b}{2a}$.

3. Results

The models for all three freestyle events and the backstroke event resulted in fixed quadratic random linear functions whereas those for the remaining three events showed the best fit as fixed quadratic random intercept functions (Table 2). The high ICC values for all the models indicated a greater variability between- rather than within-swimmers. The model for the means explained 16%–25% of the variance in the changes with age. The results from the cross validation indicated that the fixed effects of the quadratic functions for all events fell within the 95% confidence intervals (C.I.) of those of the full models, with the exception of the 100 and 200 m freestyle events (Table 2). The 1/3 and 2/3 subsamples for both of these events fell marginally outside of the C.I. of the full model for their fixed intercepts only.

Table 2. Summary of models for all events with cross validation for each of the fixed effects of the quadratic functions.

Predictor	50 m Freestyle		100 m Freestyle		200 m Freestyle		100 m Backstroke		100 m Breaststroke		100 m Butterfly		200 m Individual Medley	
	Mean	***P***	**Mean**	***P***	**Mean**	***P***	**Mean**	***P***	**Mean**	***P***	**Mean**	***P***	**Mean**	***P***
Fixed Quadratic (a)	0.21	<0.001	0.48	<0.001	0.93	<0.001	0.47	<0.001	0.50	<0.001	0.41	<0.001	0.97	<0.001
Standard error (SE)	(0.02)	–	(0.06)	–	(0.14)	–	(0.08)	–	(0.08)	–	(0.11)	–	(0.14)	–
95% C.I.	0.05	–	0.11	–	0.28	–	0.16	–	0.16	–	0.21	–	0.28	–
Cross val. 2/3 diff.	0.003	<0.001	0.051	<0.001	0.21	<0.001	0.07	<0.001	−0.068	<0.001	0.05	0.007	0.10	<0.001
Cross val. 1/3 diff.	0.03	<0.001	0.010	<0.001	0.003	0.001	−0.05	0.001	0.097	0.005	−0.13	0.001	−0.22	<0.001
Fixed Linear (b)	−2.78	<0.001	−6.38	<0.001	−12.16	<0.001	−6.37	<0.001	−6.65	<0.001	−6.40	<0.001	−12.56	<0.001
(SE)	(0.18)	–	(0.45)	–	(1.11)	–	(0.62)	–	(0.62)	–	(0.85)	–	(1.06)	–
95% C.I.	0.36	–	0.88	–	2.18	–	1.22	–	1.22	–	1.66	–	2.08	–
Cross val. 2/3 diff.	−0.04	<0.001	−0.44	<0.001	−2.01	<0.001	−0.62	<0.001	0.31	<0.001	−0.41	<0.001	−0.94	<0.001
Cross val. 1/3 diff.	−0.16	<0.001	0.28	<0.001	0.37	<0.001	0.23	<0.001	−0.22	<0.001	1.11	<0.001	1.23	<0.001
Fixed Intercept in seconds (c)	37.23	<0.001	83.81	<0.001	179.45	<0.001	95.33	<0.001	104.35	<0.001	92.79	<0.001	195.98	<0.001
(SE)	(0.38)	–	(0.99)	–	(2.39)	–	(1.37)	–	(1.12)	–	(1.65)	–	(2.21)	–
95% C.I.	0.74	–	1.94	–	4.67	–	2.68	–	2.34	–	3.23	–	4.33	–
Cross val. 2/3 diff.	0.07	<0.001	1.48	<0.001	5.36	<0.001	1.57	<0.001	0.59	<0.001	0.77	<0.001	1.86	<0.001
Cross val. 1/3 diff	0.17	<0.001	−2.47	<0.001	−3.97	<0.001	−0.88	<0.001	0.33	<0.001	−2.19	<0.001	−3.26	<0.001
Interclass correlation (ICC)	0.95		0.97		0.96		0.97		0.91		0.90		0.92	
Wald's χ^2	543.36 (df = 7)		479.95 (df = 7)		315.318 (df = 7)		298.98 (df = 7)		430.27 (df = 5)		318.57 (df = 5)		461.07 (df = 5)	
Total R^2	0.25		0.23		0.16		0.17		0.20		0.22		0.17	
n	376		280		190		178		196		132		139	

Note: Cross val. diff. is the difference between the cross validation split and the whole sample. Wald's χ^2 is Wald's chi-square.

Similar distinct trends in the trajectories of the models were observed when compared to threshold age of peak performance or a fixed age of 18 years (Figure 1). The progression of swimmers of 100 m butterfly differed from all the other events. The butterfly swimmers reached a peak performance age more than a year later than those in other events, but displayed the highest rate of improvement (Table 3). In contrast, the slowest rate of improvement and joint youngest age of peak performance occurred for swimmers of the 200 m individual medley (IM). Of the remaining events, two groups emerged; 50 and 100 m freestyle events showed very similar trajectories, as did the 100 m backstroke, breaststroke and 200 m freestyle (Figure 1, Table 3).

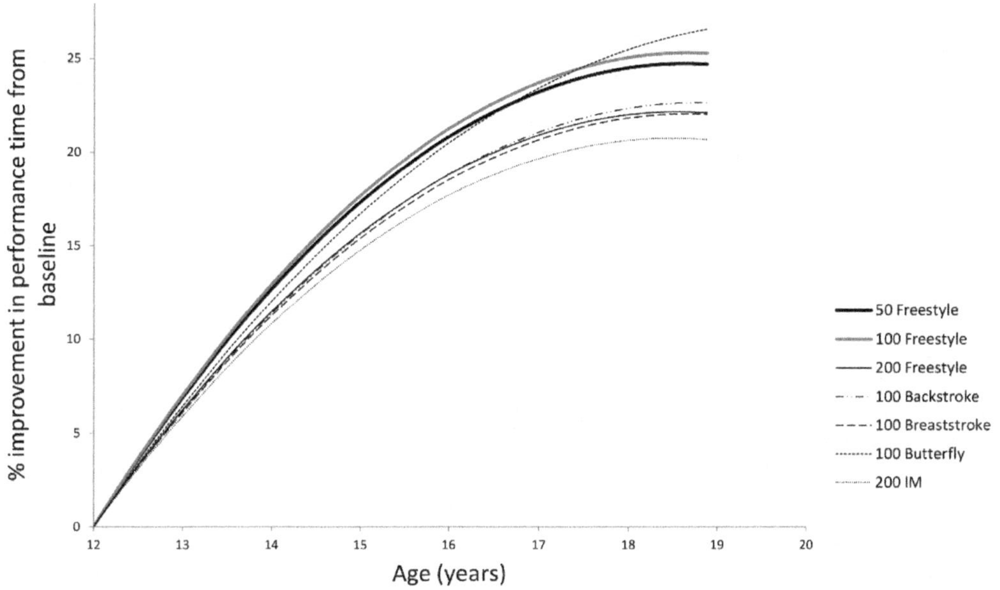

Figure 1. Quadratic functions of the progression in performance for each of the seven events modelled for males from the baseline of 12 years through to 19 years of age.

Table 3. Descriptors determined for the full models of the seven events.

Predictor	50 m Freestyle	100 m Freestyle	200 m Freestyle	100 m Backstroke	100 m Breaststroke	100 m Butterfly	200 m Individual Medley
% Rate of improvement (12 year—peak age)	24.70	25.29	22.15	22.64	22.03	26.92	20.75
% Rate of improvement (from 12 to 18.5 year)	24.70	25.28	22.15	22.60	22.02	26.16	20.75
Threshold age in peak performance (year)	18.5 (0.12)	18.7 (0.06)	18.6 (0.14)	18.7 (0.08)	18.6 (0.08)	19.8 (0.11)	18.5 (0.14)
Performance time (s) at threshold age	28.26 (0.22)	62.44 (1.53)	139.54 (9.38)	73.94 (2.07)	82.26 (2.40)	67.93 (3.09)	155.35 (9.36)

Data given as mean with standard errors shown in brackets.

4. Discussion

This is the first study to longitudinally assess the development of sub-elite adolescent male swimmers in multiple stroke techniques during competition, where the primary purpose was to generate a TI tool for young male swimmers. To achieve this, the performance progression of these swimmers was modelled to identify the mean threshold age at which they could be expected to start competing at the highest level. It was thus unsurprising that for most events, age correlated with the widely accepted age of biological maturity for males (Table 3) in agreement with previous work [21,22].

Hence it could be surmised that any further gains in performance from this point onwards, would potentially come from the biomechanical and psychological domains. However, the rate of progression in performance of male athletes, including swimmers, during adolescence is known to be attributed predominantly to the tempo of their anthropometric and physiological maturation [23].

There was a narrow range of ages (18.5–19.8 years) at which the swimmers approached their peak in performance in the seven events modelled in this study. In a retrospective study of career progression in elite swimmers, Allen, Vandenbogaerde and Hopkins [3] found ages of peak performance that were on average 6.2 years older than those for the corresponding events in this study. The discrepancy between the two studies can be explained by three factors. Firstly, Allen, Vandenbogaerde and Hopkins [3] tracked athletes back over a longer career path (from the ages of 12–30 years). Secondly, their sample only contained athletes who had already progressed to the elite level (probably through simplistic TI systems), whereas the talent pool in this study contained a wider-ranging standard of swimmers. Thirdly, the majority of their sample would have comprised athletes who grew up prior to the long-term athlete development (LTAD) generation of the post millennium era that our sample contains. But there is in fact no discordance between these two studies; they are complementary. While Allen, Vandenbogaerde and Hopkins [3] identified a potential absolute peak in performance of current and past elite swimmers, this study, based on the broad nature of the sample, provides insight into the threshold age of performance; *i.e.*, the cusp of the window of peak performance for future talented swimmers. The discrepancy between the two predicted ages therefore serves as a period of potential performance development that will come about through factors such as training interventions and increased experience, rather than maturational development. The models in Allen, Vandenbogaerde and Hopkins [3] are therefore more likely to provide coaches with a selection tool for swimmers currently in an elite squad, rather than as a means to identify future talent.

Freestyle is the most efficient stroke [24,25] and is most frequently swum in practice. It is therefore unsurprising that two of the three steepest progressions of performance occurred in freestyle events (Table 3), since this stroke contributes in excess of 30% of the events on offer at the majority of competitions [26–28]. A study by Costa, Marinho, Bragada, Silva and Barbosa [2] on elite Portuguese male freestyle swimmers, found similar rates of progression (14.36%–18.97%) between the ages of 12 and 18 years.

Vaso *et al.* [29] hypothesised that IM swimmers might peak later than those in freestyle events, due to the additional skills required in mastering all four of the recognised stroke techniques and their unique turns in this complex event. In contrast, our models suggested that male IM swimmers peaked in performance earlier than the majority of other stroke specialisms (Table 3), but showed the slowest rate of improvement from 12 to 19 years (Figure 1). There are a number of reasons that may explain this observation. Firstly, IM swimmers may have started swimming at a young age, suggesting they may have a more advanced level of biomechanical experience and learning than swimmers in other events. Nevertheless, IM swimmers may not yet have found their specialist stroke. Once they do however, these swimmers may then focus more on other events. Secondly, many LTAD-based programmes advocate that coaches discourage swimmers from specialising too early in one stroke, in favour of focusing on the continued development of all strokes [30].

The butterfly swimmers in this study reached their threshold in peak performance at a later age than all other events (Table 3). They did however demonstrate the greatest rate of improvement. The lag could be related to the need to gain sufficient experience in the stroke in order to efficiently coordinate its propulsive biomechanical actions. The butterfly stroke relies heavily on the precision of timing of its propulsive and recovery phases and consequently when these are not optimised, the rhythm becomes compromised [31]. This means that when these factors do come together, considerable performance improvements are realised.

4.1. Limitations

Being a school-level competition, the sample lacks the homogeneity of an exclusive elite-level sample, however cross validation of the models supported their generalizability. This could be seen as a limitation of the study as it does not distinguish between early and late maturers, the former of which would be more likely to have been identified as being talented within this age range [32]. But, the decision to use longitudinal competition data, so as to maximise external validity, came at the cost of collecting any corresponding anthropometric data to assess maturation.

The models fit most events well with the exception of the 100 and 200 m freestyle (Table 2). The youngest swimmers of these events were markedly variable in standard. Dormehl and Williams (2016) [33], did however find a lack of stability in the continued selection of these events by male swimmers between the ages of 12 and 19 years. Freestyle is also likely to be the stroke most favoured by inexperienced competitive swimmers, since it is the most efficient stroke with which they would be most familiar [25].

4.2. Practical Applications

Until now, quantifying deviations from average performances in adolescents has been subjective, due to the intertwined relationship between puberty, skill acquisition and underlying talent. The value of these models is that they can be used to determine if adolescent male swimmers were under- or over-performing based on their current age, because they were derived using athletes from a wide range of abilities and different stages of development. Consequently, deviations from the projected performance trajectories could be attributed to a swimmer's stage of maturational development and/or potentially the standard of coaching received. The models could be useful as a TI tool, as they estimate the age at which an average sub-elite swimmer could potentially peak. Furthermore, the expected rate of improvement would serve as a useful target-setting tool for coaches and the authors propose that this model could serve as a prototype, from which further refinements could be expected to evolve.

5. Conclusions

Separating the performance gains as a result of the combined effects of maturation and training interventions remains an elusive goal for sports scientists. This is the first study that has attempted to model the progression of sub-elite adolescent male swimmers' performances across a multitude of individual strokes and distances. These models have identified that swimmers improve at different rates and achieve peak performances at different ages in different events ranging from 18.5 and 19.6 years of age. Assessing the gap between reaching biological maturity and peak performance should however continue to be an area of interest to the research community. Effectively identifying the potential "trainability" of young but mature athletes could hold the key to further improvements in athletic performance, especially in late specialisation sports, such as swimming.

Author Contributions: S.J.D. and C.A.W designed the study, S.J.D collected the data, S.J.R. & S.J.D. statistically analysed the data, S.J.D. wrote the first draft, C.A.W. supervised the study. All authors critically reviewed, contributed to and approved the final manuscript.

Conflicts of Interest: The authors declare no conflict of interest.

References

1. Sokolovas, G. Analysis of USA swimming's all-time top 100 times. In Proceedings of the Xth International Symposium on Biomechanics and Medicine in Swimming; Vilas Boas, J.P., Alves, F., Marques, A., Eds.; University of Porto: Porto, Portugal, 2006; pp. 315–317.
2. Costa, M.J.; Marinho, D.A.; Bragada, J.A.; Silva, A.J.; Barbosa, T.M. Stability of elite freestyle performance from childhood to adulthood. *J. Sports Sci.* **2011**, *29*, 1183–1189. [CrossRef] [PubMed]
3. Allen, S.V.; Vandenbogaerde, T.J.; Hopkins, W.G. Career performance trajectories of olympic swimmers: Benchmarks for talent development. *Eur. J. Sport Sci.* **2014**, *14*, 643–651. [CrossRef] [PubMed]

4. Anderson, M.; Hopkins, W.; Roberts, A.; Pyne, D. Ability of test measures to predict competitive performance in elite swimmers. *J. Sports Sci.* **2008**, *26*, 123–130. [CrossRef] [PubMed]
5. Trewin, C.B.; Hopkins, W.G.; Pyne, D.B. Relationship between world-ranking and olympic performance of swimmers. *J. Sports Sci.* **2004**, *22*, 339–345. [CrossRef] [PubMed]
6. Pyne, D.B.; Trewin, C.B.; Hopkins, W.G. Progression and variability of competitive performance of olympic swimmers. *J. Sports Sci.* **2004**, *22*, 613–620. [CrossRef] [PubMed]
7. Avalos, M.; Hellard, P.; Chatard, J.-C. Modeling the training-performance relationship using a mixed model in elite swimmers. *Med. Sci. Sports Exerc.* **2003**, *35*, 838–846. [CrossRef] [PubMed]
8. Bergeron, M.F.; Mountjoy, M.; Armstrong, N.; Chia, M.; Côté, J.; Emery, C.A.; Faigenbaum, A.; Hall, G.; Kriemler, S.; Léglise, M.; *et al.* International olympic committee consensus statement on youth athletic development. *Br. J. Sports Med.* **2015**, *49*, 843–851. [CrossRef] [PubMed]
9. Abbott, A.; Collins, D. Eliminating the dichotomy between theory and practice in talent identification and development: Considering the role of psychology. *J. Sports Sci.* **2004**, *22*, 395–408. [CrossRef] [PubMed]
10. Martindale, R.J.J.; Collins, D.; Daubney, J. Talent development: A guide for practice and research within sport. *Quest* **2005**, *57*, 353–375. [CrossRef]
11. Lidor, R.; Côté, J.; Hackfort, D. Issp position stand: To test or not to test? The use of physical skill tests in talent detection and in early phases of sport development. *Int. J. Sport Exerci. Psychol.* **2009**, *7*, 131–146. [CrossRef]
12. Bloom, B.S. *Developing Talent in Young People*; Ballantine Books: New York, NY, USA, 1985.
13. Phillips, E.; Davids, K.; Renshaw, I.; Portus, M. Expert performance in sport and the dynamics of talent development. *Sports Med.* **2010**, *40*, 271–283. [CrossRef] [PubMed]
14. Dormehl, S.J.; Osborough, C.D. Effect of age, sex and race distance on front crawl stroke parameters in sub-elite adolescent swimmers during competition. *Pediatr. Exerc. Sci.* **2015**, *27*, 334–344. [CrossRef] [PubMed]
15. Burgess, D.J.; Naughton, G.A. Talent development in adolescent team sports: A review. *Int. J. Sports Physiol. Perform.* **2010**, *5*, 103–116. [PubMed]
16. Vaeyens, R.; Lenoir, M.; Williams, A.M.; Philippaerts, R.M. Talent identification and development programmes in sport: Current models and future directions. *Sports Med.* **2008**, *38*, 703–714. [CrossRef] [PubMed]
17. Morais, J.E.; Marques, M.C.; Marinho, D.A.; Silva, A.J.; Barbosa, T.M. Longitudinal modeling in sports: Young swimmers' performance and biomechanics profile. *Hum. Mov. Sci.* **2014**, *37*, 111–122. [CrossRef] [PubMed]
18. Costa, M.J.; Bragada, J.A.; Marinho, D.A.; Lopez, V.P.; Silva, A.J.; Barbosa, T.M. Longitudinal study in male swimmers: A hierarchical modelling of energetics and biomechanical contributions for performance. *J. Sports Sci. Med.* **2013**, *12*, 614–622. [PubMed]
19. Baxter-Jones, A.D.G.; Helms, P.; Maffulli, N.; Bainespreece, J.C.; Preece, M. Growth and development of male gymnasts, swimmers, soccer and tennis players: A longitudinal study. *Ann. Hum. Biol.* **1995**, *22*, 381–394. [CrossRef] [PubMed]
20. Witten, I.H.; Frank, E. *Data Mining: Practical Machine Learning Tools and Techniques*, 2nd ed.; Morgan Kaufmann Publishers Inc.: San Francisco, CA, USA, 2005.
21. Malina, R.M. Physical growth and biological maturation of young athletes. *Exerc. Sport Sci. Rev.* **1994**, *22*, 280–284. [CrossRef]
22. Baxter-Jones, A.D.G. Growth and development of young athletes: Should competition levels be age related? *Sports Med.* **1995**, *20*, 59–64. [CrossRef] [PubMed]
23. Beunen, G.P.; Malina, R.M. Growth and physical performance relative to the timing of the adolescent spurt. *Exerc. Sport Sci. Rev.* **1988**, *16*, 503–540. [CrossRef] [PubMed]
24. Maglischo, E.W. *Swimming Fastest*; Human Kinetics: Champaign, IL, USA, 2003; pp. 472–473.
25. Barbosa, T.M.; Fernandes, R.; Keskinen, K.L.; Colaço, P.; Cardoso, C.; Silva, J.; Vilas-Boas, J.P. Evaluation of the energy expenditure in competitive swimming strokes. *Int. J. Sports Med.* **2006**, *27*, 894–899. [CrossRef] [PubMed]
26. British Swimming & The ASA. British Swimming Championships Programme of Events. Available online: http://www.swimming.org/assets/uploads/events/British_Champs_2015_Event_Schedule3.pdf (accessed on 2 April 2015).

27. Kiehl, G. *Fina Mastbank Swimming World Cup*; Fédération Internationale de Natation: Lausanne, Switzerland, 2014.
28. International Olympic Committee. Olympic.Org. Available online: http://www.olympic.org/swimming (accessed on 25 October 2013).
29. Vaso, M.; Knechtle, B.; Rüst, C.A.; Rosemann, T.; Lepers, R. Age of peak swim speed and sex difference in performance in medley and freestyle swimming—A comparison between 200 m and 400 m in swiss elite swimmers. *J. Hum. Sport Exerc.* **2013**, *8*, 954–965. [CrossRef]
30. Amateur Swimming Association. *The Swimmer Pathway: Long Term Athlete Development*; ASA: Loughborough, UK, 2003.
31. Seifert, L.; Delignieres, D.; Boulesteix, L.; Chollet, D. Effect of expertise on butterfly stroke coordination. *J. Sports Sci.* **2007**, *25*, 131–141. [CrossRef] [PubMed]
32. Sherar, L.B.; Baxter-Jones, A.D.G.; Faulkner, R.A.; Russell, K.W. Do physical maturity and birth date predict talent in male youth ice hockey players? *J. Sports Sci.* **2007**, *25*, 879–886. [CrossRef] [PubMed]
33. Dormehl, S.J.; Williams, C.A. Stability of within-sport specialisation in competitive adolescent sub-elite swimmers. *Int. J. Perform. Anal. Sport* **2016**. in press.

12

The Age in Swimming of Champions in World Championships (1994–2013) and Olympic Games (1992–2012): A Cross-Sectional Data Analysis

Beat Knechtle [1,*], Nicola Luigi Bragazzi [2,3], Stefan König [4], Pantelis Theodoros Nikolaidis [5], Stefanie Wild [4], Thomas Rosemann [4] and Christoph Alexander Rüst [4]

1 Gesundheitszentrum St. Gallen, St. Gallen 9001, Switzerland
2 Department of Health Sciences (DISSAL), School of Public Health, University of Genoa, Genoa 16132, Italy; robertobragazzi@gmail.com
3 Department of Neuroscience, Rehabilitation, Ophthalmology, Genetics, Maternal and Child Health (DINOGMI), University of Genoa, Genoa 16132, Italy
4 Institute of Primary Care, University of Zurich, Zurich 8091, Switzerland; steven.king@gmx.ch (S.K.); stefanie.wild@gmx.ch (S.W.); thomas.rosemann@usz.ch (T.R.); christoph.ruest@bluewin.ch (C.A.R.)
5 Department of Physical and Cultural Education, Hellenic Army Academy, Vari 16673, Greece; pantelisn@phed.uoa.gr
* Correspondence: beat.knechtle@hispeed.ch

Academic Editor: Eling de Bruin

Abstract: (1) Background: We investigated the age of swimming champions in all strokes and race distances in World Championships (1994–2013) and Olympic Games (1992–2012); (2) Methods: Changes in age and swimming performance across calendar years for 412 Olympic and world champions were analysed using linear, non-linear, multi-level regression analyses and MultiLayer Perceptron (MLP); (3) Results: The age of peak swimming performance remained stable in most of all race distances for world champions and in all race distances for Olympic champions. Longer (*i.e.*, 200 m and more) race distances were completed by younger (~20 years old for women and ~22 years old for men) champions than shorter (*i.e.*, 50 m and 100 m) race distances (~22 years old for women and ~24 years old for men). There was a sex difference in the age of champions of ~2 years with a mean age of ~21 and ~23 years for women and men, respectively. Swimming performance improved in most race distances for world and Olympic champions with a larger trend of increase in Olympic champions; (4) Conclusion: Swimmers at younger ages (<20 years) may benefit from training and competing in longer race distances (*i.e.*, 200 m and longer) before they change to shorter distances (*i.e.*, 50 m and 100 m) when they become older (>22 years).

Keywords: champions; age; performance; sex difference

1. Introduction

Twenty-six years ago, Schulz and Curnow investigated the age of Olympic gold medal winners in swimming, competing between 1896 and 1980 [1]. The average age in freestyle swimming was ~18 years for women and ~21 years for men [1]. This age remained stable for almost a century [1]. Nevertheless, over time humans have undergone changes in body dimensions such as body height, body mass and slenderness, and swimming performance has improved continuously across the years [2–4].

However, there is no recent study investigating the age of today's champions and the actual change of the age of peak swimming speed over time. In recent years, new swimming records were set continuously with a peak of new records at the World Championship in 2008 due to newly introduced swimsuits [5]. The full body swimsuits were banned worldwide by 1 January 2010. Considering long course championships, the fastest performance for women and men was obtained in 50 m freestyle at the World Championship in 2009. Britta Steffen finished in 23.73 s and Cesar Cielo in 21.08 s. The most recent world records were set in 2013 for women by Katie Ledecky [6,7] in the 800 m and 1500 m freestyle at age 16, by Ruta Meilutyte [8] in the 100 m breaststroke at age 16, and by Yuliya Efimova [9,10] in the 200 m breaststroke at age 21. For men, the latest world records were set at the World Championships in 2009. In total, 11 new records were achieved in that year for men, held in different strokes by Cesar Cielo [11,12] in the 50 m and 100 m freestyle at the age of 22; Paul Biedermann [13] in the 200 m freestyle at the age of 23; Lin Zhang [14] in the 800 m freestyle at the age of 22; Brenton Rickard [15] in the 100 m breaststroke at the age of 26; Daniel Gyurta [16] in the 200 m breaststroke at the age of 20; Junya Koga [17] in the 100 m backstroke at the age of 22; Aaron Peirsol [18] in the 200 m backstroke at the age of 18; Michael Phelps [19,20] in the 100 m and 200 m butterfly at the age of 24; and Ryan Lochte [21] in the 200 m individual medley at the age of 25. No new world record was set in 2013. Regarding the Olympic Games, the most recent Olympic records were set in 2012 for women by Ranomi Kromowidjojo in the 100 m freestyle at the age of 22; Allison Schmitt [22] in the 200 m freestyle at the age of 22; Camille Muffat [23] in the 400 m freestyle at the age of 23; Melissa Franklin [24,25] in the 100 m and 200 m backstroke at the age of 17; Dana Vollmer [26,27] in the 100 m butterfly at the age of 25; and Shiwen Ye [28,29] in the 200 m and 400 m individual medley at the age of 16. For men, the latest Olympic records were set in 2012 by Yang Sun [30] in the 400 m, 800 m, and 1,500 m freestyle at the age of 21; Cameron van der Burgh [31,32] in the 100 m breaststroke at the age of 24; by Metthew Grevers [33,34] in the 100 m backstroke at the age of 27; and by Michael Phelps [35] in the 200 m individual medley at the age of 27.

This last exceptional talent has four other unbroken Olympic records from 2008 in the 200 m freestyle [36], the 100 m [37] and 200 m [38] butterfly and the 400 m individual medley [39,40] set at the age of 23. Michael Phelps (USA) won 18 Olympic gold medals, two silver medals and two bronze medals [41]. He retired after the Olympic Games in London 2012 [42]. Nevertheless, Michael Phelps returned to consistent training in November 2013 [43,44]. In 2014, he won three gold and two silver medals at the Pan Pacific Championships in August [45]. Michael Phelps intends to compete in the Olympic Games in Rio de Janeiro in 2016 [46]. That would not be the first comeback in swimming history. Ian Thorpe (AUS) retired in 2006 at the age of 23 years after he won nine Olympic medals—a gold medal in the 400 m freestyle, in the 4 × 100 m and 4 × 200 m freestyle relay in 2000 at the age of 17, a silver medal in the 200 m freestyle, and in the 4 × 100 m medley relay in 2000 at 17 years of age, a gold medal in the freestyle 200 m and 400 m, a silver medal in the freestyle relay 4 × 200 m, and a bronze medal in the 100 m freestyle in 2004 at age 21 [47]. He made his first attempt at a comeback at the Olympic Games in London in 2012 at the age of 30, but failed. Ian Thorpe won nine Olympic medals (five gold medals, three silver medals, and one bronze medal) and 13 World Championship medals (11 gold medals, one silver medal, and one bronze medal) [48]. Recently, Thorpe talked about competing in the 2016 Rio Olympics [49]. In April 2014, he suffered from a serious infection after shoulder surgery [49], but he still hopes for a comeback [50]. Another swimmer who tried to make a comeback in swimming in earlier years was Mark Spitz (USA). His aim was a comeback at the Olympic Games in 1992 at over 42 years old—20 years after his last competition at the Olympic Games in Munich in 1972 [51]. Mark Spitz won in total nine gold medals, one silver medal, and one bronze medal at Olympic Games [52]. After Michael Phelps, who won eight gold medals in one competition at the Olympic Games in 2008 (Beijing), Mark Spitz is next with seven medals won at the Olympic Games in Munich in 1972. He failed in his comeback at the Olympic Games in 1992, being two seconds slower than the required qualifying time [53]. The Olympic champion Ed Moses, a member in the 4 × 100 m medley relay and silver medal winner in the breaststroke 100 m in 2000, wanted to join the Olympic team at the age of 32 in 2012, but failed [54,55].

These data show that records at World Championships and Olympic Games were achieved in athletes age 25 and younger. Michael Phelps (born 1985) plans his comeback at the age of 31 at the

Olympic Games in 2016. The question may be raised regarding whether he will be able to perform in such a way as to win a medal at that age. For example, Dara Torres (born 1967) showed that it is possible to win a medal in a comeback at the Olympic Games. At the age of 14, Torres set her first world record. At the age of 17 she was Olympic champion in her hometown of Los Angeles in the 1984 Olympic Games in the 4 $\times$ 100 m freestyle relay. At the age of 25, she left sport, only to participate seven years later in the 2000 Olympic Games in Sydney and win five more medals. In April 2006, she gave birth to her daughter Tessa. At the 2008 Olympic Games in Beijing, at age 41, Dara Torres won three silver medals (4 $\times$ 100 m freestyle relay, 50 m freestyle, and 4 $\times$ 100 m medley relay) [56]. Inspired by the recent decisions of different swimmers to make comebacks at a competitive level, with this study we aimed to systematically investigate the age of winners of Olympic Games (1992 to 2012) and World Championships (1994 to 2013) for all race distances and strokes.

2. Materials and Methods

2.1. Ethics Approval

All procedures used in the study were approved by the Institutional Review Board of Kanton St. Gallen, Switzerland, with a waiver of the requirement for informed consent of the participants given the fact that the study involved the analysis of publicly available data.

2.2. Data Sampling and Data Analysis

All data for this study were obtained from www.swimrankings.net. This web page records all swimming race results according to events such as World Championships and Olympic Games. During data sampling and preparation for analysis, we found that data before 1992 were not complete for all strokes and distances, and we therefore started data analysis from the year 1992 onward. Full data were available going back to 1992 for 202 female and 210 male champions (*i.e.*, 412 swimmers in total), 250 in the World Championships and 162 in the Olympic Games. Prior to 2001, the 1500 m freestyle was not raced by women in the World Championships. Therefore, we have a difference of two swimmers in the number of female and male athletes. In the Olympic Games, there was a difference of six swimmers in the number of athletes between both sexes due to the missing races in the 1500 m freestyle during the whole period. All race distances which are held both in the World Championships (1994–2013) and the Olympic Games (1992–2012) were included. We excluded the 50 m breaststroke, the 50 m backstroke, and the 50 m butterfly, which were only held in the World Championships. Therefore, the following race distances were included and analysed: freestyle (50 m, 100 m, 200 m, 400 m, 800 m, and 1500 m), breaststroke (100 m, 200 m), backstroke (100 m, 200 m), butterfly (100 m, 200 m), and individual medley (200 m, 400 m). We analyzed all listed strokes and distances in both sexes and both in the World Championships and the Olympic Games for changes in the age and swimming performance of all champions over the years. Race times were converted to swimming speed using the following equation: (swimming speed ($m \cdot s^{-1}$)) = (race distance (m))/(race time (s)). The age of the athletes was calculated from the date of birth given at the web page from www.swimrankings.net.

2.3. Statistical Analysis

Descriptive values were computed as mean $\pm$ standard deviation (SD) for continuous variables. Normal distribution was tested using a D'Agostino and Pearson *omnibus* normality test and homogeneity of variances was tested using a Levene's test. A MultiLayer Perceptron (MLP), which is a feed-forward Artificial Neural Network (ANN), with the hyperbolic tangent as activation function in the input/hidden layers, and the softmax activation function in the output layer and cross-entropy as error function, was used to assess the impact of each co-variable on the swimming performance, using speed as outcome, correcting for multiple participations of some athletes to the finals at World Championships or Olympic Games. Generalized mixed models with repeated measures, thereby correcting for multiple participations, were used to analyze the data and investigate a potential impact of changes in age on swimming performance. An initial mixed model was carried out, using speed as dependent variable and age, sex, country, contest (*i.e.*, World Championships *versus* Olympic Games), type of swimming strokes (*i.e.*, freestyle, breaststroke, backstroke, butterfly, and individual medley) and calendar year as independent variables.

Then, single and multi-level regression analyses were carried out for each co-variable, correcting for age of athletes in order to prevent a misinterpretation of the "age-effect" as a "time-effect" and to avoid the impact of a cluster-effect on the results regarding the analysis of age of peak swimming performance and swimming performance. To investigate whether the trend in swimming performance over time was linear or non-linear (*i.e.*, polynomial), we additionally calculated the non-linear regression model that fits the data best. The result of the linear regression analysis was compared to the best-fit result of the non-linear analysis using Akaike's Information Criteria (AIC) and an F-test to show which model would be the most appropriate to explain the trend of the data.

Statistical analyses were performed using IBM SPSS Statistics (Version 22, IBM SPSS, Chicago, IL, USA) and GraphPad Prism (Version 6.01, GraphPad Software, La Jolla, CA, USA). Significance was accepted at $p < 0.05$ (two-sided for t-tests).

3. Results

In total, data were available for 412 performances between 1992 and 2013 with 202 women (49%) and 210 men (51%), of which 250 were competing in the World Championships and 162 in the Olympic Games. All the data (*i.e.*, age, swim speed) were characterized by normal distribution and homogeneity of variances.

3.1. *MultiLayer Perceptron Model*

MLP model proved to be a good-quality model (Figure 1). Age came out as the second variable in terms of normalized importance in predicting speed as outcome.

3.2. *Impact of Predictor Variables on Speed*

Initially, a mixed model was performed, using speed as dependent variable and all the different co-variables as independent variables, namely, sex, age, country, contest (*i.e.*, World Championship *versus* Olympic Games), type of stroke (*i.e.*, freestyle, breaststroke, backstroke, butterfly, and individual medley) and calendar year. Speed depended on all these variables but the contest ($p = 0.211$, not statistically significant) (Tables 1–3). However, in this study, we will specifically focus on the impact of age on swimming performances, while the contribution of the other co-variables will be investigated in separated contributions, currently under preparation.

3.3. *Changes in the Ages of the Champions*

The age of World champions increased over the years in the 400 m freestyle for women (Figure 2) and in the 100 m breaststroke for men (Figure 3), but remained stable (Table 4) in all other disciplines (Figures 2 and 3). Regarding the Olympic champions, the age remained stable (Table 5) in all disciplines (Figures 4 and 5). Longer race distances (*i.e.*, 200 m and over) were completed by younger champions (~20 years for women and ~22 years for men) than shorter (*i.e.*, 50 m and 100 m) race distances (~22 years for women and ~24 years for men) for each stroke and in both women and men (Tables 4 and 5). Overall, the mean ages of champions were 21 $\pm$ 3.5 years for women (minimum of 14 years, maximum of 34 years; 21 $\pm$ 3.4 at the World Championships and 21 $\pm$ 3.6 years at the Olympic Games) and 23 $\pm$ 2.8 years for men (minimum of 16 years, maximum of 32 years; 23 $\pm$ 3.0 years at the World Championships and 23 $\pm$ 2.5 years at the Olympic Games). The mean sex difference in the age of champions was ~2 years in both the World Championships and the Olympic Games, even if, when correcting for all the co-variables, the type of contest had no statistically significant impact on swimming performance (Tables 1 and 2).

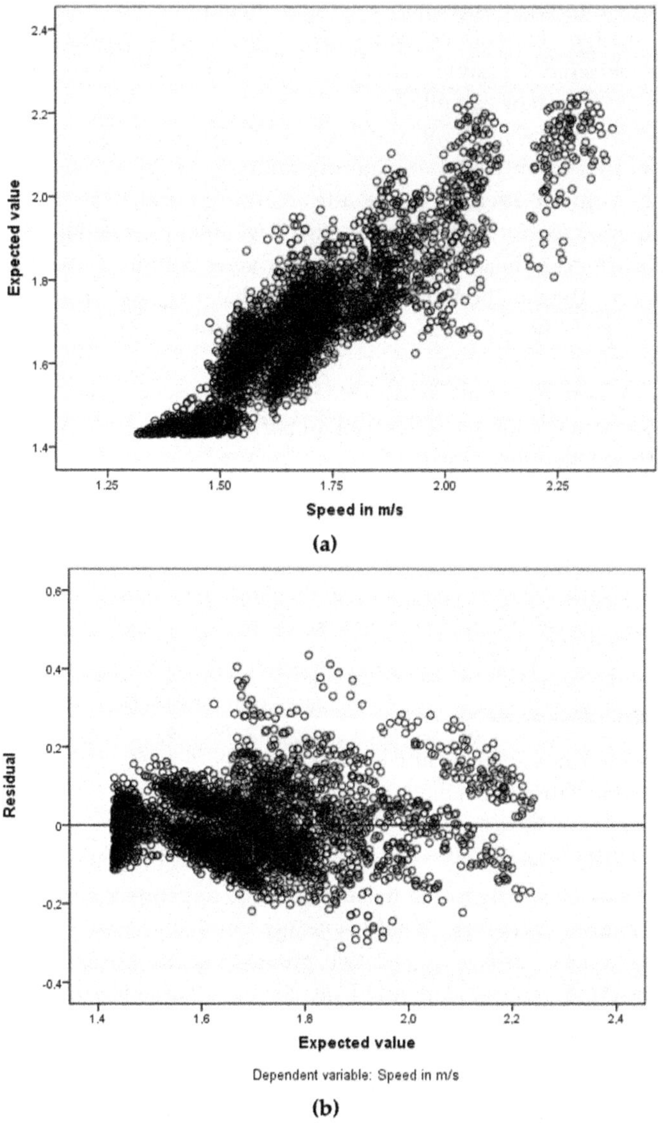

Figure 1. Quality of the MultiLayer Perceptron (MLP) model (observed values *versus* expected values scatterplot) (**a**) and quality of the MLP model (residual *versus* expected values scatterplot) (**b**).

Table 1. Importance of independent variables from the Multi-Layer Perceptron Analysis, using speed as outcome and correcting for multiple participations of athletes to finals of World Championship and Olympic Games.

Variable	Importance	Normalized Importance
Contest (*i.e.*, World Championship *versus* Olympic Games)	0.001	0.5%
Stroke (*i.e.*, freestyle, breaststroke, backstroke, butterfly, and individual medley)	0.265	100.0%
Sex	0.109	41.1%
Country	0.168	63.5%
Year	0.023	8.8%
Age	0.190	71.5%

Table 2. Fixed effects of the mixed model with speed as dependent variable and age, sex, country, calendar year, contest (*i.e.*, World Championships *versus* Olympic Games) and stroke (*i.e.*, freestyle, breaststroke, backstroke, butterfly, and individual medley) as independent variables.

Parameters	*F*-Statistics	*p*-Value
Intercept	23.958	<0.0001
World Championship *versus* Olympic Games	1.564	0.211
Contest	603.892	<0.0001
Sex	937.596	<0.0001
Country	7.685	<0.0001
Year	46.921	<0.0001
Age	167.531	<0.0001

Table 3. Estimates of the mixed model with speed as dependent variable and age, sex, country, calendar year, contest (*i.e.*, World Championship *versus* Olympic Games) and stroke (*i.e.*, freestyle, breaststroke, backstroke, butterfly, and individual medley) as independent variables.

Parameter	Estimate	SE	*T*	*p*	95% Confidence Interval	
					Lower Limit	Upper Limit
Intercept	−3.682	0.741	−4.967	<0.0001	−5.135	−2.229
World Championship	−0.006	0.005	−1.251	0.211	−0.015	0.003
Freestyle	0.245	0.007	35.561	<0.0001	0.232	0.259
Breaststroke	−0.047	0.008	−5.643	<0.0001	−0.063	−0.030
Backstroke	0.138	0.008	16.670	<0.0001	0.122	0.154
Butterfly	0.163	0.008	19.601	<0.0001	0.146	0.179
Females	−0.147	0.005	−30.620	<0.0001	−0.156	−0.137
(Country = ALG)	0.252	0.077	3.266	0.001	0.101	0.403
(Country = ARG)	−0.038	0.062	−0.616	0.538	−0.161	0.084
(Country = AUS)	0.021	0.030	0.700	0.484	−0.037	0.078
(Country = AUT)	0.011	0.037	0.284	0.777	−0.063	0.084
(Country = BAH)	0.300	0.092	3.255	0.001	0.119	0.481
(Country = BAR)	0.218	0.127	1.715	0.086	−0.031	0.467
(Country = BEL)	−0.014	0.046	−0.311	0.756	−0.105	0.076
(Country = BLR)	0.127	0.041	3.091	0.002	0.046	0.207
(Country = BRA)	0.140	0.034	4.164	<0.0001	0.074	0.206
(Country = BUL)	0.069	0.127	0.542	0.588	−0.181	0.318
(Country = CAN)	−0.014	0.031	−0.451	0.652	−0.075	0.047
(Country = CHI)	−0.196	0.068	−2.876	0.004	−0.330	−0.062
(Country = CHN)	0.023	0.030	0.758	0.449	−0.037	0.083
(Country = CRC)	−0.093	0.045	−2.078	0.038	−0.182	−0.005
(Country = CRO)	0.134	0.046	2.912	0.004	0.044	0.224
(Country = CUB)	0.060	0.053	1.136	0.256	−0.043	0.163
(Country = CZE)	−0.031	0.050	−0.625	0.532	−0.130	0.067
(Country = DEN)	−0.011	0.034	−0.322	0.747	−0.077	0.055
(Country = ESP)	−0.044	0.034	−1.288	0.198	−0.110	0.023
(Country = EST)	0.232	0.127	1.825	0.068	−0.017	0.482
(Country = EUN)	0.078	0.039	1.981	0.048	0.001	0.154
(Country = FAR)	−0.180	0.069	−2.633	0.009	−0.315	−0.046
(Country = FIN)	0.053	0.046	1.153	0.249	−0.037	0.143
(Country = FRA)	0.043	0.031	1.394	0.163	−0.018	0.104
(Country = GBR)	−0.027	0.030	−0.887	0.375	−0.086	0.032
(Country = GER)	−0.004	0.030	−0.142	0.887	−0.063	0.055
(Country = GRE)	−0.047	0.042	−1.113	0.266	−0.130	0.036

Table 3. *Cont.*

Parameter	Estimate	SE	*T*	*p*	95% Confidence Interval	
					Lower Limit	Upper Limit
(Country = HUN)	0.008	0.031	0.261	0.794	−0.052	0.068
(Country = IRL)	−0.078	0.058	−1.340	0.180	−0.192	0.036
(Country = ISL)	0.017	0.077	0.226	0.821	−0.134	0.169
(Country = ISR)	0.062	0.055	1.125	0.261	−0.046	0.170
(Country = ITA)	−0.036	0.031	−1.167	0.243	−0.097	0.025
(Country = JAM)	−0.009	0.092	−0.093	0.926	−0.190	0.172
(Country = JPN)	−0.003	0.030	−0.090	0.928	−0.061	0.056
(Country = KAZ)	−0.005	0.077	−0.067	0.947	−0.157	0.147
(Country = KEN)	0.147	0.069	2.135	0.033	0.012	0.281
(Country = KOR)	−0.044	0.045	−0.979	0.328	−0.133	0.044
(Country = LTU)	0.100	0.046	2.164	0.031	0.009	0.190
(Country = MAS)	0.063	0.127	0.497	0.619	−0.186	0.312
(Country = MDA)	−0.051	0.092	−0.551	0.582	−0.232	0.130
(Country = NED)	0.115	0.032	3.625	<0.0001	0.053	0.177
(Country = NOR)	−0.015	0.049	−0.302	0.763	−0.110	0.081
(Country = NZL)	−0.058	0.037	−1.555	0.120	−0.131	0.015
(Country = PNG)	0.100	0.127	0.783	0.434	−0.150	0.349
(Country = POL)	−0.004	0.033	−0.110	0.912	−0.068	0.061
(Country = PUR)	0.176	0.059	3.020	0.003	0.062	0.291
(Country = ROU)	−0.066	0.034	−1.957	0.050	−0.132	0.000
(Country = RSA)	0.071	0.033	2.187	0.029	0.007	0.135
(Country = RUS)	0.031	0.031	1.011	0.312	−0.029	0.091
(Country = SIN)	0.124	0.127	0.975	0.330	−0.125	0.373
(Country = SLO)	−0.043	0.047	−0.912	0.362	−0.135	0.050
(Country = SRB)	0.065	0.055	1.176	0.240	−0.043	0.173
(Country = SUI)	−0.091	0.049	−1.872	0.061	−0.187	0.004
(Country = SUR)	0.079	0.092	0.855	0.393	−0.102	0.260
(Country = SVK)	0.073	0.041	1.790	0.074	−0.007	0.154
(Country = SWE)	0.133	0.033	3.986	<0.0001	0.068	0.199
(Country = TCH)	−0.088	0.127	−0.693	0.488	−0.338	0.161
(Country = TPE)	0.006	0.127	0.050	0.960	−0.243	0.256
(Country = TRI)	0.250	0.055	4.547	<0.0001	0.142	0.358
(Country = TUN)	−0.129	0.041	−3.168	0.002	−0.208	−0.049
(Country = UKR)	0.019	0.033	0.585	0.559	−0.045	0.084
(Country = USA)	0.033	0.029	1.142	0.254	−0.024	0.091
(Country = VEN)	0.072	0.055	1.301	0.193	−0.036	0.180
(Country = YUG)	0.194	0.127	1.522	0.128	−0.056	0.443
(Country = ZIM) *reference*	–	–	–	–	–	–
Year	0.003	0.000	6.850	<0.0001	0.002	0.003
Age	0.009	0.002	12.943	<0.0001	0.008	0.010

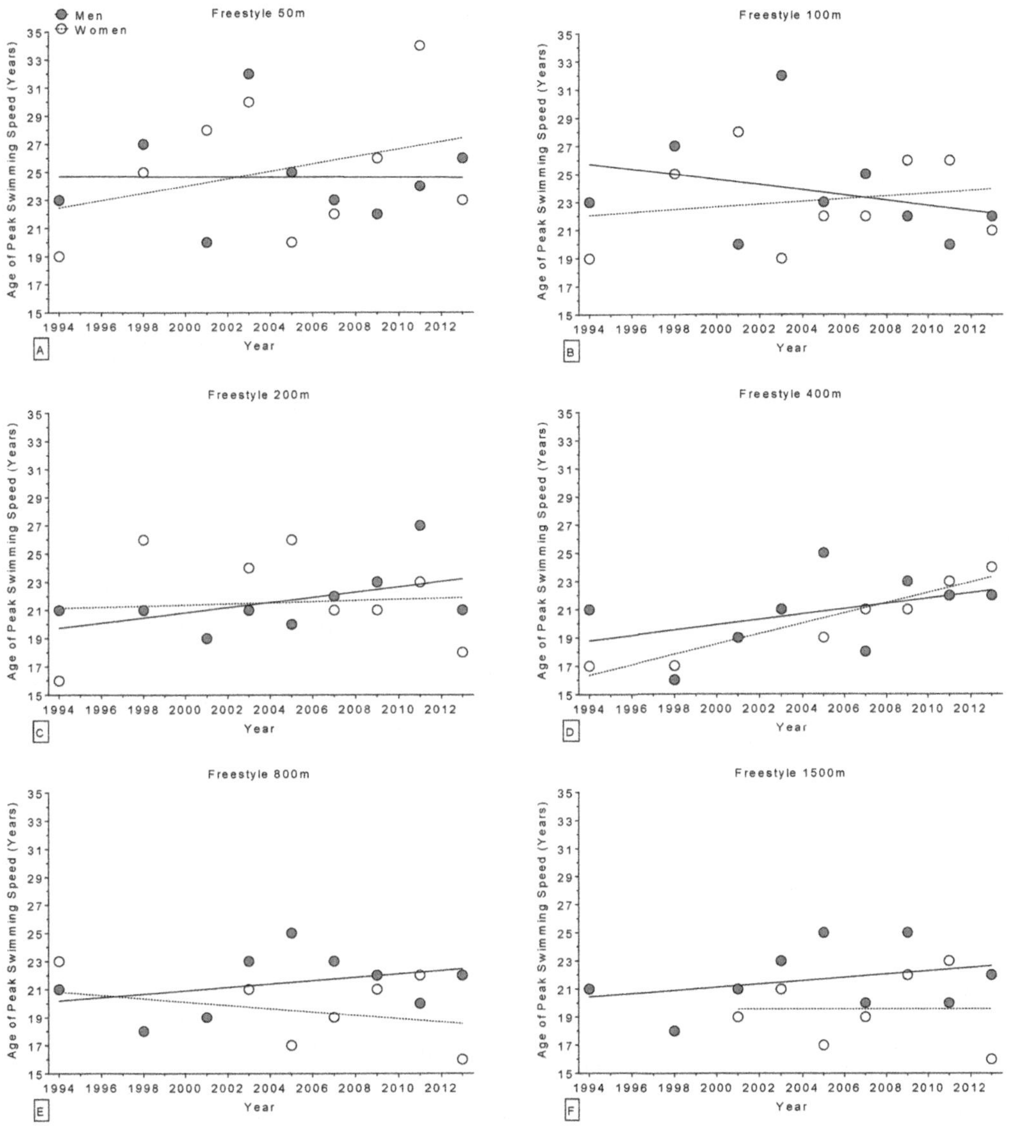

Figure 2. Change in the age of world champions (1994–2013) over time for freestyle 50 m (**Panel A**); 100 m (**Panel B**); 200 m (**Panel C**); 400 m (**Panel D**); 800 m (**Panel E**); and 1500 m (**Panel F**).

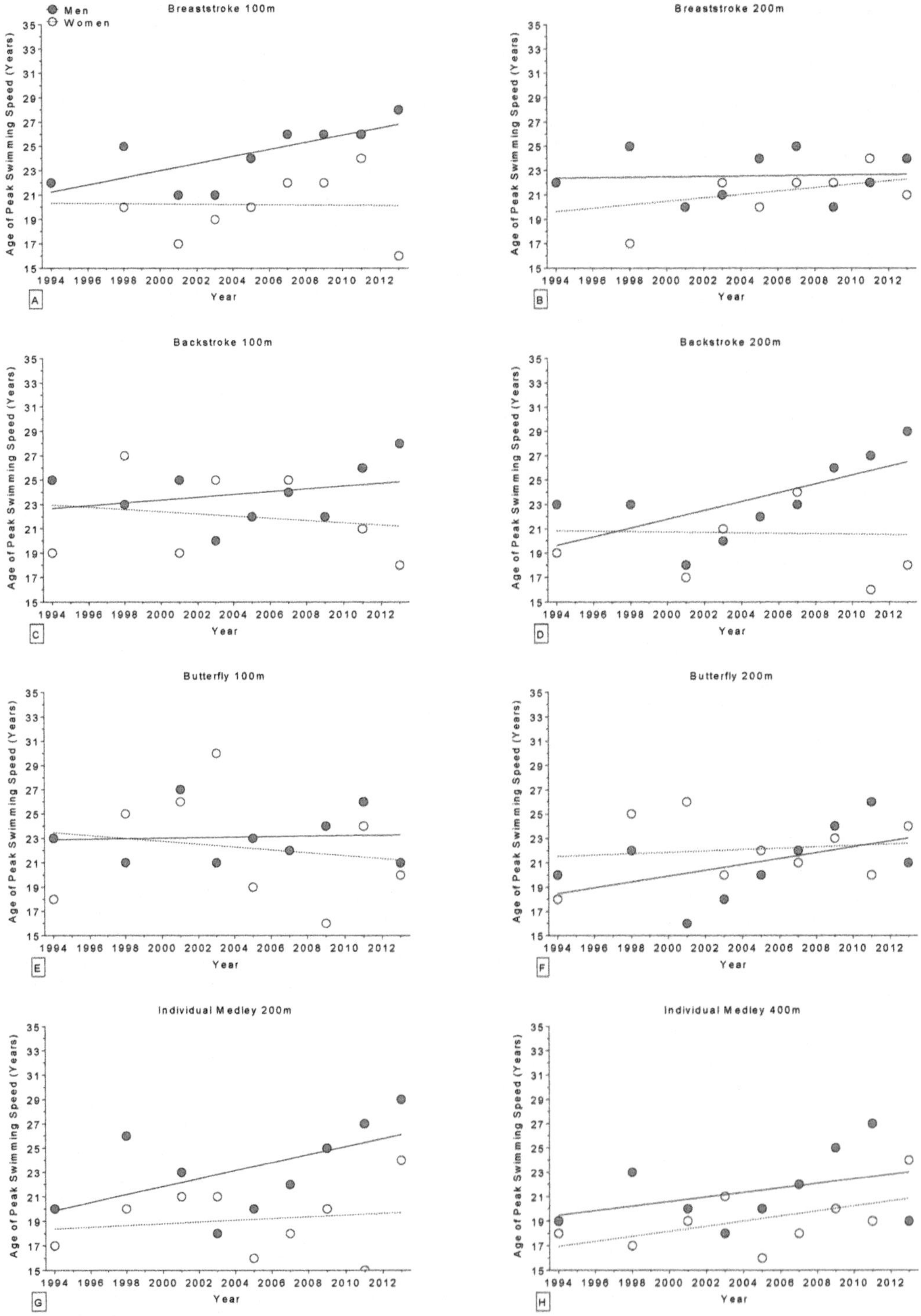

Figure 3. Change in the age of world champions (1994–2013) over time for 100 m breaststroke (**Panel A**); 200 m breaststroke (**Panel B**); 100 m backstroke (**Panel C**); 200 m backstroke (**Panel D**); 100 m butterfly (**Panel E**); 200 m butterfly (**Panel F**); 200 m individual medley (**Panel G**); and 400 m individual medley (**Panel H**).

Table 4. Changes in the age (years) of World champions over time.

Stroke and Distance	Sex	1994	Age	2013
		Freestyle		
50 m	Women	†	24.0 ± 2.1	†
	Men	†	22.6 ± 1.5	†
100 m	Women	†	22.8 ± 1.3	†
	Men	†	24.2 ± 1.0	†
200 m	Women	†	21.7 ± 1.2	†
	Men	†	22. ± 0.7	†
400 m	Women	21.6 ± 0.9	–	21.6 ± 0.9
	Men	†	22.3 ± 1.4	†
800 m	Women	†	20.9 ± 1.1	†
	Men	†	21.8 ± 3.1	†
1500 m	Women	†	21.8 ± 4.7	†
	Men	†	21.9 ± 1.1	†
		Breaststroke		
100 m	Women	†	21.3 ± 1.6	†
	Men	23.0 ± 2.2	–	25.3 ± 3.8
200 m	Women	†	21.8 ± 4.7	†
	Men	†	22.9 ± 0.3	†
		Backstroke		
100 m	Women	†	21.4 ± 0.9	†
	Men	†	23.2 ± 1.2	†
200 m	Women	†	20.3 ± 1.2	†
	Men	†	23.2 ± 1.0	†
		Butterfly		
100 m	Women	†	22.2 ± 1.2	†
	Men	†	22.5 ± 2.6	†
200 m	Women	†	20.0 ± 2.7	†
	Men	†	21.0 ± 2.3	†
		Individual Medley		
200 m	Women	†	21.2 ± 0.8	†
	Men	†	23.7 ± 1.5	†
400 m	Women	†	20.4 ± 1.0	†
	Men	†	22.1 ± 0.9	†

Note: † = no change between 1992 and 2013.

Table 5. Changes in the age (years) of Olympic champions over time.

Stroke and Distance	Sex	1992	Age	2012
		Freestyle		
50 m	Women	†	26.9 ± 5.1	†
	Men	†	27.1 ± 3.6	†
100 m	Women	†	23.3 ± 2.0	†
	Men	†	24.3 ± 1.0	†
200 m	Women	†	21.3 ± 1.6	†
	Men	†	22.5 ± 0.5	†
400 m	Women	†	21.7 ± 1.0	†
	Men	†	22.3 ± 1.0	†
800 m	Women	†	21.2 ± 1.8	†
	Men	†	22.3 ± 0.8	†
1500 m	Women	–	–	–
	Men	†	22.3 ± 0.8	†
		Breaststroke		
100 m	Women	†	21.5 ± 1.0	†
	Men	†	26.4 ± 3.3	†
200 m	Women	†	20.3 ± 4.5	†
	Men	†	23.3 ± 1.6	†
		Backstroke		
100 m	Women	†	18.0 ± 2.3	†
	Men	†	23.8 ± 1.2	†
200 m	Women	†	21.2 ± 0.8	†
	Men	†	23.3 ± 1.2	†
		Butterfly		
100 m	Women	†	23.0 ± 2.9	†
	Men	†	23.5 ± 1.0	†
200 m	Women	†	21.7 ± 1.4	†
	Men	†	21.3 ± 3.2	†
		Individual Medley		
200 m	Women	†	22.0 ± 1.3	†
	Men	†	23.7 ± 2.1	†
400 m	Women	†	20.0 ± 0.9	†
	Men	†	22.7 ± 1.4	†

Note: † = no change between 1992 and 2012.

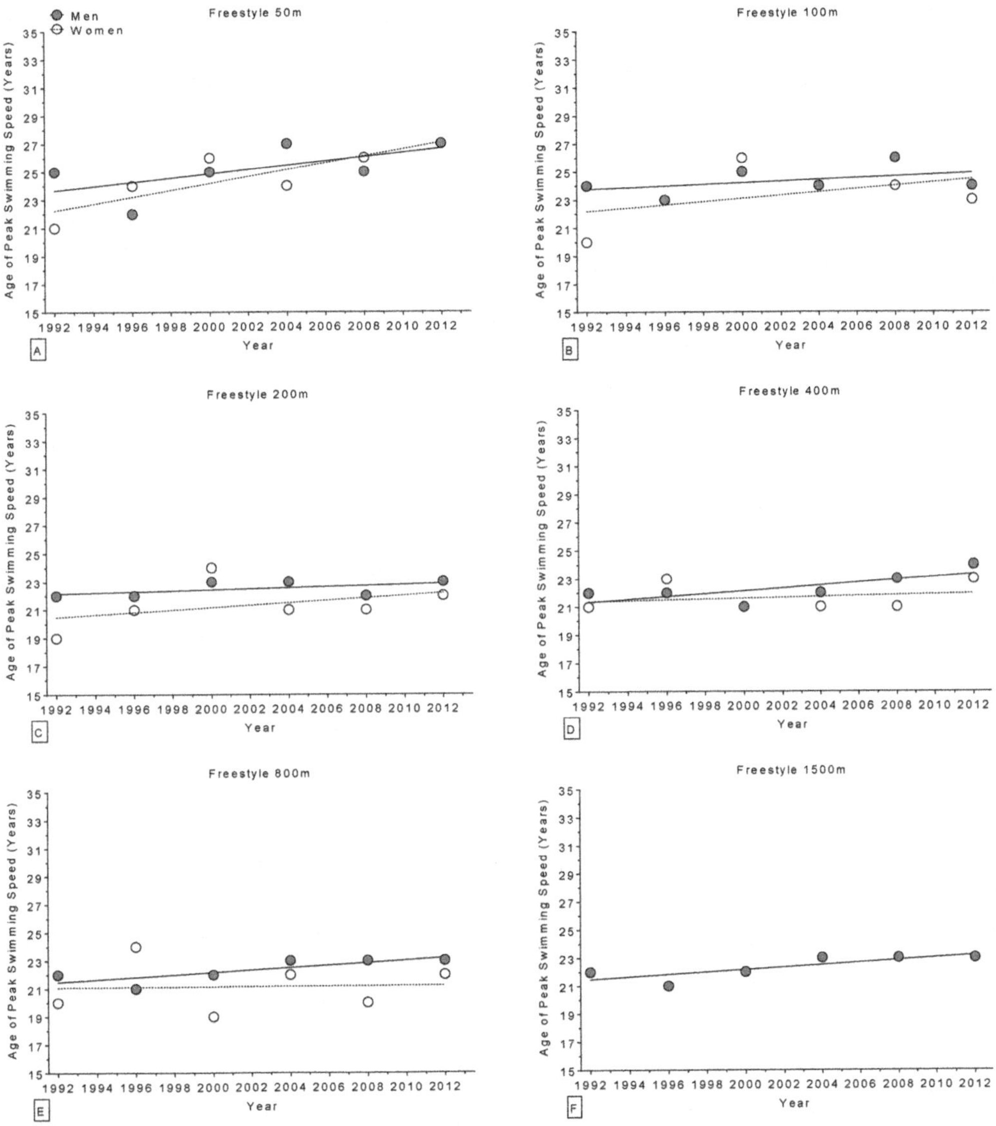

Figure 4. Change in the age of Olympic champions (1992–2012) over time in freestyle for 50 m (**Panel A**); 100 m (**Panel B**); 200 m (**Panel C**); 400 m (**Panel D**); 800 m (**Panel E**); and 1500 m (**Panel F**).

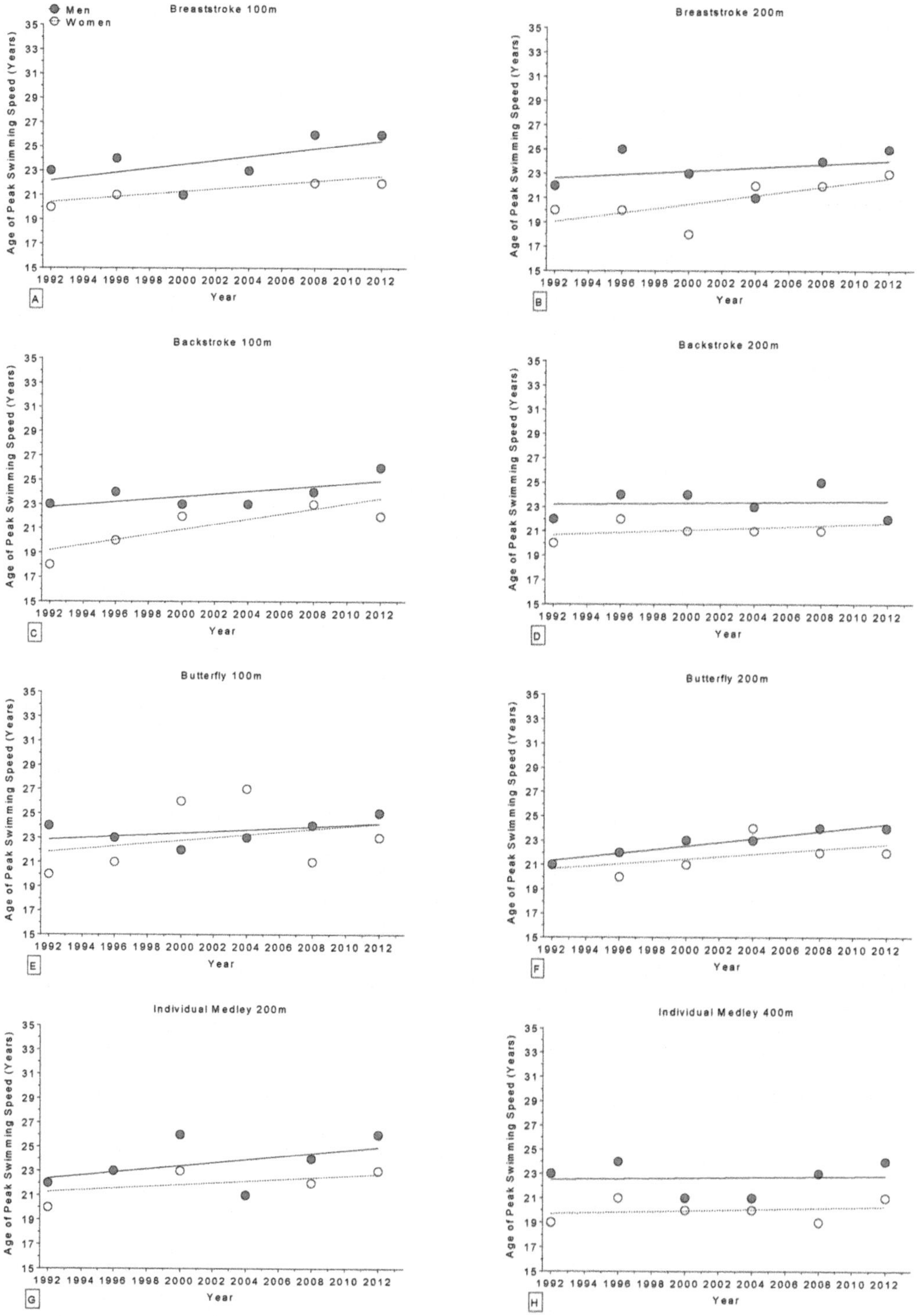

Figure 5. Change in the age of Olympic champions (1992–2012) over time for 100 m breaststroke (**Panel A**); 200 m breaststroke (**Panel B**); 100 m backstroke (**Panel C**); 200 m backstroke (**Panel D**); 100 m butterfly (**Panel E**); 200 m butterfly (**Panel F**); 200 m individual medley (**Panel G**); and 400 m individual medley (**Panel H**).

3.4. Changes in Swimming Performances across the Years

In world champions, swimming performance improved linearly and significantly across calendar years (Table 6) in 21 of 28 distances of freestyle (Figure 6), breaststroke, backstroke, butterfly and individual medley (Figure 7), with the exception of one non-linear increase in the 200 m backstroke for women. Regarding the Olympic champions, swimming performance improved significantly across calendar years (Table 7) in 16 of 27 distances of freestyle (Figure 8), breaststroke, backstroke, butterfly and individual medley (Figure 9). All results were corrected for co-variables and remained unmodified.

Table 6. Multi-level regression analyses for change in swimming performance of world champions using speed as dependent variable (values broken down for stroke and sex) and correcting for multiple participations and the other co-variables.

Stroke and Distance	Sex	*B*	SE (*B*)	Stand. ß	*T*	*p*
			Freestyle			
50 m	Women	0.004	0.002	0.693	2.206	0.070
	Men	0.006	0.001	0.846	3.997	0.007
100 m	Women	0.004	0.001	0.755	2.747	0.033
	Men	0.004	0.001	0.768	3.293	0.017
200 m	Women	0.003	0.001	0.694	2.844	0.029
	Men	0.004	0.002	0.846	2.797	0.031
400 m	Women	0.005	0.002	1.282	2.335	0.058
	Men	0.001	0.001	0.259	0.672	0.527
800 m	Women	0.003	0.000	0.985	7.017	<0.001
	Men	0.002	0.001	0.593	1.754	0.130
1500 m	Women	0.003	0.001	0.906	4.285	0.013
	Men	0.001	0.001	0.514	1.478	0.190
			Breaststroke			
100 m	Women	0.005	0.001	0.943	7.108	<0.001
	Men	0.005	0.001	1.126	6.187	0.001
200 m	Women	0.004	0.000	1.022	8.260	<0.001
	Men	0.004	0.000	0.926	9.188	<0.001
			Backstroke			
100 m	Women	0.004	0.001	0.800	3.970	0.007
	Men	0.006	0.001	1.003	8.373	<0.001
200 m	Women	0.003	0.001	0.730	2.646	0.038
	Men	0.005	0.001	0.854	3.346	0.016
			Butterfly			
100 m	Women	0.004	0.000	0.905	9.760	<0.001
	Men	0.006	0.002	0.827	3.590	0.011
200 m	Women	0.002	0.001	0.769	3.002	0.024
	Men	0.003	0.001	0.687	2.049	0.086
			Individual medley			
200 m	Women	0.003	0.001	0.754	2.930	0.026
	Men	0.006	0.001	1.037	4.527	0.004
400 m	Women	0.003	0.001	0.902	4.589	0.004
	Men	0.002	0.001	0.761	2.697	0.036

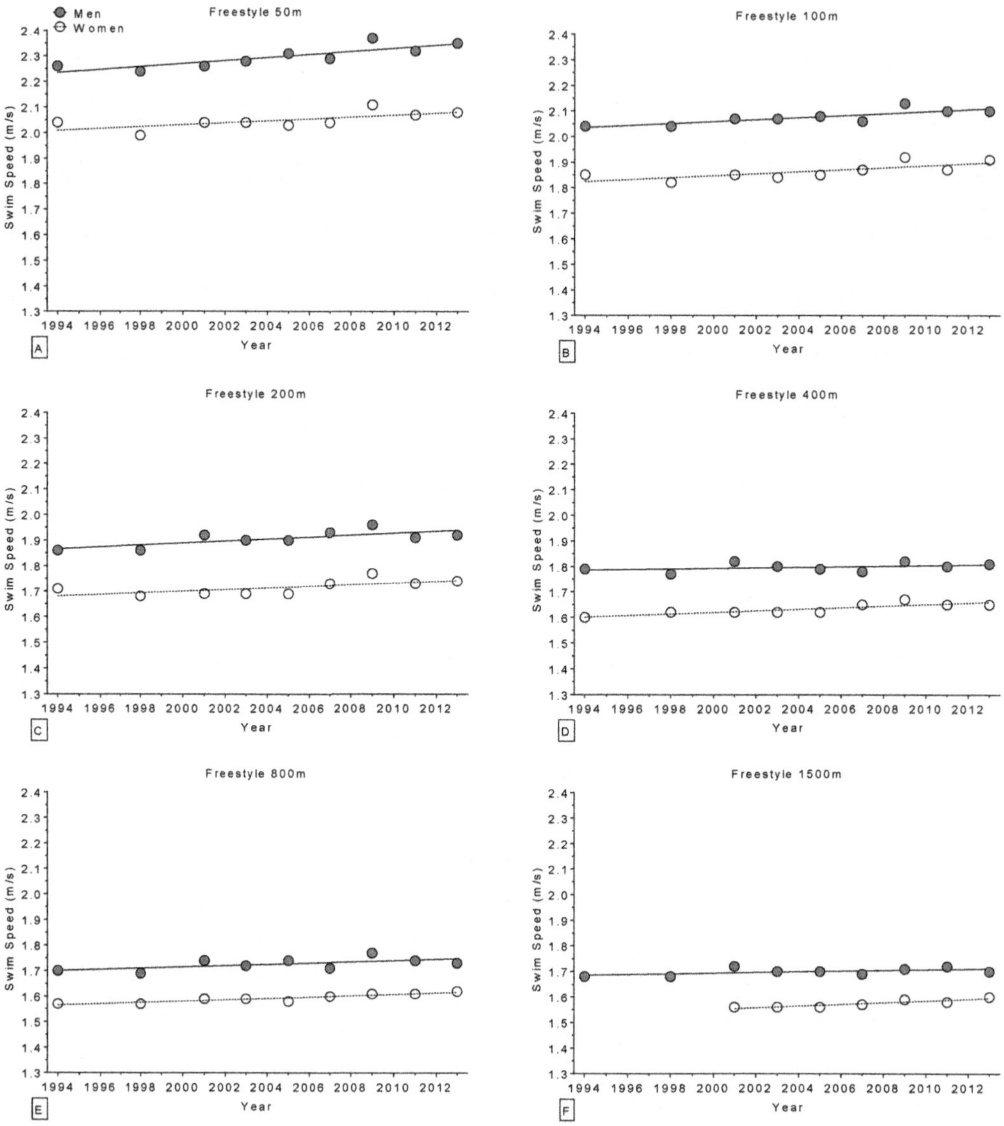

Figure 6. Change in freestyle swimming speed over time in world champions (1994–2013) for 50 m (**Panel A**); 100 m (**Panel B**); 200 m (**Panel C**); 400 m (**Panel D**); 800 m (**Panel E**); and 1500 m (**Panel F**).

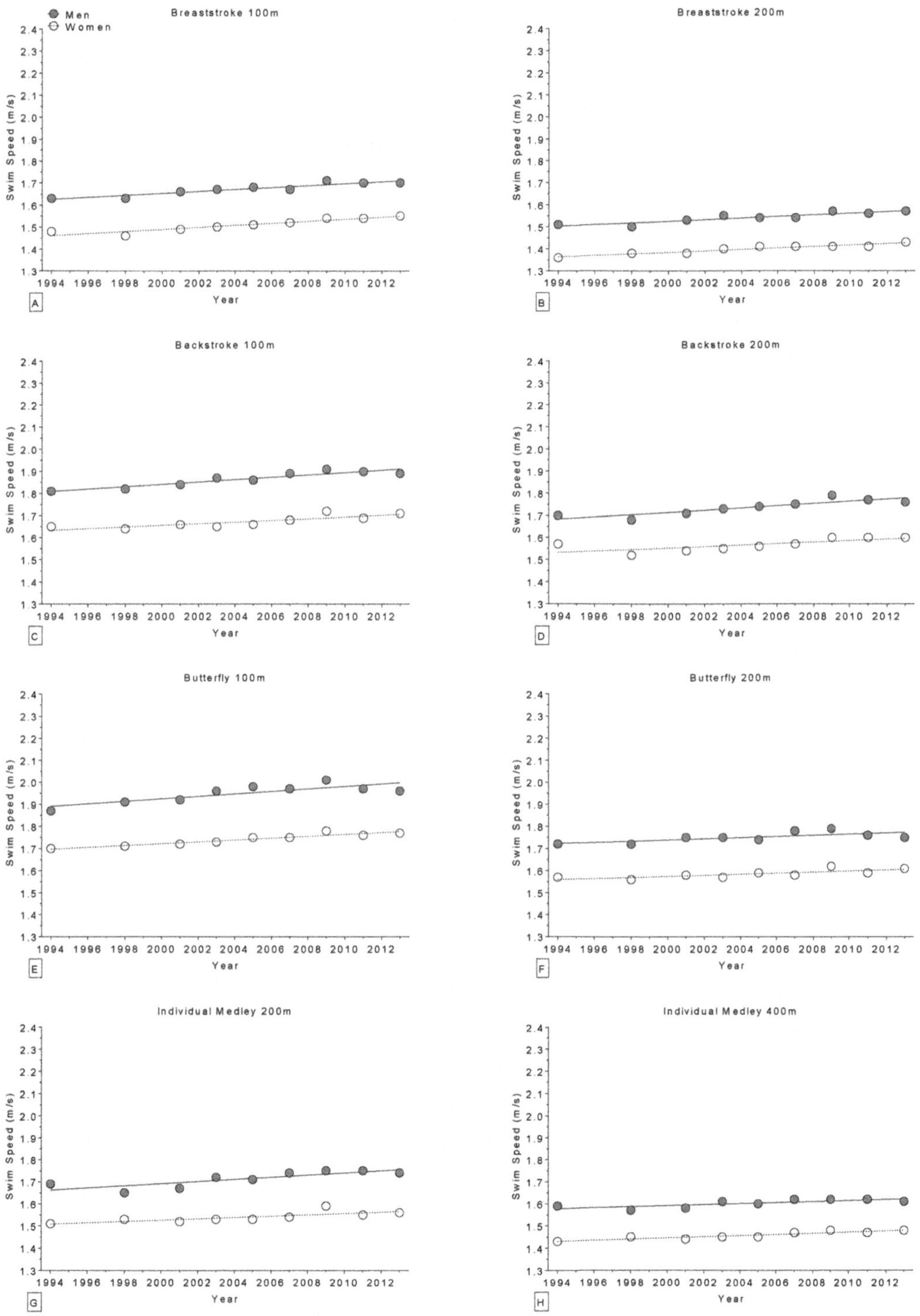

Figure 7. Change in swimming speed over time in world champions (1994–2013) for 100 m breaststroke (**Panel** A); 200 m breaststroke (**Panel B**); 100 m backstroke (**Panel C**); 200 m backstroke (**Panel D**); 100 m butterfly (**Panel E**); 200 m butterfly (**Panel F**); 200 m individual medley (**Panel G**); and 400 m individual medley (**Panel H**).

Table 7. Multi-level regression analyses for change in swimming performance of the Olympic champions using speed as dependent variable (values broken down for stroke and sex) and correcting for multiple participations and the other co-variables

Stroke and Distance	Sex	*B*	SE (*B*)	Stand. *ß*	*T*	*p*
			Freestyle			
50 m	Women	0.004	0.001	0.884	2.822	0.067
	Men	0.004	0.001	0.826	2.862	0.064
100 m	Women	0.003	0.000	0.914	8.164	0.004
	Men	0.004	0.001	0.909	3.496	0.040
200 m	Women	0.003	0.001	0.737	2.468	0.090
	Men	0.004	0.001	0.923	4.636	0.019
400 m	Women	0.002	0.000	1.010	4.756	0.018
	Men	0.003	0.001	0.847	2.710	0.073
800 m	Women	0.002	0.001	0.891	3.354	0.044
	Men	0.001	0.001	0.483	1.083	0.358
1500 m	Women	–	–	–	–	–
	Men	0.002	0.001	0.898	2.561	0.083
			Breaststroke			
100 m	Women	0.003	0.000	1.003	8.998	0.003
	Men	0.003	0.001	0.758	5.260	0.013
200 m	Women	0.004	0.001	1.053	3.885	0.030
	Men	0.003	0.001	0.798	2.410	0.095
			Backstroke			
100 m	Women	0.003	0.001	0.839	2.966	0.059
	Men	0.003	0.001	0.769	4.159	0.025
200 m	Women	0.002	0.001	0.684	1.604	0.207
	Men	0.004	0.001	0.961	6.540	0.007
			Butterfly			
100 m	Women	0.004	0.002	0.778	2.057	0.132
	Men	0.004	0.001	0.844	4.513	0.020
200 m	Women	0.003	0.001	0.958	5.700	0.011
	Men	0.004	0.001	1.030	3.669	0.035
			Individual medley			
200 m	Women	0.002	0.001	0.500	2.025	0.136
	Men	0.005	0.001	0.956	6.424	0.008
400 m	Women	0.002	0.000	0.696	6.724	0.007
	Men	0.004	0.001	0.962	5.072	0.015

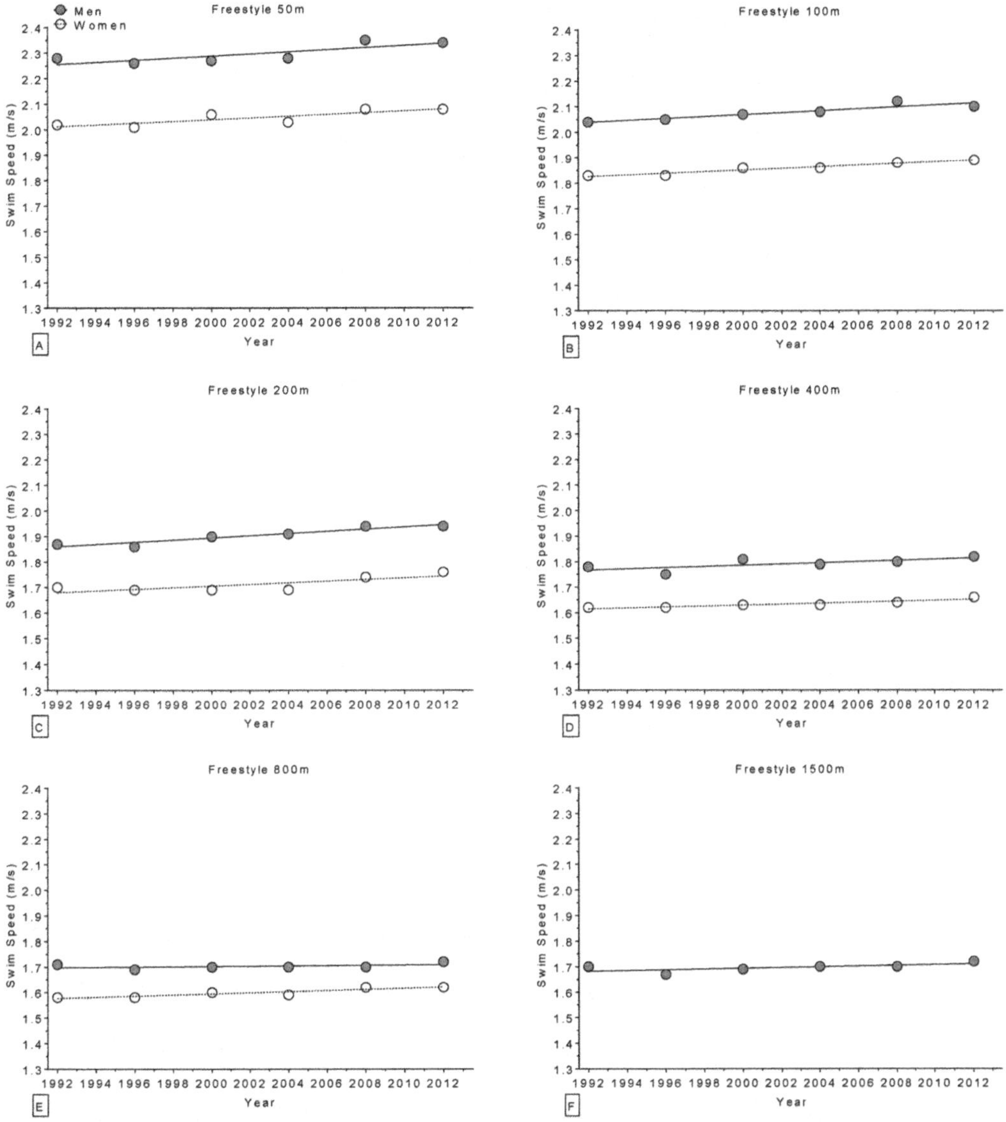

Figure 8. Change in freestyle swimming speed over time in Olympic champions (1992–2012) for 50 m (**Panel A**); 100 m (**Panel B**); 200 m (**Panel C**); 400 m (**Panel D**); 800 m (**Panel E**); and 1500 m (**Panel F**).

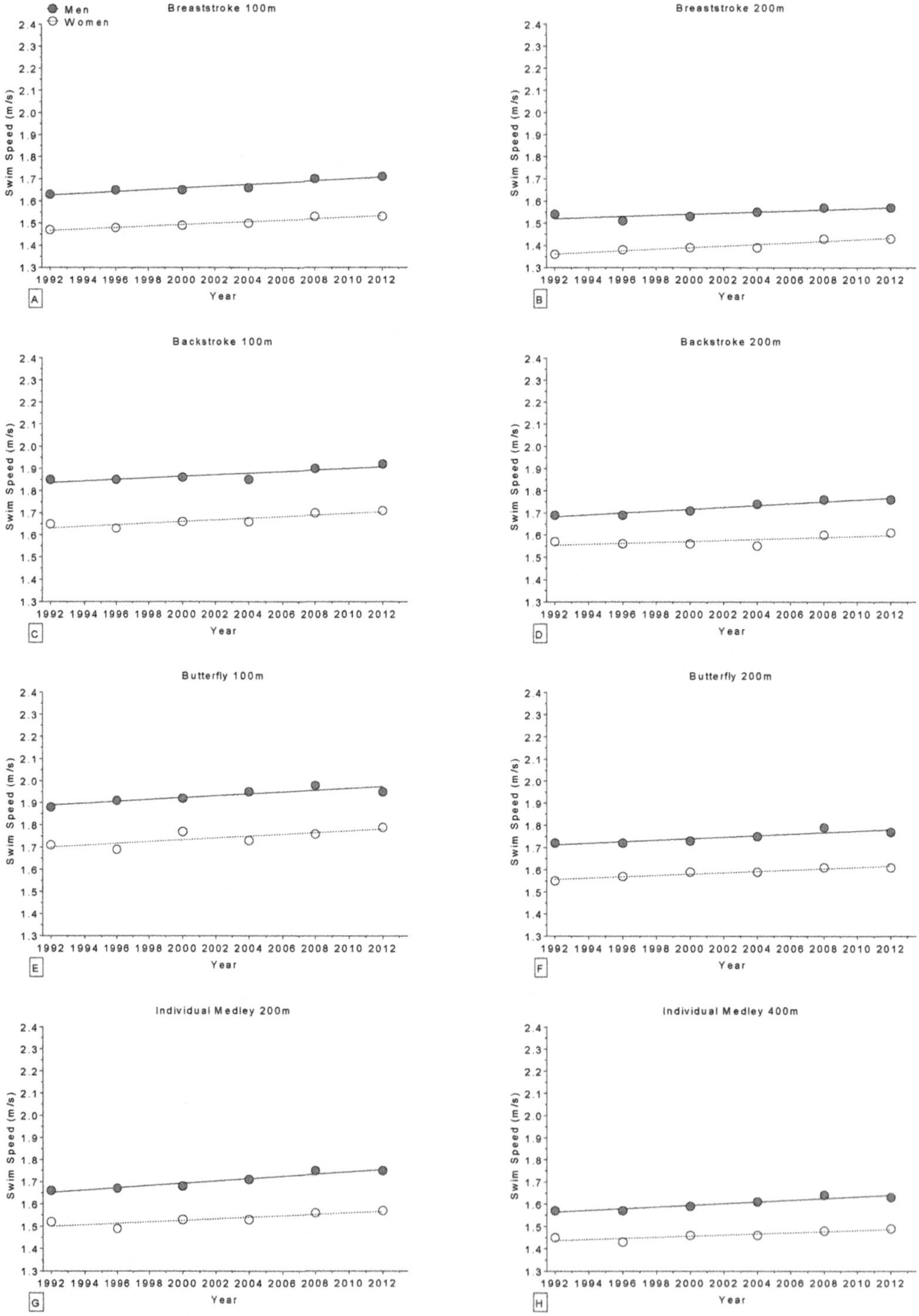

Figure 9. Change in swimming speed over time in Olympic champions (1992–2012) for 100 m breaststroke (**Panel A**); 200 m breaststroke (**Panel B**); 100 m backstroke (**Panel C**); 200 m backstroke (**Panel D**); 100 m butterfly (**Panel E**); 200 m butterfly (**Panel F**); 200 m individual medley (**Panel G**); and 400 m individual medley (**Panel H**).

4. Discussion

The present study examined the changes in age and swimming performance of female and male world and Olympic champions for all strokes and race distances in indoor, long course pools. The main findings were: (1) the age of champions remained stable in most race distances; (2) longer race distances (*i.e.*, 200 m and over) were completed by younger champions than shorter race distances (*i.e.*, 50 m and 100 m) for each stroke, and in both women and men; (3) female champions were ~2 years younger than male champions with a mean age of ~21 and ~23 years for women and men, respectively; (4) swimming performance improved in most race distances for world and Olympic champions, but remained stable in several race distances.

4.1. Unchanged Age of Peak Swimming Performance in Champions over Time

A first important finding was that the age of peak swimming performance for champions at the world class level remained stable in most strokes and race distances. The only increases in the age of world champions were found in the freestyle 400 m for women and in the breaststroke 100 m for men. Schulz and Curnow described the age of peak performance of Olympic gold medal winners as unchanged at ~18 years for women and ~21 years for men for almost a century [1]. In comparison with this, the present champions competing in the last ~20 years are ~2–3 years older, with a mean age of 21 $\pm$ 3.5 years in women and 23 $\pm$ 2.8 years in men.

Nevertheless, there are no more studies investigating the champions. However, several studies focus on top swimmers [57–63] for different strokes and distances. For example, Allen *et al.* focused on the top 16 pool events held at the 2008 and 2012 Olympic Games [57]. They presented a result for the age of the top 16, which is comparable to the age of champions in the present study, with a difference of approximately one year for the older swimmers in the study by Allen *et al.* [57]. Interestingly, Allen *et al.* reported that the age for the freestyle 50 m was also higher in women than in men, as is the case in the present study [57]. In all the other distances, the results were reversed, with higher ages in men compared to women [57].

Moreover, there seems to be a trend of an increase in the age of finalists over time as it was described recently for the same time period, strokes and competitions [3]. König *et al.* [3] reported in the case of the World Championships that the age of the finalists increased for all strokes and distances with the exception of the 200 m backstroke in women, and the 400 m freestyle and the 200 m breaststroke in men, where the age of the finalists decreased. In the Olympic Games, the age of the finalists increased for all strokes and distances with the exception of the 800 m freestyle in women and the 400 m individual medley in men. This finding for finalists in elite swimming competitions is in line with other sports disciplines such as running and triathlon [64,65], where the increase in the age was attended by a continuous improvement in performance. Examples were given for the "Ironman Hawaii" in the study by Gallmann *et al.*, with an increase from ~26 years to ~35 years for women and from ~27 years to ~34 years for men in the time period of 1983 to 2012 [65]. During the same period, race times of the elite athletes decreased [65].

Thus, is there any chance for a previous top swimmer like Michael Phelps to win another medal in a competition at the world class level in a comeback after his retirement? The mean age of champions is far below 30 years. Nevertheless, three male champions (*i.e.*, Aleksandr Vladimirovich Popov, 50 m freestyle at the World Championships in 2003; Roland Schoeman, 50 m freestyle at the World Championships in 2013; and Jason Lezak, 100 m freestyle at the Olympic Games in 2008) and six female champions (*i.e.*, Claudia Poll, 400 m freestyle at the World Championships in 2005; Dara Torres, 50 m freestyle, 100 m freestyle and 100 m butterfly at the Olympic Games in 2000; Marleen Veldhuis, 50 m freestyle at the Olympic Games in 2012; and Svitlana Bondarenko, 100 m breaststroke at the Olympic Games in 2004) were 33 years old [65]. There was even one female champion (Therese Alshammar) who won in 2011 at the World Championships in the 50 m freestyle at the age of 34 [66]. Aleksandr Vladimirovich Popov from Russia showed that it is possible to win a gold medal in swimming after age 30. In 1992 (at age 20) at the Barcelona Olympics, he won the 50 m freestyle with a time of 21.91 s.

In 2003 (at age 31) in the same pool in Barcelona at the World Championships, he won the 50 m freestyle with a time of 21.92 s [67]. It is also worth mentioning that Dara Torres won the silver medal in 50 m freestyle at the 2008 Olympic Games in Beijing at the age of 41 [56]. Moreover, in other sports disciplines such as running there are some exceptional athletes who surprised with their outstanding performance. For example, a 90-year old marathon runner officially became the first person to finish a whole marathon at this age [68]. His official finishing time was 6 h, 48 min and 55 s. Müller *et al.* investigated the physiological alterations in that exceptional race [69]. Therefore, we assume that there is also still a certain chance to win a gold medal at the world class level for swimmers over 30 years of age and for athletes intending to make a comeback at that age.

4.2. Younger Swimmers Were Faster in Longer Race Distances

In accordance to other studies investigating the association of age and race distances [1,3,58,59,61,62], we also came to a second important finding that longer race distances were associated with younger swimmers' age for all strokes and in both women and men. Tanaka and Seals assumed that this phenomenon was based on the different energy-producing pathways in skeletal muscle involved with diverse intensities [70].

This important finding could be explained through physiological and biological factors.

For sprint distances (e.g., 50 m freestyle), an athlete's body uses an energy-pathway that is fast enough to deliver the required energy in a foreseeable time. That can be achieved by anaerobic metabolism [71,72]. Aerobic metabolism delivers the needed energy for endurance sports disciplines and endurance swimming distances (e.g., 1500 m freestyle) [73]. Furthermore, Larsson *et al.* reported that there is an increase of isometric and dynamic strength until the age of ~30 years [74]. An improvement in swimming performance until the age of ~30 years can be assumed for sprint distances. For endurance distances, a decrease in metabolic rates, longer response times, poorer coordination and a reduced maximum oxygen uptake (VO_2 max) after the age of ~20 might explain the younger swimmers' age [75–77].

4.3. Female Champions Were Younger than Male Champions

A third important finding was that female champions were younger than male champions with a difference of ~2 years. That is in line with other studies reporting a sex difference of ~2 years. Schulz and Curnow examined Olympic champions from 1896 to 1980 [1]. They reported a constant sex difference in the age of peak swimming performance of ~2 years. Different reasons have been assumed to explain that sex difference. König *et al.* pointed to the different maturation processes during puberty [3]. Most important parameter in this context is body height [2], growth velocity that was not reached until the age of ~12 years in girls and ~14 years in boys [78], the different onset of puberty at ~11 years in girls and ~13 years, expressed as the skeletal/biological age [79], different bone growth (*i.e.*, metacarpal thickness, width, length and medullary diameter) between girls and boys.

4.4. Increase of Peak Swimming Performance across the Years

In 1997, Tanaka and Seals [70] described an interaction between age and sex in freestyle swimming. They concluded that the rate of decline with advancing age appeared to be associated with the length of the performance (*i.e.*, from 50 to 1500 m) and with the sex. These female and male world and Olympic champions improved swimming performance in most race distances with a larger trend of improvement observed in Olympic champions, although the age of peak swimming performance remained stable in most race distances for World champions and in all race distances for Olympic champions. These findings differ from recent findings for finalists competing in World Championships and Olympic Games where performance improved and age increased [3]. Additionally, when freestyle swimmers competing at national level were investigated (*i.e.*, Swiss swimmers between 1994 and 2012), the age of peak swimming speed was younger in women compared to men for the 50 m to the 800 m freestyle. For women, the age of peak swimming speed increased over time in the 50 m but decreased over time in the 1500 m freestyle. For men, the age of peak swimming speed decreased over time in the 50 m freestyle [80].

As Schulz and Curnow reported, swimming performance changed "dramatically" between 1896 and 1980 [1]. They explained this enormous increase in performance by external factors such as improved training programs and diets, better equipment, larger population bases from which athletes are selected, as well as more efficient selection strategies. We can only agree with this. All those factors changed over time. The equipment (e.g., swimsuits), to a certain extent, helps swimmers reach peak swimming speed [5]. It has been shown that wearing a full-body suit or a waist-to-ankle suit significantly reduced passive drag. The reduction in drag was associated with a decreased energy cost of sub-maximal swimming and an increased distance per stroke, at the same stroke rates, and reduced freestyle performance time [81].

Different studies investigating peak swimming performance showed controversial results concerning its evolution over time [59,82]. Buhl *et al.* [59] described a limit in performance at the international level for freestyle, while they showed that there was an increase of up to 5.3% at national (*i.e.*, Switzerland) level. Koch-Ziegenbein *et al.* showed an increase in swimming performance of 1.2%–5.2% at international level for breaststroke [82]. The results in the present study are more stable concerning the swimming performance, compared to the results from the study of König *et al.* describing swimming performance in finalists [3]. This might strengthen the prediction of a limit in swimming performance. However, as König *et al.* already reported, the trend in progression of peak swimming performance remains a controversial question and needs further investigation [3].

As a result of newly introduced swimsuits [5], numerous word records were set in 2009. Some investigations showed that swimming performance would reach its limit [4,58,83]. Berthelot described that swimming performance may soon reach its limit [58]. Nevill *et al.* analyzed front-crawl swimming from 1957 to 2007 [83]. They proclaimed that a non-linear, flattened S-shaped logistic curve would fit the data best. In the present study we assumed that linear regression would describe the data best. We also might not have investigated a time period which is long enough to assess progression in swimming performance [3].

4.5. Strengths and Limitations of this Study and Implications for Future Research

A strength of the present study is first that all distances and all strokes of freestyle, breaststroke, backstroke, butterfly and individual medley were included. Second, the topic from this study is up to date and interesting for today's world class swimmers. Nevertheless, the present study is limited in terms of missing variables such as anthropometric [2,84–86], biological [1,74–76], and physiological factors [67,70,83,84,87,88]. For calculating the age of champions at the particular event, the year of birth and the exact date of event were considered. It was not possible to find all the exact dates of birth for each swimmer. The website from where the data analyzed in the present study were retrieved [89] provides only the year of birth of the athletes, but the exact date of events. Thus, we accepted this lack of precision on the assumption that the differences will compensate one another by a normal distribution. Consequently further research is needed on the age of peak swimming performance, its change over the years, and its comportment in different strokes and race distances as in the present study, in recent years and also at the international level. A further limitation is that we did not consider whether or not athletes were wearing non-textile suits/full-body suits during this period [90], a factor that might influence race time through its effect on passive drag [81,91]. Furthermore, beginning with the season 2013–2014, the Fédération Internationale de Natation (FINA) changed the rules for breaststroke swimming and, therefore, the new rule changes are likely to see faster swims [92].

4.6. Practical Applications

In swimming, longer race distances were completed at younger ages than shorter race distances. The opposite is true for running where older athletes were faster in longer races [93]. The knowledge about the changes in the age of champions over time could be of great interest for swimmers competing at the world class level, as well as for their coaches and sports managers.

5. Conclusions

These findings suggest, first, that female (~21 years) swimming champions were ~2 years younger compared to male (~23 years) champions for all strokes and distances competing at the world class level. Second, longer (200 m and over) race distances were completed by younger champions (~20–22 years) compared to shorter (50 m and 100 m) race distances (~22–24 years). Third, the age of champions remained stable over time in most strokes and distances. Fourth, swimming performance improved in all strokes and distances.

Author Contributions: Beat Knechtle drafted the manuscript, Stefan König collected the data, created the design of the study and helped drafting the manuscript, Stefanie Wild helped in collecting the data and drafting the manuscript, Thomas Rosemann participated in the design of the study and helped to draft, and Pantelis Theodoros Nikolaidis, Nicola Luigi Bragazzi and Christoph Alexander Rüst performed the statistical analyses and helped drafting the manuscript. All authors read and approved the final version of the manuscript.

Conflicts of Interest: The authors declare no conflict of interest.

References

1. Schulz, R.; Curnow, C. Peak performance and age among superathletes: Track and field, swimming, baseball, tennis, and golf. *J. Gerontol.* **1988**, *43*, P113–P120. [CrossRef] [PubMed]
2. Charles, J.D.; Bejan, A. The evolution of speed, size and shape in modern athletics. *J. Exp. Biol.* **2009**, *212*, 2419–2425. [CrossRef] [PubMed]
3. König, S.; Valeri, F.; Wild, S.; Rosemann, T.; Rüst, C.A.; Knechtle, B. Change of the age and performance of swimmers across world championships and olympic games finals from 1992 to 2013—A cross-sectional data analysis. *SpringerPlus* **2014**, *3*. [CrossRef] [PubMed]
4. Stanula, A.; Maszczyk, A.; Roczniok, R.; Pietraszewski, P.; Ostrowski, A.; Zajac, A.; Strzała, M. The development and prediction of athletic performance in freestyle swimming. *J. Hum. Kinet.* **2012**, *32*, 97–107. [CrossRef] [PubMed]
5. O'Connor, L.M.; Vozenilek, J.A. Is it the athlete or the equipment? An analysis of the top swim performances from 1990 to 2010. *J. Strength Cond. Res.* **2011**, *25*, 3239–3241. [CrossRef] [PubMed]
6. Zaccardi, N. Katie Ledecky Breaks Another World Record 2014. Available online: http://olympictalk.nbcsports.com/2014/06/22/katie-ledecky-800-world-record-swimming-olympics (accessed on 29 December 2015).
7. Keith, B. Katie Ledecky Breaks World Record in Women'S 1500 M Freestyle 2014. Available online: https://swimswam.com/katie-ledecky-breaks-world-record-womens-1500-meter-freestyle (accessed on 2 March 2016).
8. Hope, N. World Swimming Championships: Ruta Meilutyte Storms to Record 2013. Available online: http://www.bbc.com/sport/0/swimming/23491784 (accessed on 29 December 2015).
9. Meilutyte Sets World Record in 50 Meters Breaststroke. Available online: http://www.reuters.com/article/us-swimming-world-meilutyte-record-idUSBRE97208Y20130803 (accessed on 2 March 2016).
10. Rogers, I. Russia's Efimova Wins 200 m Breaststroke Gold 2013. Available online: http://www.reuters.com/article/us-swimming-world-women-breaststroke-idUSBRE9710Y020130802 (accessed on 2 March 2016).
11. Memorable Moments. Available online: http://www.cesarcielo.com.br/home/en/?page_id=61 (accessed on 29 December 2015).
12. Wires, N. Brazil's Cesar Cielo Breaks 50 m Freestyle World Record 2009. Available online: http://www.france24.com/en/20091218-brazil-swimming-cesar-cielo-freestyle-world-record-frederick-bousquet (accessed on 29 December 2015).
13. 200 m Freestyle World Record 2014. Available online: http://www.yourswimlog.com/200m-freestyle-world-record (accessed on 29 December 2015).

14. Zhang Lin Breaks World Record and Swimsuit Matters 2009. Available online: http://www.chinahush.com/2009/07/30/zhang-lin-of-china-broke-the-world-record-becomes-the-first-chinese-male-swimmer-won-the-world-championship-gold-and-swimsuit-matters/ (accessed on on 2 March 2016).
15. Jeffery, N. Brenton Rickard Wins Breaststroke Gold for Australia at World Swimming Championships 2009. Available online: http://www.news.com.au/entertainment/celebrity-life/brenton-rickard-wins-breaststroke-gold-for-australia-at-world-swimming-championships/story-e6frfmqr-1225755358351 (accessed on 29 December 2015).
16. Gennaro, T. Daniel Gyurta Lowers His scm 200 Breaststroke World Record in Dubai. Available online: http://swimswam.com/daniel-gyurta-lowers-scm-200-breaststroke-world-record-dubai (accessed on 29 December 2015).
17. Japan's Junya Koga Wins Men's 100 m Backstroke Final 2009. Available online: http://english.sina.com/sports/2009/0728/259022.html (accessed on 29 December 2015).
18. Flash! Aaron Peirsol Reclaims World Record, Smashes 52-s Barrier 2009. Available online: http://www.swimmingworldmagazine.com/news/usa-swimming-national-championships-flash-aaron-peirsol-reclaims-world-record-smashes-52-second-barrier-swimmingworld-tv-interview-included (accessed on 29 December 2015).
19. 2009 Fina World Championships in Rome, Michael Phelps v Milorad Cavic in the 100 Butterfly. Available online: http://swimswam.com/10-michael-phelps-world-record-races-video (accessed on 29 December 2015).
20. Crouse, K. Phelps Grabs Record in 100 Butterfly 2009. Available online: http://www.nytimes.com/2009/08/02/sports/02swim.html?_r=1 (accessed on 2 March 2016).
21. Ryan Lochte Sets World Record in 200 IM. Available online: http://www.usatoday.com/story/sports/olympics/2012/12/15/ryan-lochte-world-record-200-meter-im/1770995/ (accessed on 2 March 2016).
22. Schmitt, A. Commemorating this Day in London 2012: Allison Schmitt 2013. Available online: http://www.teamusa.org/News/2013/July/31/Commemorating-This-Day-In-London-2012-Allison-Schmitt (accessed on 29 December 2015).
23. 400 m Freestyle Women. Available online: http://www.olympic.org/swimming-400m-freestyle-women (accessed on 29 December 2015).
24. Missy Franklin Biography. Available online: http://www.biography.com/people/missy-franklin-20903291 (accessed on 29 December 2015).
25. Crouse, K. Franklin, Racing between Races, Squeezes in Gold 2012. Available online: http://www.nytimes.com/2012/07/31/sports/olympics/monday-olympics-swimming.html?pagewanted=all (accessed on 2 March 2016).
26. Dana Vollmer Gets Gold with World Record 100-m. Butterfly. Available online: http://www.cbsnews.com/news/dana-vollmer-gets-gold-with-world-record-100-m-butterfly/ (accessed on 2 March 2016).
27. Brady, E. American Dana Vollmer Sets World Record in 100 Fly 2012. Available online: http://usatoday30.usatoday.com/sports/olympics/london/swimming/story/2012-07-29/dana-vollmer-world-record-butterfly-olympics/56575462/1 (accessed on 29 December 2015).
28. Thompson, N. Ye Shiwen's "Unbelievable" Swims Are Talk of Olympics 2012. Available online: http://edition.cnn.com/2012/07/31/sport/olympics-china-ye-shiwen-profile (accessed on 29 December 2015).
29. Xinhua. Ye Breaks World Record and Wins Women's 400 m Medley Gold 2012. Available online: http://english.cntv.cn/20120729/101020.shtml (accessed on 29 December 2015).
30. Xinhua. Sun Yang Breaks World Record in 1500 m Freestyle 2012. Available online: http://www.chinadaily.com.cn/2012olympics/2012-08/05/content_15645095.htm (accessed on 29 December 2015).
31. Cameron van der Burgh Takes Gold in Men's 100 m Breaststroke Final 2012. Available online: http://mg.co.za/article/2012-07-29-cameron-van-der-burgh-takes-gold-in-mens-100m-breaststroke-final (accessed on 29 December 2015).
32. Olympics Swimming: Cameron van der Burgh Wins 100 m Breaststroke 2012. Available online: http://www.bbc.com/sport/0/olympics/18904545 (accessed on 29 December 2015).
33. London 2012 Swimming: Usa's Matt Grevers Wins 100 m Backstroke Gold Medal 2012. Available online: http://sports.ndtv.com/swimming/news/194428-london-2012-swimming-usas-matt-grevers-wins-100m-backstroke-gold-medal (accessed on 29 December 2015).

34. Men's 100 m Backstroke 2012. Available online: http://www.bbc.co.uk/sport/olympics/2012/sports/swimming/events/mens-100m-backstroke (accessed on 29 December 2015).
35. Bull, A. London 2012: Phelps Beats Lochte to Win Olympic 200 m Individual Medley 2012. Available online: http://www.theguardian.com/sport/2012/aug/02/michael-phelps-beats-ryan-lochte (accessed on 29 December 2015).
36. Beijing 2008 Olympic Swimming 200 m Free Gold Medal Final 2008. Available online: http://www.olympic.org/videos/beijing-2008-olympic-swimming-200m-free-gold-medal-final (accessed on 29 December 2015).
37. Beijing 2008: Men's 100 m Fly 2008. Available online: http://sportsscientists.com/2008/08/beijing-2008-mens-100-m-fly (accessed on 29 December 2015).
38. Xinhua. Phelps Wins Olympic Men's 200 m Butterfly Gold in World Record Time 2008. Available online: http://news.xinhuanet.com/english/2008-08/13/content_9244696.htm (accessed on 29 December 2015).
39. Michael Phelps Wins First Gold in Beijing 2008. Available online: http://www.olympic.org/videos/michael-phelps-wins-first-gold-in-beijing (accessed on 29 December 2015).
40. Michael Phelps Breaks Games Record in Heats of 400 m Individual Medley—Olympics 2008. Available online: http://www.telegraph.co.uk/sport/olympics/2529210/Michael-Phelps-breaks-Games-record-in-heats-of-400m-individual-medley-Olympics-2008.html (accessed on 29 December 2015).
41. Auerbach, N. Bored in Retirement, Michael Phelps Happy to Be back at U.S. Nationals 2014. Available online: http://www.usatoday.com/story/sports/olympics/2014/08/04/michael-phelps-us-national-swimming-championships/13574029 (accessed on 29 December 2015).
42. Park, A. After Ending Career with a Gold, Is Phelps the Greatest Olympian of All Time? Available online: http://olympics.time.com/2012/08/04/after-ending-career-with-a-gold-is-phelps-the-greatest-olympian-of-all-time (accessed on 29 December 2015).
43. Michael pheLps Plans His Comeback 2014. Available online: http://espn.go.com/olympics/swimming/story/_/id/10946394/michael-phelps-solidifies-training-plan-leading-two-biggest-events-2014 (accessed on 29 December 2015).
44. Forde, P. Reinvigorated Michael Phelps to Return to Pool with Eye on 2016 Olympics 2014. Available online: http://sports.yahoo.com/news/reinvigorated-michael-phelps-ends-retirement-with-eye-on-2016-olympics-172959662.html (accessed on 29 December 2015).
45. Arrowsmith, R. Michael Phelps set to Take a Break from Swimming to "Better Understand Myself" Following Arrest for Drink Driving 2014. Available online: http://www.dailymail.co.uk/sport/othersports/article-2781380/Michael-Phelps-set-break-swimming-following-arrest-drink-driving.html (accessed on 29 December 2015).
46. Predicting the 2016 U.S. Olympic Team by Age, Experience. Available online: https://swimswam.com/predicting-2016-u-s-olympic-team-age-experience/ (accessed on 14 February 2015).
47. Ian Thorpe. Available online: http://www.databaseolympics.com/players/playerpage.htm?ilkid=THORPIAN01 (accessed on 29 December 2015).
48. Thorpe risks reputation by jumping back in the pool. Available online: http://blogs.reuters.com/sport/2011/02/03/thorpe-risks-reputation-by-jumping-back-in-the-pool/ (accessed on 2 March 2016).
49. Mason, P. Heroes of Swimming: Ian Thorpe 2014. Available online: http://www.theguardian.com/lifeandstyle/the-swimming-blog/2014/apr/15/heroes-of-swimming-ian-thorpe (accessed on 29 December 2015).
50. Haack, M. Ian Thorpe Über Ein Comeback—"Sag Niemals Nie" 2014. Available online: http://www.welt.de/sport/article131338158/Ian-Thorpe-ueber-ein-Comeback-Sag-niemals-nie.html (accessed on 29 December 2015).
51. Reed, S.; Bennet, L. Superswimmer Mark Spitz, 39, Aims for the '92 Olympics 1990. Available online: http://connection.ebscohost.com/c/articles/9001151412/superswimmer-mark-spitz-39-aims-the-92-olympics (accessed on 2 March 2016).
52. Mark Spitz. Available online: http://www.olympic.org/mark-spitz (accessed on 29 December 2015).
53. Top 10 Failed Comeback Attempts 2011. Available online: http://www.nzherald.co.nz/sport/news/article.cfm?c_id=4&objectid=10767646 (accessed on 29 December 2015).
54. Zaccardi, N. Swimmer Ed Moses Attempts Comeback; and Moreolympic Notes 2011. Available online: http://www.si.com/more-sports/2011/06/13/ed-mosesolympiccomeback (accessed on 29 December 2015).

55. Watkins, M. Catching up with Ed Moses 2013. Available online: http://www.usaswimming.org/ViewNewsArticle.aspx?TabId=1801&itemid=5674&mid=13305 (accessed on 29 December 2015).
56. Dara Torres, Race Results. Available online: http://www.sports-reference.com/olympics/athletes/to/dara-torres-1.html (accessed on 14 February 2015).
57. Allen, S.V.; Vandenbogaerde, T.J.; Hopkins, W.G. Career performance trajectories of olympic swimmers: Benchmarks for talent development. *Eur. J. Sport Sci.* **2014**, *14*, 643–651. [CrossRef] [PubMed]
58. Berthelot, G.; Len, S.; Hellard, P.; Tafflet, M.; Guillaume, M.; Vollmer, J.C.; Gager, B.; Quinquis, L.; Marc, A.; Toussaint, J.F. Exponential growth combined with exponential decline explains lifetime performance evolution in individual and human species. *Age* **2012**, *34*, 1001–1009. [CrossRef] [PubMed]
59. Buhl, C.; Knechtle, B.; Rust, C.A.; Rosemann, T.; Lepers, R. A comparison of medley and freestyle performance for national and international swimmers between 1994 and 2011. *Open Access J. Sports Med.* **2013**, *4*, 79–87. [PubMed]
60. Kollarz, C.; Knechtle, B.; Rüst, C.; Rosemann, T.; Lepers, R. Comparison of age of peak swimming speed in elite backstroke swimmers at national and international level. *OA Sports Med.* **2013**, *1*. [CrossRef]
61. Kollarz, C.; Knechtle, B.; Rüst, C.A.; Rosemann, T.; Lepers, R. The age difference in peak performance of backstroke swimming between men and women: A cross sectional data analysis of backstroke and freestyle swimming in elite swiss swimmers from 2006 to 2010. *Adapt. Med.* **2013**, *5*, 171–180.
62. Wolfrum, M.; Knechtle, B.; Rüst, C.A.; Rosemann, T.; Lepers, R. Sex-related differences and age of peak performance in breaststroke *versus* freestyle swimming. *BMC Sports Sci. Med. Rehabil.* **2013**, *5*. [CrossRef] [PubMed]
63. Vaso, M.; Knechtle, B.; Rüst, C.A.; Rosemann, T.; Lepers, R. Age of peak swim speed and sex difference in performance in medley and freestyle swimming—A comparison between 200 m and 400 m in swiss elite swimmers. *J. Hum. Sport Exerc.* **2013**, *8*, 954–965. [CrossRef]
64. Lepers, R.; Cattagni, T. Do older athletes reach limits in their performance during marathon running? *Age* **2012**, *34*, 773–781. [CrossRef] [PubMed]
65. Gallmann, D.; Knechtle, B.; Rüst, C.A.; Rosemann, T.; Lepers, R. Elite triathletes in "ironman hawaii" get older but faster. *Age* **2014**, *36*, 407–416. [CrossRef] [PubMed]
66. Fina. Available online: http://www.fina.org (accessed on 29 December 2015).
67. Alexsandr Popow, Race Results. Available online: http://www.sports-reference.com/olympics/athletes/po/aleksandr-popov-2.html (accessed on 14 February 2015).
68. Leichtathletik: Der 90-Jährige Marathonmann 2014. Available online: http://www.srf.ch/player/tv/sportaktuell/video/leichtathletik-der-90-jaehrige-marathonmann?id=6af06f30-49b7-45ea-a1be-1d5c4027258f (accessed on 29 December 2015).
69. Mueller, S.M.; Knechtle, B.; Knechtle, P.; Toigo, M. Physiological alterations after a marathon in the first 90-year-old male finisher: Case study. *SpringerPlus* **2014**, *3*. [CrossRef] [PubMed]
70. Tanaka, H.; Seals, D.R. Age and gender interactions in physiological functional capacity: Insight from swimming performance. *J. Appl. Physiol.* **1997**, *82*, 846–851. [PubMed]
71. Ramsbottom, R.; Nevill, A.M.; Nevill, M.E.; Newport, S.; Williams, C. Accumulated oxygen deficit and short-distance running performance. *J. Sports Sci.* **1994**, *12*, 447–453. [CrossRef] [PubMed]
72. Spriet, L.L. Anaerobic metabolism in human skeletal muscle during short-term, intense activity. *Can. J. Physiol. Pharmacol.* **1992**, *70*, 157–165. [CrossRef] [PubMed]
73. Ghosh, A.K. Anaerobic threshold: Its concept and role in endurance sport. *Malays. J. Med. Sci.* **2004**, *11*, 24–36. [PubMed]
74. Larsson, L.; Grimby, G.; Karlsson, J. Muscle strength and speed of movement in relation to age and muscle morphology. *J. Appl. Physiol. Respir. Environ. Exerc. Physiol.* **1979**, *46*, 451–456. [PubMed]
75. Lata, H.; Walia, L. Ageing: Physiological aspects. *JK Sci.* **2007**, *9*, 111–115.
76. Rodrigues, A.N.; Perez, A.J.; Carletti, L.; Bissoli, N.S.; Abreu, G.R. Maximum oxygen uptake in adolescents as measured by cardiopulmonary exercise testing: A classification proposal. *J. Pediatria* **2006**, *82*, 426–430. [CrossRef]
77. Maximal Oxygen Uptake Norms. Available online: http://www.topendsports.com/testing/norms/vo2max.htm (accessed on 29 December 2015).
78. Wheeler, M.D. Physical changes of puberty. *Endocrinol. Metab. Clin. N. Am.* **1991**, *20*, 1–14.

79. Tanner, J.M.; Whitehouse, R.H.; Marshall, W.A.; Carter, B.S. Prediction of adult height from height, bone age, and occurrence of menarche, at ages 4 to 16 with allowance for midparent height. *Arch. Dis. Child.* **1975**, *50*, 14–26. [CrossRef] [PubMed]
80. Rüst, C.A.; Knechtle, B.; Rosemann, T.; Lepers, R. The changes in age of peak swim speed for elite male and female swiss freestyle swimmers between 1994 and 2012. *J. Sports Sci.* **2014**, *32*, 248–258. [CrossRef] [PubMed]
81. Chatard, J.C.; Wilson, B. Effect of fastskin suits on performance, drag, and energy cost of swimming. *Med. Sci. Sports Exerc.* **2008**, *40*, 1149–1154. [CrossRef] [PubMed]
82. Koch-Ziegenbein, P.; Knechtle, B.; Rüst, C.; Rosemann, T.; Lepers, R. Differences in swimming speed on short course and long course for female and male breaststroke swimmers—A comparison of swimmers at national and international level. *OA Sports Med.* **2013**, *1*, 18. [CrossRef]
83. Nevill, A.M.; Whyte, G.P.; Holder, R.L.; Peyrebrune, M. Are there limits to swimming world records? *Int. J. Sports Med.* **2007**, *28*, 1012–1017. [CrossRef] [PubMed]
84. Lätt, E.; Jürimäe, J.; Mäestu, J.; Purge, P.; Rämson, R.; Haljaste, K.; Keskinen, K.L.; Rodriguez, F.A.; Jürimäe, T. Physiological, biomechanical and anthropometrical predictors of sprint swimming performance in adolescent swimmers. *J. Sports Sci. Med.* **2010**, *9*, 398–404. [PubMed]
85. Siders, W.A.; Lukaski, H.C.; Bolonchuk, W.W. Relationships among swimming performance, body composition and somatotype in competitive collegiate swimmers. *J. Sports Med. Phys. Fit.* **1993**, *33*, 166–171.
86. Zampagni, M.L.; Casino, D.; Benelli, P.; Visani, A.; Marcacci, M.; De Vito, G. Anthropometric and strength variables to predict freestyle performance times in elite master swimmers. *J. Strength Cond. Res.* **2008**, *22*, 1298–1307. [CrossRef] [PubMed]
87. Jürimäe, J.; Haljaste, K.; Cicchella, A.; Lätt, E.; Purge, P.; Leppik, A.; Jürimäe, T. Analysis of swimming performance from physical, physiological, and biomechanical parameters in young swimmers. *Pediatr. Exerc. Sci.* **2007**, *19*, 70–81. [PubMed]
88. Zamparo, P. Effects of age and gender on the propelling efficiency of the arm stroke. *Eur. J. Appl. Physiol.* **2006**, *97*, 52–58. [CrossRef] [PubMed]
89. Worldwide swimming ranking. Available online: www.swimrankings.net (accessed on 2 March 2016).
90. Fina Approved Swimwear. Available online: http://www.fina.org/content/fina-approved-swimwear (accessed on 14 February 2015).
91. Cortesi, M.; Fantozzi, S.; Di Michele, R.; Zamparo, P.; Gatta, G. Passive drag reduction using full-body swimsuits: The role of body position. *J. Strength Cond. Res./Natl. Strength Cond. Assoc.* **2014**, *28*, 3164–3171. [CrossRef] [PubMed]
92. Fina Announces Another Rules Change to Breaststroke Pullouts. Available online: https://swimswam.com/fina-announces-another-rules-change-breaststroke-pullouts/ (accessed on 14 February 2015).
93. Knechtle, B.; Valeri, F.; Zingg, M.A.; Rosemann, T.; Rüst, C.A. What is the age for the fastest ultra-marathon performance in time-limited races from 6 h to 10 days? *Age* **2014**, *36*, 9715. [CrossRef] [PubMed]

Self-Reported Use and Reasons among the General Population for Using Sports Nutrition Products and Dietary Supplements

Floris Wardenaar [1,*], Remko van den Dool [2], Ingrid Ceelen [1], Renger Witkamp [3] and Marco Mensink [3]

[1] HAN University of Applied Sciences, Nijmegen 6525 AJ, The Netherlands; Ingrid.ceelen@han.nl
[2] *Mulier Instituut*, Utrecht 3584 AA, The Netherlands; r.vandendool@mulier.nl
[3] Wageningen University, Wageningen 6700 EV, The Netherlands; Renger.witkamp@han.nl (R.W.); Marco.mensink@wur.nl (M.M.)
* Correspondence: Floris.wardenaar@han.nl

Academic Editor: Beat Knechtle
Received: 23 April 2016; Accepted: 3 June 2016; Published: 7 June 2016

Abstract: The purpose of the present study was to determine the prevalence of dietary supplements (DS's) and sport nutrition product (SNPs) among the general population, to identify differences for gender, age, and exercise frequency, and to determine the main reasons for use. The study was designed as a web-based questionnaire in a representative sample (n = 1544) of the Dutch population. Sixty-two percent (n = 957) of the respondents reported having used DS's, SNPs, or both in the last twelve months. Women and older people reported the highest DS use. The highest use of SNPs was reported by regular exercising men and younger people with improving sporting performance as their main objective. Most frequently reported DS's were multivitamins (28%) and vitamin C (19%)—for SNPs, energy drinks (22%) and isotonic drinks (19%). Health considerations were the most important motivation (DS's 90% and SNPs 52%), but also performance was substantially reported (DS's 14% and SNPs 35%). A substantial group of sedentary respondents also reported the use of SNPs. This study confirms that DS's, SNPs, or both are widely used among the general population. Both health as performance are important reasons for use. It can be questioned whether the use of SNPs fits all respondents' physical activity needs.

Keywords: nutritional supplements; sports dietetics; exercise; health; performance

1. Introduction

Nutritional supplements such as dietary supplements (DS's) and sports nutrition products (SNPs) are commonly used by athletes to maximize their performance, to accelerate recovery, to prevent nutrient deficiencies, and to maintain good general health [1–4]. However, these arguments give the impression that they are also often used by physically less active people and that these products are actively promoted by suppliers aiming to reach a wider target group [5,6].

The majority of the literature investigating DS and SNP use does combine both as nutritional supplements or only focuses on dietary supplements, despite the fact that SNPs do not only contain macronutrients but also micronutrients. Moreover, SNPs are increasingly found on the shelves of supermarkets, making these types of products easily accessible for the general population. Thus, from a nutritional perspective, it is necessary to include SNPs in dietary analysis.

Consumers of both DS's and SNPs may use these preparations with the intention of maintaining good health [5], often unaware of the supporting scientific evidence—or lack thereof [6]. Further, it can be questioned whether they also use these type of products for performance reasons. Surveys on dietary supplement consumption by the general population generally focus on the use of multivitamins or other micro-nutrient products, but often make no distinction between sport-specific DS's and SNPs, or make no mention of them at all [7]. Until now, this has only been investigated in small groups of non-athletes included as controls to compare their use with the nutritional supplement use of elite athletes [1,6,8]. However, two of these three studies did not provide a clear insight into the contribution of sport-specific SNPs used in the non-athletes group [1,8]; therefore, obtaining additional information in a large sample of a general population can be seen as valuable.

From an earlier pilot survey among general consumers in the Netherlands, we concluded that a typical user of sports supplements and sports nutrition products is a young (<35 years) male, who regularly takes part in sports (>once/week) and is a member of a sports club [5]. When subjects were asked about their reasons for using DS's and SNPs, we found a lower prevalence of sports-oriented use (5.8% for DS's and 21.6% for SNPs) compared to other studies [6,8].

Therefore, as part of the Dutch National Sport Study [9], we investigated the self-reported use and the main reasons for use of DS's and SNPs. The objectives of this survey were (a) to determine the prevalence in the Dutch general population of dietary supplement and sports nutrition product use, in general and for specific DS's and SNPs; (b) to identify differences in use for gender, age, and exercise frequency; and (c) to determine the main reasons for using DS's, SNPs, or both, particularly for physical performance purposes in comparison to general health purposes. Knowledge of the prevalence and motivation for use of DS's and SNPs, especially in non-athletes, is of relevance for (sports) dieticians and health professionals giving dietary advice.

2. Materials and Methods

2.1. Study Design

The present study was part of the Dutch Sport nutrition and Supplement Study (DSSS), which had been approved by the Ethics Board of Wageningen University. To obtain insight in nutritional supplement use of a representative sample of the general population questions were integrated in the Dutch National Sport Study (NSO). GfK Panel Services Benelux BV (GfK) conducted the survey between 22 November 22 and 4 December 2013 using an Internet-based questionnaire (Bellview, Pulse Train, North Palm Beach, FL, USA). To reduce selection bias, the questionnaire was given a neutral title: "Health and exercise". Moreover, those respondents submitting a completed questionnaire were rewarded with an incentive (bonus points with a value of €1.60 that could be spent within the GfK panel rewarding system), which encouraged those respondents that were not primarily interested in health and exercise to participate. The average duration for filling out the total NSO questionnaire was 16 min, with 2 min for the sport-specific nutrition questions.

2.2. Study Population

Out of a panel of 10,000 representative households, 2350 participants received an invitation to fill out the questionnaire. Within thirteen days, 1544 questionnaires were returned (response percentage of 66%), which was considered to deliver a representative sample of the population in the Netherlands for example in terms of age (15–80 years), gender (50%–50% men and women), education level (35% lower education; 42% middle-education; 23% higher education), and ethnicity (80% autochthonous; 8% Western-immigrant; 12% non-Western immigrant).

2.3. Questions

To investigate the prevalence of dietary supplement and sports nutrition product use, in general and for specific DS and SNP subcategories, a questionnaire was developed that examined the self-reported use of DS's and SNPs in the previous 12 months. All products questioned are shown in Table 1. Dietary supplements were products classified as supplements that prevent or treat a perceived nutrient deficiency, *i.e.*, vitamins, minerals, and essential fatty acids. Ergogenic supplements were also included in this category, because they could be used for health purposes as well as performance improvement. Sport nutrition products were macronutrient containing beverages, *i.e.*, sports drinks (electrolyte- and carbohydrate-containing drinks for rehydration and refuelling and energy drinks containing mainly carbohydrate for refuelling) and recovery drinks (containing a combination of carbohydrate and protein aiming to optimize post-exercise recovery), to provide a more convenient form of nutrients in situations where everyday foods are not practical—particularly to address the nutritional needs/goals of an exercise session. All DS's that could be selected were pre-defined, with an option to indicate "none" or "other" use; in case of SNPs, the option "none of these supplements" was included.

The questions asked were: (1) Which dietary supplements have you used in the last twelve months? (pre-selected options); (2) Which sports nutrition products have you used in the last twelve months? (pre-selected options); (3) and (4) Please indicate the main reason for using these products (DS's and(or) SNPs). Subjects were asked to select only one option: for health purposes, for physical performance purposes, to improve both, or for other purposes. Gender and sporting frequency were detected as part of the general questionnaire. Respondents were asked to select one or more sports out of a pre-specified list of 44 sports and an "other" option. The exercise frequency (per year) was obtained by an open question that was part of the annual NSO questionnaire: How many times have you exercised in the last twelve months?

Table 1. Prevalence of use of dietary supplements and sports nutrition products.

	Total	Gender		Age (Years)					Sporting Frequency per Year				
		Men	Women	15–20	21–35	36–50	51–65	66–80	0	1–11	12–59	60–119	>120
		(*n* = 791)	(*n* = 753)	(*n* = 111)	(*n* = 358)	(*n* = 400)	(*n* = 422)	(*n* = 253)	(*n* = 401)	(*n* = 137)	(*n* = 484)	(*n* = 275)	(*n* = 247)
		A	B	C	D	E	F	G	H	I	J	K	L
Dietary supplements													
Multivitamins/ minerals	28 (26–30)	23 (20–26)	32 (29–35) a	26 (18–34)	32 (27–37) f,g	29 (25–31)	25 (21–29)	23 (18–28)	22 (18–26)	24 (17–31)	27 (23–31)	34 (28–40) h,i,j	34 (28–40) h,i,j
Vitamin C	19 (17–21)	17 (14–20)	21 (18–24)	20 (13–27)	23 (19–27) g	19 (15–23)	19 (15–23)	13 (9–17)	15 (11–19)	17 (11–23)	20 (16–24)	22 (17–27) h	22 (17–27) h
Vitamin D	16 (14–18)	12 (10–14)	20 (17–23) a	13 (7–19)	17 (13–21)	12 (9–15)	16 (12–18)	21 (16–26) e	14 (10–18)	16 (10–22)	15 (12–18)	17 (13–21)	18 (13–23)
Calcium	8 (7–9)	5 (3–7)	11 (9–13) a	7 (2–12)	6 (3–9)	5 (3–7)	11 (8–14) d,e	14 (10–18) c,d,e	7 (5–9)	7 (3–11)	6 (4–8)	9 (5–13)	13 (9–17) h,j
Magnesium	7 (6–8)	3 (2–4)	10 (8–12) a	10 (4–16) d,e	5 (3–7)	4 (2–6)	9 (6–12) d,e	9 (5–13) e	7 (5–9)	5 (1–9)	5 (3–7)	6 (3–9)	11 (7–15) h,j,k
Essential fatty acids/fish oil	5 (4–6)	3 (2–4)	6 (4–8) a	6 (2–10)	4 (2–6)	5 (3–7)	6 (4–8)	3 (1–5)	3 (1–5)	4 (1–7)	6 (4–8)	6 (3–9)	4 (1–7)
Iron	5 (4–6)	4 (3–5)	7 (5–9) a	8 (3–13)	7 (4–10)	5 (3–7)	4 (2–6)	5 (2–8)	4 (2–6)	6 (2–10)	5 (3–7)	7 (4–10)	8 (5–11) h
Caffeine	5 (4–6)	6 (4–8)	5 (4–6)	16 (9–23) d,e,f,g	8 (5–11) e,f,g	3 (1–5)	3 (1–5)	2 (0–4)	3 (1–5)	3 (0–6)	6 (4–8) h	6 (3–9) h	8 (5–11) h
Probiotics	7 (6–8)	4 (3–5)	9 (7–11) a	7 (2–12)	7 (4–10)	7 (5–9)	7 (5–9)	5 (2–8)	5 (3–7)	5 (2–8)	7 (5–9)	8 (5–11)	7 (4–10)
Zinc	3 (2–4)	3 (2–4)	2 (1–3)	2 (0–4)	3 (1–5)	2 (0–4)	3 (1–5)	3 (1–5)	1 (0–2)	4 (1–7)	3 (1–5)	2 (0–4)	4 (1–7) h
Creatine	1 (0–2)	1 (0–2)	1 (0–2)	1 (−1–3)	2 (1–3) f	1 (0–2) f	0	1 (1–3)	0	0	1 (0–2)	0	4 (1–7) h,j
B-alanine	1 (0–2)	1 (0–2)	1 (0–2)	1 (−1–3)	1 (0–2)	0	1 (0–2)	1 (0–2)	0	1 (0–2)	1 (0–2)	0	2 (0–4) h
Beetroot juice/nitrate	1 (0–2)	1 (0–2)	1 (0–2)	0	0	2 (1–3)	1 (0–2)	2 (0–4)	0	1 (0–2)	1 (0–2)	2 (0–4)	2 (0–4)
Sodium bicarbonate	1 (0–2)	1 (0–2)	1 (0–2)	1 (−1–3)	0	1 (0–2)	1 (0–2)	1 (0–2)	1 (0–2)	1 (0–2)	0	1 (0–2)	1 (0–2)
HMB *	0	1 (0–2)	0	2 (0–4)	0	1 (0–2)	0	0	0	1 (0–2)	1 (0–2)	0	1 (0–2)
Quercetin	0	0	0	0	0	1 (0–2)	0	0	0	1 (0–2)	0	0	0
Other than these DS's	4 (3–5)	3 (2–4)	5 (3–7) a	5 (0–10)	6 (3–9) e,f	3 (1–5)	3 (1–5)	3 (1–5)	3 (1–5)	5 (2–8)	3 (2–4)	5 (2–8)	7 (4–10) h,j
None	51 (50–52)	57 (56–58)	44 (42–46)	55 (41–59)	43 (40–46)	53 (51–55)	52 (50–54)	54 (52–56)	59 (57–61)	49 (46–52)	50 (49–51)	47 (44–50)	44 (41–47)
Sports nutrition products													
Energy drinks	22 (20–24)	27 (24–30) a	16 (13–19)	43 (34–52) e,f,g	36 (31–41) e,f,g	21 (17–25) f,g	13 (10–16) g	2 (0–4)	10 (7–13)	21 (14–28) h	25 (21–29) h	26 (5) h	29 (6) h
Isotonic drinks	19 (17–21)	23 (20–26) a	15 (12–18)	37 (28–46) d,e,f,g	27 (22–32) e,f,g	21 (17–25) f,g	11 (8–14) g	5 (2–8)	5 (3–7)	17 (11–23) h	20 (16–24) h	28 (5) h,i,j	30 (6) h,i,j
Protein shakes	5 (4–6)	5 (3–7)	5 (3–8)	7 (2–12) f,g	10 (7–13) e,f,g	6 (4–8) f,g	3 (2–4)	2 (0–4)	2(1–3)	3 (0–6)	5 (3–7) h	7 (3) h	14 (4) h,i,j,k
Recovery drinks	3 (2–4)	5 (3–7) a	1 (0–2)	7 (2–12) f	5 (3–7) f	3 (1–5)	1 (−1–3)	0	0	1 (-1–3)	3 (1–5)	4 (2)	8 (3) i,j,k
Energy gels	1 (0–2)	1 (0–2)	1 (0–2)	1 (−1–3)	1 (0–2)	2 (1–3) f	0	0	0	1 (0–2)	0	1 (1)	4 (2) j,k
None of these SNPs	66 (64–68)	61 (58–64)	72 (69–75)	38 (37–39)	49 (48–50)	64 (63–65)	80 (76–84)	92 (88–96)	86 (85–87)	67 (66–68)	64 (60–68)	55 (54–56)	52 (51–53)

Sample size n = 1544, and sample size per subgroup was given as (n). All data is presented as a percentage and 95 CI. Capital letters are used as a label for subgroups within categories for gender, age, and sporting frequency. Lower case letters displayed below a specific value indicate that this value is significantly larger than the corresponding capital letters. * HMB: beta-hydroxy-beta-methylbutyrate.

2.4. Statistical Analysis

After terminating the registration period results were entered into SPSS (IBM SPSS Statistics, version 20, IBM Corporation, New York, United States). All self-reported results are given as percentages. For each value, a 95% confidence interval was estimated and expressed as a percentage based on the following formula $\sqrt{(p(1-p)/n)}$, of which p is the sample proportion and n is the sample size. Individual (2 × 2) chi-square tests were used to assess whether there was a difference in the expected distribution of DS and SNP use within tied subcategories such as gender, age, and sporting frequency. Results were considered significantly different at $P \leqslant 0.05$. No correction was calculated for multiple comparisons because of the relatively small number of equations between each subcategory.

3. Results

A response rate of 66% within 13 days resulted in a sample size of $n = 1544$ with comparable numbers of men ($n = 791$) and women ($n = 753$). The largest proportion, 76% of the sample, was aged between 21 and 65 years. Of the total study population, 35% reported that they were not engaged in any sporting activity or only 1–11 times a year in the last twelve months and are considered sedentary, while 31% of the population exercised between 12 and 59 times a year. One third of the study population (33%) indicated that they were a member of a sports club, and most of the subjects performed recreational sports without a competitive element (77%). Table 1 contains numbers (n) of participants in specific subgroups.

3.1. Prevalence

The most reported DS's were multivitamin/mineral supplements, vitamin C, and vitamin D. The most frequently reported SNPs were energy drinks and isotonic drinks (Table 1). With regard to total prevalence of DS and SNP use in total, 62% (95% CI: 60–64) of the study population reported the use of DS's, SNPs, or both. The percentage use of products categorized as DS's or SNPs was only 28% (95% CI: 26–30) and 12% (95% CI: 10–14), respectively. In total, 38% (95% CI: 36–40) did not report using any type of product (Table 2).

As shown in Table 1, men reported using more SNPs, such as energy drinks, isotonic drinks, and recovery drinks, than women, except for protein shakes and energy gels. Women reported a higher proportion of vitamin and mineral supplements, essential fatty acids, probiotics, and other DS's than did men. No differences between men and women were seen for the use of ergogenic supplements, such as caffeine and creatine.

The use of dietary supplements was different between age categories, as can be seen in Table 1. For example, vitamin D and calcium supplement use was higher in the oldest age category of 66–80 years. Moreover, magnesium was high in both the youngest age group of 15–20 years and the oldest age groups of 51–65 and 66–80 years. The sport-specific use of caffeine (defined as tablet/capsule, energy drink/sport nutrition product, coffee, or an equivalent) was especially high in the two youngest age groups of 15–20 and 21–35 years old. Regarding SNPs, energy drink, isotonic drink, and protein shake prevalence was the highest in the two youngest age categories of 15–20 and 21–35 years. The prevalence of the use of recovery drinks declined as age increased. In general, some differences between age groups existed, resulting in a higher prevalence in the use of SNPs or in the combination of DS's and SNPs (*i.e.*, using both) in the younger categories (15–20 years and 21–35 years) compared with the older age categories (51–65 years and 66–80 years), as shown in Table 2.

The part of the population that exercised >60 times a year reported the greatest consumption of SNPs. This group also reported the highest percentages for the single product use of multivitamin and minerals, vitamin C, isotonic drinks, energy drinks, protein drinks, recovery drinks, and energy gels (Table 1). People who did not exercise, or who exercised less than 11 times a year, reported the highest non-use (51%) of DS's and SNPs (Table 2). This percentage was significantly higher than all categories with active participation in sports. Nevertheless, of those participants reporting no exercise, a relatively large number still indicated using SNPs (8%, (95% CI: 5–11)) or a combination of DS's and SNPs (7%, (95% CI: 5–9)). The frequency of SNP use found in those not exercising was equal to those exercising 1–11 times a year in the case of those reporting only the use of SNPs (8% (95% CI: 5–11) *vs.* 9% (95% CI: 4–14)). This was not the case for combined use of DS's and SNPs between those not active and those exercising 1–11 times a year (7% (95% CI: 5–9) *vs.* 24% (95% CI: 17–31)). Overall, this resulted in a relative large group of sedentary individuals using SNPs.

3.2. Reasons

Most subjects reported health reasons as the main motivation for using DS's, with a range of 61–89% among categories (Table 3). Improvement of physical performance was not frequently selected as a single reason for use (range 1–8% for different subcategories), although the combined reason (health *and* performance) was reported frequently in some but not all groups. This was most frequently seen in the age group of 15–20 years (25% (95% CI: 19–31)), and the group exercising >120 times a year (22% (95% CI: 18–26)). Furthermore, for SNP use, health reasons were more frequently indicated than performance reasons, with, for health, a range of 17–43% among categories (Table 3), although "other reasons" was answered more frequently (range: 24%–67%). The group exercising >120 times, in comparison with other subcategories, most frequently reported "physical performance purposes" as reasons for use: 23% (95% CI: 19–27] indicated performance as the sole reason, while 34% (95 CI: 29–39) indicated the combined reason of health and performance as the main argument for use.

Women more frequently reported health reasons as their motivation for DS use than men (84% (95% CI: 80–88) *vs.* 72% (95% CI: 69–75)), but not for SNPs (33% (95% CI: 31–35) *vs.* 25% (95% CI: 23–27)). Men reported higher percentages for physical performance purposes and a combination of health and physical performance purposes as the most important reason for DS and SNP use than women.

Table 2. Combined prevalence of use or non-use of dietary supplements and sports nutrition products or both for different groups.

		Age (Years)					Sporting Frequency per Year				
	Total	15–20	21–35	36–50	51–65	66–80	0	1–11	12–59	60–119	>120
		(*n* = 111)	(*n* = 358)	(*n* = 400)	(*n* = 422)	(*n* = 253)	(*n* = 401)	(*n* = 137)	(*n* = 484)	(*n* = 275)	(*n* = 247)
		C	D	E	F	G	H	I	J	K	L
DS's	28 (26–30)	10 (4–16)	22 (18–26) c	23 (19–27) c	38 (34–42) c,d,e	40 (34–46) c,d,e	35 (30–40) j,k,l	27 (19–35)	27 (24–31)	24 (19–29)	25 (20–30)
SNPs	12 (10–14)	27 (19–35) d,e,f,g	16 (12–20) f,g	13 (10–16) g	9 (6–12) g	2 (0–4)	8 (5–11)	9 (4–14)	12 (9–15) h	16 (12–18) h,i	17 (12–22) h,i
Both	21 (19–23)	35 (26–44) e,f,g	35 (30–40) e,f,g	24 (20–28) f,g	11 (7–15) g	6 (3–9)	7 (5–9)	24 (17–31) h	24 (20–28) h	29 (24–33) h	31 (25–37) h,j
None	38 (36–40)	28 (20–36)	27 (22–32)	41 (36–47) c,d	43 (38–48) c,d	52 (46–58) c,d,e,f	51 (46–56) i,j,k,l	40 (32–48)	37 (33–41)	31 (25–36)	27 (21–33)

Sample size *n* = 1544, and sample size per subgroup was given as (*n*). All data is presented as a percentage and 95 CI. DS = dietary supplement; SNP = sports nutrition product. Capital letters are used as a label for subgroups within categories for gender, age, and sporting frequency. Lower case letters displayed below a specific value indicate that this value is significantly larger than the corresponding capital letters.

Table 3. Percentage of health or performance reasons for the use of dietary supplements and sports nutrition products.

		Gender		Age (Years)					Sporting Frequency per Year				
	Total	Men	Women	15–20	21–35	36–50	51–65	66–80	0	1–11	12–59	60–119	>120
		(*n* = 791)	(*n* = 753)	(*n* = 111)	(*n* = 358)	(*n* = 400)	(*n* = 422)	(*n* = 253)	(*n* = 401)	(*n* = 137)	(*n* = 484)	(*n* = 275)	(*n* = 247)
		A	B	C	D	E	F	G	H	I	J	K	L
Dietary supplements													
Health	79 (77–81)	72 (69–75)	84 (80–88) a	61 (53–69)	74 (69–79)	81 (76–86) c	85 (80–90) c,d	85 (79–91) c,d	89 (84–94) i,j,k,l	79 (71–87) i	79 (75–83) i	80 (74–86) i	66 (60–72)
Performance	3 (2–4)	5 (4–6) b	1 (0–2)	4 (1–7)	4 (2–6) f	4 (3–5) f	1 (0–2)	1 (0–2)	0	8 (5–11)	3 (2–4)	2 (1–3)	3 (1–5)
Both	11 (10–12)	17 (15–19) b	7 (6–8)	25 (19–31) d,c,f,g	12 (9–15)	9 (7–11)	9 (7–11)	9 (7–11)	1 (0–2)	7 (4–10) h	11 (9–13) h	14 (11–17) h	22 (18–26) h,i,j
Other	7 (6–8)	6 (5–7)	9 (7–11)	10 (6–14)	11 (9–13)	6 (4–8)	6 (4–8)	5 (3–7)	10 (8–12) k	6 (3–9)	8 (6–10)	4 (2–6)	9 (6–12)
Sports nutrition products													
Health	29 (27–31)	25 (23–27)	33 (31–35)	17 (11–23)	25 (22–28)	32 (29–35) c	40 (37–43) c,d	43 (41–45) c	31 (29–33) i	35 (30–40) i	29 (26–32) i	33 (29–37) i	18 (14–22)
Performance	12 (11–13)	15 (13–17) b	7 (6–8)	8 (4–12)	16 (13–19) f	12 (10–14) f	4 (3–5)	5 (4–6)	0	9 (6–12)	10 (8–12)	10 (7–13)	23 (19–27) i,j,k
Both	23 (22–24)	28 (26–30) b	17 (15–29)	28 (21–35) d	17 (14–20)	24 (21–27)	29 (27–31) d	29 (27–31)	2 (1–3)	11 (8–14) h	26 (23–29) h,i	23 (19–27) h	34 (29–39) h,i
Other	37 (35–39)	32 (30–34)	43 (41–45) a	46 (38–54) e,f	41 (37–44) f	32 (29–35)	27 (25–29)	24 (22–26)	67 (64–70)	45 (39–51)	34 (31–37)	33 (29–37)	25 (21–29)

Sample size *n* = 1544, and sample size per subgroup was given as (*n*). All data is presented as a percentage and 95 CI. Capital letters are used as a label for subgroups within categories for gender, age and sporting frequency. Lower case letters displayed below a specific value indicate that this value is significantly larger than the corresponding capital letters.

4. Discussion

Almost two-thirds of the respondents indicated having used DS's, SNPS, or both in the previous twelve months. DS's were used more frequently than SNPs, with improving health being the most important motivating factor. The most frequently reported products used were, for DS's, vitamin and mineral supplements, and, for SNPs, energy drinks. DS use was most frequently reported by women and older people. On the other hand, men, young people, and those exercising most frequently reported the highest use of SNPs. Women tended to indicate general health considerations more frequently compared to men as their main reason, whereas men reported physical performance purposes as their main reason for use more often than women. Remarkably, even sedentary respondents reported a relatively high prevalence of SNP use.

4.1. *Prevalence and Reasons*

Combined use of DS and SNP intake of specific groups and populations has been previously reported, ranging from 22% to 98% based on different methods [1–4,6,8,10–18], while we measured a substantial percentage of 61% (combining both DS's and SNPs) in the current study. Only a few studies have focused on the sport-specific use of DS's and SNPs in non-athletes [1,6,14]. Although the combined DS and SNP use in the present study is lower than in most recent studies with athletes [2–4], it is much higher than the reported 4.8% in a small group of non-athletic controls (n = 60) as presented previously [1]. This may be explained by geographical differences indicating the relevance of this type of study for specific regions worldwide.

Overall DS use in this Dutch sample (49%) is similar to DS use of a representative sample of the US population (*i.e.*, 52% [19]) and data based on the latest Dutch Food Consumption Survey (VCP) [20]. This VCP was also questioning dietary supplement use throughout the year, and showed a range of 26–36% for men and 34–54% for women across different age groups. The results of the present study are at the upper end of the results of the VCP, most likely due to including or not including specific types of DS's (for example ergogenic supplements), but also reflecting some of the differences in our population with those of the VCP (maybe as a result of including those interested in a questionnaire about health and exercise), despite the fact that we included a representative sample of the Dutch population. As observed previously, multivitamins, vitamin C, and vitamin D were most frequently reported [19–21].

Gender differences found in the present study are in line with results found earlier in a study including 1689 non-athletes as controls of an athletic population [8]. These authors reported a difference in total nutritional supplement use—a combination of DS's and SNPs—between men (32%) and women (52%) [8]. We found a similar gender difference although the total prevalence of DS and SNP use was higher in our study, and the difference between both groups was much smaller: 60% *vs.* 64% for men and women, respectively. Interestingly, the women in our study reported higher DS use compared with men (36% *vs.* 20%), while men reported a higher prevalence of SNPs. This gender difference was also previously detected by others [2,8,13,22]. An explanation might be that DS's are more frequently linked to health, whereas SNPs are more frequently associated with physical performance. This would be in line with our observations that women reported "health" more often as the reason for use, while men reported "physical performance." In contrast, some studies did not find a gender difference [3] or in fact found the opposite [1,12], which may also depend on the definitions used for DS's and SNPs.

It is interesting to note that, compared with older respondents, younger respondents use more SNPs or both SNPs and DS's. This contrasts with some previous investigations that indicated a higher prevalence of nutritional supplement use in adult athletes compared with adolescents [23,24]. It can be speculated that SNPs, such as sports drinks and energy drinks, have become increasingly popular among younger individuals in recent years. This might be attributed to marketing strategies of companies producing these type of products that are appealing to young athletes, resulting, for example, in parents buying these drinks at the supermarket for their children to replenish energy and fluid at half-time during their sports activities on the weekend.

Our findings are also in line with the National Health and Nutrition Examination Study. That study revealed comparable trends for those being active (>120 times a year in the present study *vs.* vigorous in NHANES), reporting the highest percentages for total DS use, but also for the top ranked products like multivitamin/mineral and vitamin C [19].

4.2. Strengths and Limitations

The novelty of this paper is that we examined the use of DS's and SNPs in a representative sample of a general population in relation to reasons for use, *i.e.*, health purposes, physical performance purposes, both, or other reasons, for the total category of DS's, SNPs, or combined use of DS's and SNPs. To the best of our knowledge, this is the first study investigating the general reason for use (health, performance, or both) of both DS's and SNPs in a general population. Besides this, we used a sound sampling strategy with a strong response rate.

An important added value of the present study is that it evaluated the prevalence of intake of DS's and SNPs separately, as well as the different types of products used—an insight which has generally not been provided in other large cohort publications [19–21,25,26]. For example, there does not seem to be any nutritional substantiation for energy-containing SNPs used by the majority of the non-exercising population. Combining DS's and SNPs will not provide this insight.

The estimated proportions with a confidence interval (CI) of 95% are relatively small, which increases the likelihood that the true value of the respondents will actually lay close to the reported average percentage.

As we did not investigate frequency of use or quantity, this should be investigated in the near future. As a consequence, our results reflect the total prevalence of respondents using a product at least once in this period. This may inflate the results for prevalence of use; on the other hand, others have questioned nutritional supplement use in the last 12 months [27], which can be seen as indicative for the (absolute) prevalence of this type of product and the difference in proportion between products and categories.

Since we were limited by the number of questions that could be included in the questionnaire, we chose to pre-select the most relevant types of DS's and SNPs. In the case of SNPs, sports energy bars are missing in this category because we focused on fluid-based SNPs; therefore, the prevalence of SNP use in our study could be underestimated, but should at least give a representative picture of fluid-based SNP use. It could be debated why, for example, ergogenic supplements such as creatine and B-alanine were classified as DS's, as others would put these in the SNPs category because of their sports-performance-enhancing claims. On the other hand, some but not all of these ergogenic supplements could be used for health purposes as well. For example, there is a relation between the nitrate in beetroot juice and blood pressure. Quercitin is a polyfenol that could also be related to health and caffeine and seen from a healthy life style perspective, for example, to stimulate energy metabolism to enhance body weight loss. As there is not a single definition, either legal or within nutritional science, of what constitutes a dietary supplement [28], we chose to combine all supplements based on tablets, capsules, drops, and so on in small doses, mostly defined in mg or mcg. As the included sport nutrition products were defined as those delivering substantial energy, macronutrients, fluid, or a combination of the three. In this case, classifying ergogenics as DS's could affect the prevalence of sport-specific use as a reason. On the other hand, the prevalence of the reason for physical performance regarding DS's is only 14%, compared with 79% using DS's for health purposes. The contribution of these ergogenic supplements on sport-specific use can be stated as limited. Still, this can be seen as a limitation that could have been prevented if we divided these categories beforehand.

As health is the main reason for use of DS's, SNPs, or both, these observations suggest that the general population has the impression that both DS's and SNPs are considered a healthy choice. An obvious question is whether the majority of this population needs these products, and whether the products used actually enhanced their sporting performance or influenced their health.

5. Conclusions

This study shows a high prevalence of DS and SNP use among the general population. Dietary supplement use was most frequently reported by women and older people, while men, young people, and those exercising most frequently reported the highest use of SNPs. Next to improving health, improvement of physical performance appears to be an important objective for both DS's and SNPs, and the combined use of these products. It can be questioned whether the use of SNPs fits all respondents' physical activity needs and in particular for those classified as being sedentary.

Acknowledgments: The Dutch National Sport Study (NSO) was partly funded by a grant from the Ministry of Health, Welfare and Sport. The writing of this article as part of the Dutch Sport nutrition and Supplement Study was made possible by a regional government grant as part of the Eat2Move project of the province of Gelderland, the Netherlands. Special thanks to Jeanne de Vries and Andy Maytum for giving feedback on the manuscript.

Author Contributions: F.W. and R.v.d.D. designed the research; R.v.d.D. and F.W. conducted the research; R.v.d.D., F.W., I.C., and M.M. analyzed the data and performed statistical analysis; R.W. and M.M. had primary responsibility for the final content. All authors have read and approved the manuscript.

Conflicts of Interest: All authors declare no conflicts of interest.

Abbreviations

The following abbreviations are used in this manuscript:

DS's	Dietary Supplements
SNPs	Sport Nutrition Products
NSO	Dutch National Sport Study (in Dutch: Nationaal SportOnderzoek)
DSSS	Dutch Sport nutrition and Supplement Study

References

1. Giannopoulou, I.; Noutsos, K.; Apostolidis, N.; Bayios, I.; Nassis, G.P. Performance level affects the dietary supplement intake of both individual and team sports athletes. *J. Sports Sci. Med.* **2013**, *12*, 190–196. [PubMed]
2. Kang, M.; Kim, D.W.; Baek, Y.J.; Moon, S.H.; Jung, H.J.; Song, Y.J.; Paik, H.Y. Dietary supplement use and its effect on nutrient intake in Korean adult population in the korea national health and nutrition examination survey iv (2007–2009) data. *Eur. J. Clin. Nutr.* **2014**, *68*, 804–810. [CrossRef] [PubMed]
3. Tavani, A.; Colombo, P.; Scarpino, V.; Zuccaro, P.; Pacifici, R.; La Vecchia, C. A survey of dietary supplement use among Italian sporting club athletes. *Nutrafoods* **2014**, *13*, 29–34. [CrossRef]
4. Wiens, K.; Erdman, K.A.; Stadnyk, M.; Parnell, J.A. Dietary supplement usage, motivation, and education in young, Canadian athletes. *Int. J. Sport Nutr. Exerc. Metab.* **2014**, *24*, 613–622. [CrossRef] [PubMed]
5. Wardenaar, F.C.; Ceelen, I.J.M.; Van den Dool, R.; Witkamp, R.; Mensink, M. Het gebruik van voedingssupplementen en sportvoeding door meer en minder actieve nederlanders—Een inventarisatie op basis van het nationaal sport onderzoek 2012 onder de nederlandse bevolking (use of dietary supplemenets and sport nutrition products in the dutch general population). *Ned. Tijdschri. Voeding Diet.* **2014**, *69*, S1–S9. (In Dutch)
6. Kristiansen, M.; Levy-Milne, R.; Barr, S.; Flint, A. Dietary supplement use by varsity athletes at a Canadian university. *Int. J. Sport Nutr. Exerc. Metab.* **2005**, *15*, 195–210. [PubMed]
7. Sette, S.; Le Donne, C.; Piccinelli, R.; Arcella, D.; Turrini, A.; Leclercq, C.; Group, I.-S.S. The third Italian national food consumption survey, inran-scai 2005-06—Part 1: Nutrient intakes in Italy. *Nutr. Metab. Cardiovasc. Dis.* **2011**, *21*, 922–932. [CrossRef] [PubMed]
8. Sundgot-Borgen, J.; Berglund, B.; Torstveit, M.K. Nutritional supplements in Norwegian elite athletes—Impact of international ranking and advisors. *Scand. J. Med. Sci. Sports* **2003**, *13*, 138–144. [CrossRef] [PubMed]
9. Mulier Instituut. Nationaal Sportonderzoek 2013. Available online: http://www.mulierinstituut.nl/projecten/sportdeelname/nationaal-sportonderzoek-nso/2013-2/ (accessed on 23 April 2016).
10. Chen, S.; Binns, C.W.; Maycock, B.; Liu, Y.; Zhang, Y. Prevalence of dietary supplement use in healthy pre-school chinese children in Australia and China. *Nutrients* **2014**, *6*, 815–828. [CrossRef] [PubMed]

11. De Silva, A.; Samarasinghe, Y.; Senanayake, D.; Lanerolle, P. Dietary supplement intake in national-level Sri Lankan athletes. *Int. J. Sport Nutr. Exerc. Metab.* **2010**, *20*, 15–20.
12. Evans, M.W.J.; Ndetan, H.; Perko, M.; Williams, R.; Walker, C. Dietary supplement use by children and adolescents in the united states to enhance sport performance: Results of the national health interview survey. *J. Prim. Prev.* **2012**, *33*, 3–12. [CrossRef] [PubMed]
13. Froiland, K.; Koszewski, W.; Hingst, J.; Kopecky, L. Nutritional supplement use among college athletes and their sources of information. *Int. J. Sport Nutr. Exerc. Metab.* **2004**, *14*, 104–120. [PubMed]
14. Heikkinen, A.; Alaranta, A.; Helenius, I.; Vasankari, T. Dietary supplementation habits and perceptions of supplement use among elite finnish athletes. *Int. J. Sport Nutr. Exerc. Metab.* **2011**, *21*, 271–279. [PubMed]
15. MacKay, D.; Wallace, T.C. Re: Dietary supplement use by children and adolescents in the united states to enhance sport performance: Results of the national health interview survey. *J. Prim. Prev.* **2012**, *33*, 225–227. [CrossRef] [PubMed]
16. Petroczi, A.; Naughton, D.P.; Pearce, G.; Bailey, R.; Bloodworth, A.; McNamee, M. Nutritional supplement use by elite young uk athletes: Fallacies of advice regarding efficacy. *J. Int. Soc. Sports Nutr.* **2008**, *5*, 22. [CrossRef] [PubMed]
17. Scofield, D.E.; Unruh, S. Dietary supplement use among adolescent athletes in central nebraska and their sources of information. *J. Strength Cond. Res.* **2006**, *20*, 452–455. [PubMed]
18. Yu, S.M.; Kogan, M.D.; Huang, Z.J. Vitamin-mineral supplement use among US women, 2000. *J. Am. Med. Women's Assoc.* **2003**, *58*, 157–164.
19. Radimer, K.; Bindewald, B.; Hughes, J.; Ervin, B.; Swanson, C.; Picciano, M.F. Dietary supplement use by us adults: Data from the national health and nutrition examination survey, 1999–2000. *Am. J. Epidemiol.* **2004**, *160*, 339–349. [CrossRef] [PubMed]
20. Van Rossum, C.T.M.; Fransen, H.P.; Verkaik-Kloosterman, J.; Buurma-Rethans, E.J.M.; Ocké, M.C. *Dutch National Food Consumption Survey 2007–2010: Diet of Children and Adults Aged 7 to 69 Years*; RIVM Report 350050006; National Institute for Public Health and the Environment: Bilthoven, The Netherlands, 5 October 2011; pp. 521–522.
21. Timbo, B.B.; Ross, M.P.; McCarthy, P.V.; Lin, C.T. Dietary supplements in a national survey: Prevalence of use and reports of adverse events. *J. Am. Diet. Assoc.* **2006**, *106*, 1966–1974. [CrossRef] [PubMed]
22. Huang, S.H.; Johnson, K.; Pipe, A.L. The use of dietary supplements and medications by Canadian athletes at the atlanta and sydney olympic games. *Clin. J. Sport Med.* **2006**, *16*, 27–33. [CrossRef] [PubMed]
23. Braun, H.; Koehler, K.; Geyer, H.; Kleiner, J.; Mester, J.; Schanzer, W. Dietary supplement use among elite young german athletes. *Int. J. Sport Nutr. Exerc. Metab.* **2009**, *19*, 97–109. [PubMed]
24. McDowall, J.A. Supplement use by young athletes. *J. Sports Sci. Med.* **2007**, *6*, 337–342. [PubMed]
25. Millen, A.E.; Dodd, K.W.; Subar, A.F. Use of vitamin, mineral, nonvitamin, and nonmineral supplements in the united states: The 1987, 1992, and 2000 national health interview survey results. *J. Am. Diet. Assoc.* **2004**, *104*, 942–950. [CrossRef] [PubMed]
26. Schaffer, D.M.; Gordon, N.P.; Jensen, C.D.; Avins, A.L. Nonvitamin, nonmineral supplement use over a 12-month period by adult members of a large health maintenance organization. *J. Am. Diet. Assoc.* **2003**, *103*, 1500–1505. [CrossRef] [PubMed]
27. Slater, G.; Tan, B.; Teh, K.C. Dietary supplementation practices of Singaporean athletes. *Int. J. Sport Nutr. Exerc. Metab.* **2003**, *13*, 320–332. [PubMed]
28. Maughan, R.J.; Greenhaff, P.L.; Hespel, P. Dietary supplements for athletes: Emerging trends and recurring themes. *J. Sports Sci.* **2011**, *29* (Suppl. S1), S57–S66. [CrossRef] [PubMed]

14

Effects of Short-Term Dynamic Constant External Resistance Training and Subsequent Detraining on Strength of the Trained and Untrained Limbs: A Randomized Trial

Pablo B. Costa [1,*], Trent J. Herda [2,†], Ashley A. Herda [2,†] and Joel T. Cramer [3]

1 Exercise Physiology Laboratory, Department of Kinesiology, California State University, Fullerton, CA 92831, USA
2 Department of Health, Sport and Exercise Sciences, University of Kansas, Lawrence, KS 66045, USA; t.herda@ku.edu (T.J.H.); a.herda@ku.edu (A.A.H.)
3 Department of Nutrition and Health Sciences, University of Nebraska—Lincoln, Lincoln, NE 68583, USA; jcramer@unl.edu
* Correspondence: pcosta@fullerton.edu
† These authors contributed equally to this work.

Academic Editor: Eling de Bruin

Abstract: Short-term resistance training has been shown to increase isokinetic muscle strength and performance after only two to nine days of training. The purpose of this study was to examine the effects of three days of unilateral dynamic constant external resistance (DCER) training and detraining on the strength of the trained and untrained legs. Nineteen men were randomly assigned to a DCER training group or a non-training control group. Subjects visited the laboratory eight times, the first visit was a familiarization session, the second visit was a pre-training assessment, the subsequent three visits were for training sessions (if assigned to the training group), and the last three visits were post-training assessments 1, 2, and 3 (*i.e.*, 48 h, 1 week, and 2 weeks after the final training session). Strength increased in both trained and untrained limbs from pre- to post-training assessment 1 for the training group and remained elevated at post-training assessments 2 and 3 ($p \leqslant 0.05$). No changes were observed in the control ($p > 0.05$). Possible strength gains from short-term resistance training have important implications in clinical rehabilitation settings, sports injury prevention, as well as other allied health fields such as physical therapy, occupational therapy, and athletic training.

Keywords: training-induced; neuromuscular adaptation; isotonic; muscle mechanics; unilateral; cross education

1. Introduction

Allied health professionals, such as physical therapists, occupational therapists, and athletic trainers, may benefit from rapid increases in strength of a patient or athlete recovering from injury [1–3]. In theory, if an individual's strength can be increased within a short period of time, an alternative to more expensive and invasive medical procedures may be offered [1,2]. In addition, they are more likely to comply with a rehabilitation program and perhaps decrease the risk of reinjury [3]. Consequently, short-term resistance training has been shown to increase isokinetic muscle strength and performance after only two to nine days of training [1,2,4,5]. This short time course for strength adaptations may conveniently coincide with the commonly limited rehabilitation treatments due to minimal insurance coverage or lack of compliance [1,2], or the time demands for return to play in sports. If patients do not improve quickly, the risk of injury reoccurrence may increase [1]. This potential for short-term resistance training to improve muscular performance in a relatively shorter period of time would have important implications for professionals working in rehabilitation settings [1–3].

Evidence has shown that improvements in muscle performance can be observed in a shorter period than what is typically used in longer traditional training programs [1,2,6,7]. For example, Prevost *et al.*, (1999) investigated velocity-specific short-term training for two days and reported 22.1% increases in peak torque (PT) at $270° \cdot s^{-1}$ after training at $270° \cdot s^{-1}$, but no changes for training at 30 and $150° \cdot s^{-1}$ at the testing velocities of 30 and $150° \cdot s^{-1}$ [4]. Similarly, Coburn *et al.*, (2006) compared short-term resistance training effects after three sessions of slow- or fast-velocity and found that PT increased for both training groups [2]. However, the slower velocity training group increased PT at both velocities whereas PT increased only at the faster velocity for the faster velocity training group [2]. No changes in PT were observed for the control group and no changes in EMG amplitude were reported for any of the groups at any of the velocities. The authors concluded three sessions of slow or fast velocity isokinetic resistance training were sufficient to increase PT and the lack of EMG amplitude changes suggested increases in leg extension PT were not caused by increases in muscle activation [2].

The principle of training called reversibility, or detraining, occurs when a complete cessation or substantial reduction in training causes a partial or complete reversal of the adaptations induced by training [8,9]. Detraining occurs after an individual discontinues a training program [8–15]. Most of the increases in strength found with resistance training are lost after several weeks of detraining [10–14,16,17]. However, Colliander and Tesch (1992) showed that a resistance training program incorporating combined concentric and eccentric leg extension exercise retained more of the novel strength gains than a concentric-only training program [16]. In addition, Farthing (2003) found eccentric muscle action training elicited greater strength gains than concentric training [18]. Because isokinetic muscle actions are typically concentric, it is unknown whether dynamic constant external resistance (DCER) training, which uses coupled concentric and eccentric muscle actions, and isokinetic training would affect detraining differently.

Isokinetic muscle actions have been traditionally used in rehabilitation and testing scenarios. Several studies have examined the effects of isokinetic training on strength and/or muscle cross-sectional area (CSA) [1,2,4,5] and isokinetic training allows development of maximum tension throughout the range of motion [7]. However, DCER training would offer a more accessible, convenient, cost-effective, and practical method of training, in addition to perhaps providing a greater stimulus to elicit increases in strength [19]. Furthermore, no studies have investigated the effects of short term resistance training on the contralateral untrained limb or on detraining. Therefore, the purpose of this study was to examine the effects of three days of DCER training and subsequent detraining on isokinetic on strength of the trained and untrained contralateral leg extensors during maximal leg extension muscle actions.

2. Method

2.1. Subjects

Nineteen apparently healthy untrained men (mean ± SD age = 21.6 ± 3.4 years; body mass = 77.9 ± 14.0 kg; height = 173.9 ± 4.1 cm) were randomly assigned to a DCER training group or control group. Participants were minimally active and naïve to the intent of the study. Individuals with a history of chronic resistance training (>1 day/week) in the previous 12 months or those who reported engaging in one or more lower-body resistance training exercise for six months prior to the start of the study were excluded from participating. Prior to any testing, all subjects read and signed an informed consent form and completed a health status questionnaire. Individuals with any degenerative neuromuscular or joint disorders, or who sustained injuries distal to the waist within six months prior to screening were also excluded from the study. Subjects were asked to maintain their daily activities, but refrain from any exercise and/or nutritional supplements throughout the course of the study. Individuals who had been taking nutritional supplements three months prior to screening were not permitted to participate. This study was approved by the university's Institutional Review Board for the Protection of Human Subjects.

2.2. Research Design

A mixed factorial design was used to examine the effects of three days of short-term unilateral resistance training and subsequent detraining on strength. Subjects visited the laboratory on eight separate occasions. The first visit was a familiarization session, the second visit was a pre-training assessment, the subsequent three visits were for training (if assigned to the training group), and the last three visits were the post-training assessments (*i.e.*, 48 h, 1 week, and 2 weeks after the final training session). Pre-training assessments were performed 48 h prior to the start of training. Testing included assessments of DCER strength. The training group performed DCER leg extension exercise with the dominant leg in each of the three days of training whereas the control group did not take part in the training intervention. After the three training sessions, post-training assessments were performed in an identical manner to the pre-training assessments. In order to examine the time course of the effects of training, post-training assessments were performed 48 h, 1 week, and 2 weeks after the final training session. All pre- and post-training assessments were conducted at approximately the same time of day.

2.3. Dynamic Constant External Resistance Assessments

The maximal strength of the leg extensors were assessed using a DCER Nautilus leg extension machine (Nautilus, Inc., Vancouver, WA, USA). The input axis of the machine was aligned with the axis of rotation of the knee. The distal anterior portion of the leg superior to the ankle was used as the load bearing point. Three submaximal warm-up sets of increasing tester-selected intensities (*i.e.*, 6–8, 3–5, and 1–2 repetitions) preceded the maximal strength attempt. When one attempt was successful, the load was increased by 2–5 kg until a failed repetition occurred. A failed repetition was defined as the inability to complete the full range of motion with the assigned load. During the tests, loud verbal encouragement was provided by the investigator. Each subject was instructed to provide maximal effort throughout the entire range of motion. The greatest load moved through a complete leg extension range of motion was considered the one repetition maximum (1-RM). A 1-min rest was allowed between each successive attempt [20,21].

2.4. Dynamic Constant External Resistance Training Protocol

After a rest period of 48 h following the pre-training assessment, the training group took part in three DCER training sessions separated by 48 h. Participants in the training group performed 4 sets of 10 repetitions. Each training session began with ten warm-up repetitions at approximately 25% of the resistance used for the DCER training session. Approximately 80% of the 1-RM obtained during the DCER maximal strength assessment was used as the starting load for the DCER group. A 2-min rest period was allowed between each training set. Training load for the DCER group was continually increased and adjusted by approximately 1.14 kg as each participant was able to tolerate a given load with ease in order to ensure that the subject reached failure at approximately the 10th repetition. All participants taking part in the DCER training intervention were supervised during all training sessions.

2.5. Rating of Perceived Exertion

Rating of perceived exertion (RPE) was used to compare effort among the DCER training days and sets [22–26]. Prior to the start of the study, subjects received instructions on how to use the RPE scale to rate their perceived exertion. A Category-Ratio scale (CR-10) was used, where "0" is classified as rest (no effort) and "10" is classified as maximal effort (most stressful exercise ever performed). The CR-10 has been slightly modified to reflect American English (e.g., easy and hard instead of light and strong, respectively) [24]. Subjects were asked to provide a number on the scale to rate their overall effort immediately after each set was completed and after the entire training session. The RPE assessments were conducted during each session by showing the scale and asking subjects "How would you rate your effort?" and "How would you rate your entire workout?" immediately after each set of training and after each training session, respectively. Therefore, in this study, "set RPE" was defined as the RPE reported by the subject after each set, while "session RPE" was defined as the RPE reported each day after the training session was completed.

2.6. Statistical Analyses

A three-way mixed factorial ANOVA (time (pre- *vs.* post-training assessment 1 *vs.* post-training assessment 2 *vs.* post-training assessment 3) × group (DCER *vs.* control) × limb (trained *vs.* untrained) was used to analyze the 1-RM data. A two-way repeated measured ANOVA (time [training session 1 *vs.* training session 2 *vs.* training session 3) × set (1 *vs.* 2 *vs.* 3 *vs.* 4)) was used to analyze RPE assessed after each set during training. A one-way repeated measures ANOVA (time (training session 1 *vs.* training session 2 *vs.* training session 3)) was used to analyze training session RPE. When appropriate, follow-up analyses were performed using lower-order two- and one-way repeated measured ANOVAs, and paired sample *t*-tests. An alpha level of $p \leqslant 0.05$ was considered statistically significant for all comparisons. Predictive Analytics SoftWare (PASW) version 18.0.0 (SPSS Inc., Chicago, IL, USA) was used for all statistical analyses.

3. Results

3.1. Dynamic Constant External Resistance Assessments

Table 1 contains the means (±SE) for 1-RM strength in the trained and untrained leg. There was no three-way interaction for time × group × limb ($p = 0.11$). However, there was a significant two-way interaction for time × group ($p = 0.001$). Post-hoc pairwise comparisons for the marginal means indicated that 1-RM increased in both trained and untrained limbs from pre- to post-training assessment 1 for the DCER group ($p < 0.001$) (Figure 1). There were no differences in 1-RM strength for the DCER group among post-training assessments 1, 2, and 3 ($p > 0.05$) (Figure 2). No significant changes were found for the control group ($p > 0.05$).

Table 1. Means (±SE) for leg extension 1-RM.

	Group		Pre-Training Assessment 1	Post-Training Assessment 1	Post-Training Assessment 2	Post-Training Assessment 3
1-RM (kg)	DCER (n = 10)	Trained	43.0 ± 3.0	52.6 ± 3.8 *	50.5 ± 3.5 *	50.2 ± 3.2 *
		Untrained	41.9 ± 2.7	48.9 ± 4.2 *	48.9 ± 3.8 *	48.6 ± 3.5 *
	CONT (n = 9)	Trained	41.7 ± 2.2	41.9 ± 2.1	41.8 ± 1.9	42.7 ± 1.6
		Untrained	41.9 ± 2.1	41.8 ± 1.9	41.7 ± 2.0	42.2 ± 1.7

Notes: 1-RM = 1 repetition maximum; DCER = dynamic constant external resistance; CONT = control. * Denotes significant change from pre- to post-assessments.

3.2. Rating of Perceived Exertion

Table 2 contains the means (±SE) for set and session RPE from the training group. There was no two-way interaction for time × set for set RPE ($p = 0.41$). However, there was a significant main effect for set ($p < 0.001$). Post-hoc pairwise comparisons for the marginal means (collapsed across time) indicated a significant main effect for set RPE ($p < 0.05$). RPE increased significantly from the first until the last set within each session ($p < 0.05$). For session RPE, there was no main effect for time ($p = 0.55$).

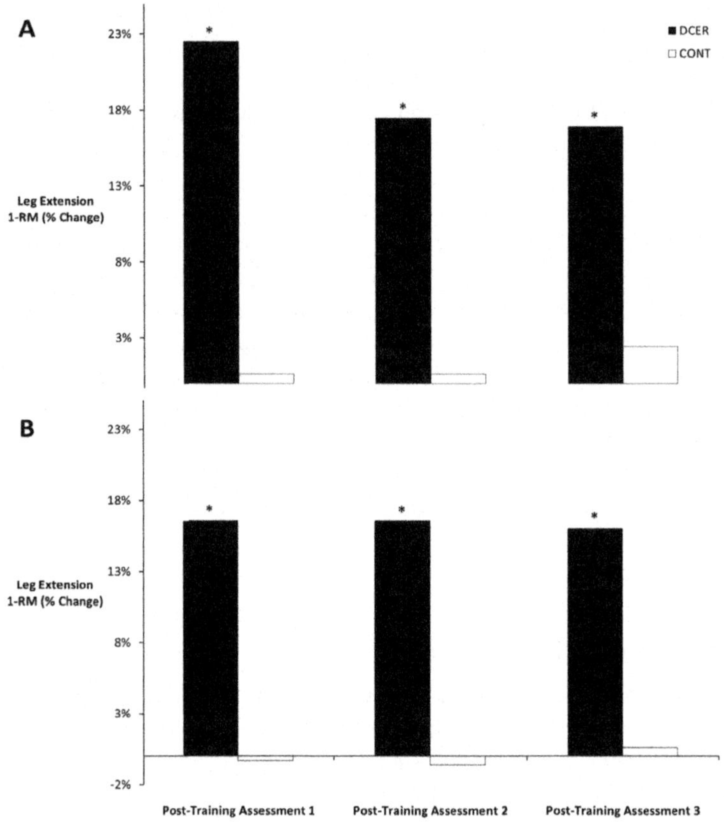

Figure 1. Means of percent change for leg extension 1-RM for the trained (**A**) and untrained (**B**) legs. * Denotes significant difference from the pre-test for the DCER group. DCER = dynamic constant external resistance; CONT = control.

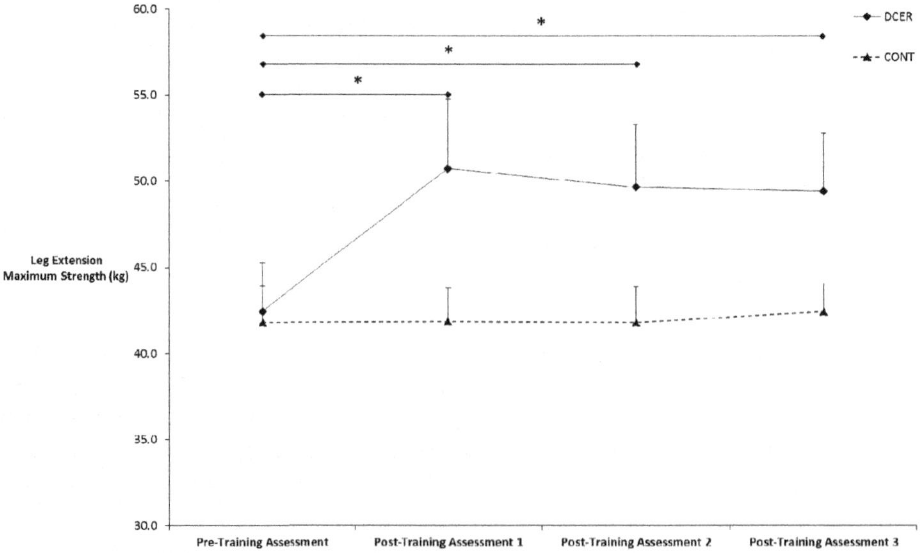

Figure 2. Means (±SE) for leg extension 1-RM collapsed across limb. * Denotes significant difference from the pre-test for the DCER group. DCER = dynamic constant external resistance; CONT = control.

Table 2. Means (±SE) for set and session rating of perceived exertion for the DCER group.

Training Session	1st Set	2nd Set	3rd Set	4th Set	Session
Session 1	6.4 ± 0.54	7.3 ± 0.63 *	8.3 ± 0.45 *	8.6 ± 0.37 *	7.6 ± 0.48
Session 2	5.4 ± 0.37	6.9 ± 0.31 *	7.8 ± 0.29 *	8.6 ± 0.43 *	7.1 ± 0.35
Session 3	5.8 ± 0.33	6.9 ± 0.43 *	7.9 ± 0.50 *	8.5 ± 0.48 *	7.5 ± 0.40

Notes: DCER = dynamic constant external resistance. * Denotes significant change over sets within each training session.

4. Discussion

Perhaps the most important finding of the present study was the increase in DCER strength acquired by the training group. DCER strength increased from pre- to post-training assessment 1 in the trained and untrained legs for the DCER training group and remained elevated during post-training assessments 2 and 3. To our knowledge, this was the first study to report DCER strength gains with short-term resistance training while also considering the detraining period of two weeks. These findings are in agreement with previous studies reporting PT increases after short-term isokinetic training [1,2]. In addition, the DCER group retained the strength gains during post-training assessments 2 and 3. That is, DCER strength remained elevated over a two-week period. Typical increases in strength obtained in longer resistance training programs are diminished after several weeks of detraining [10–14,16]. Colliander and Tesch (1992) compared the effects of resistance training and detraining using concentric-only and combined concentric and eccentric muscle actions of the leg extensors and reported that the group performing coupled concentric and eccentric muscle actions had a greater overall increase in PT after training and detraining than the concentric-only group [16]. These authors suggested strength decreases observed during detraining are not likely due to atrophy, but perhaps a reduction in neural drive or motor unit activation and hypothesized eccentric muscle actions are capable of inducing greater motor unit activation than concentric muscle actions [16]. Thus, it was suggested a resistance training program incorporating combined concentric and eccentric repetitions of leg extension can retain more of the obtained strength gains than the training program with concentric-only repetitions [16]. Likewise, Farthing (2003) found eccentric-only muscle action training elicited greater strength gains than concentric-only training [18]. Similarly, Knight *et al.*, (2001) suggested that isotonic muscle actions may be more effective at increasing torque because isokinetic resistance is accommodating, hence, it decreases with fatigue [19]. These findings [16,18,19], along with the findings of the current study may indicate an advantage of DCER over isokinetic resistance training programs when conducted over a relatively short period of time.

For the DCER training group, despite training only one leg, strength increased on the contralateral limb and was maintained over the two-week detraining period. Unilateral resistance training of a limb can increase the strength of the contralateral limb through a concept termed cross-education [27]. Increases in strength of the contralateral, untrained limb, have been extensively reported in the literature [27,28]. Possibly an important finding of the current study is that short-term resistance training also elicited the cross-education effect. This has important implications for injury rehabilitation, where in the initial period post-injury strength gains on an injured limb can conceivably be obtained with short-term contralateral resistance training. Contralateral strength gains have been hypothesized to be attributed to central neural adaptations (*i.e.*, excitation of the cortex), increased motoneuron output, and improved postural stabilization [27–29]. Accordingly, structural changes in the brain have been reported after only four weeks of unilateral resistance training concomitant with strength increases in trained and untrained limb [30]. In fact, strength gains may not be restricted to the contralateral untrained muscle, but might be observed in the contralateral untrained antagonist muscle [31]. Therefore, future studies should investigate the effects of short-term resistance training on contralateral antagonist muscles.

Strength gains were also maintained during the two-week detraining period in the DCER group. Although in the present study subjects were untrained, these findings were similar to those of Hortobagyi *et al.*, (1993), who found that two weeks of detraining of resistance-trained athletes did not cause a significant decrease in maximal bench press, squat, isometric, or concentric isokinetic strength [32]. Similarly, Shaver (1975) reported that recently acquired strength can be maintained in both trained and untrained limb for up to one week [33]. To our knowledge, the current study is the first to demonstrate short-term increases in strength can be maintained for a two-week period and in untrained limbs. In contrast, other authors have suggested strength gains that have been recently acquired may diminish faster than in strength-trained athletes [9,33]. Thus, the experience with resistance training (novice *vs.* well-trained athletes) should be considered when interpreting the results of a short-term resistance training program and its potential lasting effects.

The neuromuscular system undergoes numerous adaptations following a resistance training program [6,7,34–38]. Short-term resistance training has been shown to increase muscle strength and isokinetic performance after only a few days of training. Increases in muscular strength following a resistance training program can be attributed to neural and hypertrophic factors [6,34–37,39]. Therefore, voluntary strength increases due to not only the CSA and quality of muscle mass but also to the extent in which the muscle mass is able to activate [39]. In general, neural factors are believed to account for most of the increases in strength in the early stages of a resistance training program, whereas hypertrophic factors gradually become prevalent after several weeks of training [6,36,38–42]. Research suggests early adaptations to resistance training programs are related to improvements in neuromuscular efficiency, which perhaps indicates an increased capacity to activate skeletal muscle voluntarily [1,2,4,7,42]. Hence, initial improvements in strength and muscular performance reported following short-term resistance training are generally attributed to neural adaptations rather than muscle fiber hypertrophy [6,7]. However, the specific mechanisms of such adaptations in short-term training are not fully understood [2]. For example, Akima *et al.*, (1999) reported increases in PT after two weeks of resistance training but no changes in muscle CSA or fiber area suggesting strength increases occurred without muscle hypertrophy [7]. Similarly, Prevost *et al.*, (1999) reported velocity-specific increases in PT training at $270^{\circ}{\cdot}s^{-1}$ after increases in PT after two days of isokinetic training but not with training at 30 and $150^{\circ}{\cdot}s^{-1}$ [4]. Because improvements were only seen in one velocity, and muscle hypertrophy would most likely yield strength increases at the other velocities, investigators suggested that neural adaptations play a major role in strength improvements which are specific to a training velocity [4]. Beck *et al.*, (2007) suggested that responses to training might be influenced by the number of training sessions, training volume, and muscle(s) being tested [3]. Nevertheless, Akima *et al.*, (1999) and Costa *et al.*, (2013) suggested future studies should investigate the precise mechanisms underlying strength gains obtained with short-term resistance training [7,43].

The results revealed there were no differences in RPE as acknowledged by the subjects among the DCER training sessions. However, RPE increased from the first to the fourth set within each training session. These results are similar to those found by Egan *et al.*, (2006), who reported mean session RPE values of 7.3 for six sets of six repetitions of traditional resistance training using squats at an intensity of 80% of 1-RM [22]. Likewise, Sweet *et al.*, (2004) reported mean RPE values between 6.8 and 8.2 for 70 and 90% of leg press 1-RM, respectively [23]. Thus, perceived effort from a short-term resistance training program in the current study was similar to previous studies and was not lower because of the shorter training program duration.

5. Conclusions

The primary finding of this study was that DCER strength increased in the trained and untrained limbs with three days of contralateral training. This has important implications for injury rehabilitation, where in the initial period post-injury, strength gains on an injured limb can possibly be obtained with short-term resistance training. Furthermore, research has shown the feasibility and benefits of preoperative resistance training prior to surgical intervention to decrease the odds of inpatient rehabilitation, reduce the length of hospital stay, and promote overall postoperative recovery [44–47]. It is believed the increases were due to an unidentified factor because of strength gains observed in the untrained limb after DCER resistance training. Future studies should investigate the precise physiological components responsible for short-term contralateral strength gains. The findings of the current study may indicate an advantage of DCER over isokinetic resistance training programs when conducted over a relatively short period of time. These findings have important implications in clinical rehabilitation settings, sports injury prevention, as well as in other allied health fields such as physical therapy, occupational therapy, and athletic training. To our knowledge, the current study is the first to demonstrate recently-acquired strength can be maintained for a two-week period in untrained limbs. Therefore, future studies should examine the effects of short-term resistance training on injury prevention and rehabilitation.

Author Contributions: Pablo B. Costa was involved in the study concept and design, and was the primary manuscript writer, and carried out data acquisition, data analysis, and data interpretation. Trent J. Herda and Ashley A. Herda were significant contributors to data acquisition, read and approved the final manuscript, and were manuscript reviewers/revisers. Joel T. Cramer was the primary manuscript reviewer/reviser, a substantial contributor to concept and design, contributed to data analysis and interpretation, and was involved in manuscript revision.

Conflicts of Interest: The authors declare no conflict of interest.

References

1. Cramer, J.T.; Stout, J.R.; Culbertson, J.Y.; Egan, A.D. Effects of creatine supplementation and three days of resistance training on muscle strength, power output, and neuromuscular function. *J. Strength Cond. Res.* **2007**, *21*, 668–677. [PubMed]
2. Coburn, J.W.; Housh, T.J.; Malek, M.H.; Weir, J.P.; Cramer, J.T.; Beck, T.W.; Johnson, G.O. Neuromuscular responses to three days of velocity-specific isokinetic training. *J. Strength Cond. Res.* **2006**, *20*, 892–898. [PubMed]
3. Beck, T.W.; Housh, T.J.; Johnson, G.O.; Weir, J.P.; Cramer, J.T.; Coburn, J.W.; Malek, M.H.; Mielke, M. Effects of two days of isokinetic training on strength and electromyographic amplitude in the agonist and antagonist muscles. *J. Strength Cond. Res.* **2007**, *21*, 757–762. [PubMed]
4. Prevost, M.C.; Nelson, A.G.; Maraj, B.K.V. The effect of two days of velocity-specific isokinetic training on torque production. *J. Strength Cond. Res.* **1999**, *13*, 35–39.
5. Brown, L.E.; Whitehurst, M. The effect of short-term isokinetic training on force and rate of velocity development. *J. Strength Cond. Res.* **2003**, *17*, 88–94. [PubMed]
6. Moritani, T.; deVries, H.A. Neural factors *versus* hypertrophy in the time course of muscle strength gain. *Am. J. Phys. Med.* **1979**, *58*, 115–130. [PubMed]
7. Akima, H.; Takahashi, H.; Kuno, S.Y.; Masuda, K.; Masuda, T.; Shimojo, H.; Anno, I.; Itai, Y.; Katsuta, S. Early phase adaptations of muscle use and strength to isokinetic training. *Med. Sci. Sports Exerc.* **1999**, *31*, 588–594. [CrossRef] [PubMed]
8. Mujika, I.; Padilla, S. Muscular characteristics of detraining in humans. *Med. Sci. Sports Exerc.* **2001**, *33*, 1297–1303. [CrossRef] [PubMed]
9. Mujika, I.; Padilla, S. Detraining: Loss of training-induced physiological and performance adaptations. Part i: Short term insufficient training stimulus. *Sports Med.* **2000**, *30*, 79–87. [CrossRef] [PubMed]
10. Hakkinen, K.; Komi, P.V.; Tesch, P.A. Effects of combined concentric and eccentric strength training and detraining on force-time, muscle fiber and metabolic characteristics of leg extensor muscles. *Scand. J. Sports Sci.* **1981**, *3*, 50–58.
11. Hakkinen, K.; Alen, M.; Komi, P.V. Changes in isometric force- and relaxation-time, electromyographic and muscle fibre characteristics of human skeletal muscle during strength training and detraining. *Acta Physiol. Scand.* **1985**, *125*, 573–585. [CrossRef] [PubMed]
12. Houston, M.E.; Froese, E.A.; Valeriote, S.P.; Green, H.J.; Ranney, D.A. Muscle performance, morphology and metabolic capacity during strength training and detraining: A one leg model. *Eur. J. Appl. Physiol. Occup. Physiol.* **1983**, *51*, 25–35. [CrossRef] [PubMed]

13. Narici, M.V.; Roi, G.S.; Landoni, L.; Minetti, A.E.; Cerretelli, P. Changes in force, cross-sectional area and neural activation during strength training and detraining of the human quadriceps. *Eur. J. Appl Physiol. Occup. Physiol.* **1989**, *59*, 310–319. [CrossRef] [PubMed]
14. Thorstensson, A. Observations on strength training and detraining. *Acta Physiol. Scand.* **1977**, *100*, 491–493. [CrossRef] [PubMed]
15. Andersen, L.L.; Andersen, J.L.; Magnusson, S.P.; Aagaard, P. Neuromuscular adaptations to detraining following resistance training in previously untrained subjects. *Eur. J. Appl. Physiol.* **2005**, *93*, 511–518. [CrossRef] [PubMed]
16. Colliander, E.B.; Tesch, P.A. Effects of detraining following short term resistance training on eccentric and concentric muscle strength. *Acta Physiol. Scand.* **1992**, *144*, 23–29. [CrossRef] [PubMed]
17. Faigenbaum, A.D.; Westcott, W.L.; Micheli, L.J.; Outerbridge, A.R.; Long, C.J.; LaRosa-Loud, R.; Zaichkowsky, L.D. The effects of strength training and detraining on children. *J. Strength Cond. Res.* **1996**, *10*, 109–114. [CrossRef]
18. Farthing, J.P.; Chilibeck, P.D. The effects of eccentric and concentric training at different velocities on muscle hypertrophy. *Eur. J. Appl Physiol.* **2003**, *89*, 578–586. [CrossRef] [PubMed]
19. Knight, K.; Ingersoll, C.; Bartholomew, J. Isotonic contractions might be more effective than isokinetic contractions in developing muscle strength. *J. Sport Rehabil.* **2001**, *10*, 124–131.
20. Weir, J.P.; Wagner, L.L.; Housh, T.J. The effect of rest interval length on repeated maximal bench presses. *J. Strength Cond. Res.* **1994**, *8*. [CrossRef]
21. Matuszak, M.E.; Fry, A.C.; Weiss, L.W.; Ireland, T.R.; McKnight, M.M. Effect of rest interval length on repeated 1 repetition maximum back squats. *J. Strength Cond. Res.* **2003**, *17*, 634–637. [PubMed]
22. Egan, A.; Winchester, J.; Foster, C.; McGuigan, M. Using session rpe to monitor different methods of resistance exercise. *J. Sports Sci. Med.* **2006**, *5*, 289–295.
23. Sweet, T.W.; Foster, C.; McGuigan, M.R.; Brice, G. Quantitation of resistance training using the session rating of perceived exertion method. *J. Strength Cond. Res.* **2004**, *18*, 796–802. [PubMed]
24. Foster, C.; Florhaug, J.A.; Franklin, J.; Gottschall, L.; Hrovatin, L.A.; Parker, S.; Doleshal, P.; Dodge, C. A new approach to monitoring exercise training. *J. Strength Cond. Res.* **2001**, *15*, 109–115. [PubMed]
25. Day, M.L.; McGuigan, M.R.; Brice, G.; Foster, C. Monitoring exercise intensity during resistance training using the session rpe scale. *J. Strength Cond. Res.* **2004**, *18*, 353–358. [PubMed]
26. Douris, P.C. The effect of isokinetic exercise on the relationship between blood lactate and muscle fatigue. *J. Orthop. Sports Phys. Ther.* **1993**, *17*, 31–35. [CrossRef] [PubMed]
27. Munn, J.; Herbert, R.D.; Gandevia, S.C. Contralateral effects of unilateral resistance training: A meta-analysis. *J. Appl. Physiol.* **2004**, *96*, 1861–1866. [CrossRef] [PubMed]
28. Carroll, T.J.; Herbert, R.D.; Munn, J.; Lee, M.; Gandevia, S.C. Contralateral effects of unilateral strength training: Evidence and possible mechanisms. *J. Appl. Physiol.* **2006**, *101*, 1514–1522. [CrossRef] [PubMed]
29. Rutherford, O.M.; Jones, D.A. The role of learning and coordination in strength training. *Eur. J. Appl. Physiol. Occup. Physiol.* **1986**, *55*, 100–105. [CrossRef] [PubMed]
30. Palmer, H.S.; Haberg, A.K.; Fimland, M.S.; Solstad, G.M.; Moe Iversen, V.; Hoff, J.; Helgerud, J.; Eikenes, L. Structural brain changes after 4 weeks of unilateral strength training of the lower limb. *J. Appl. Physiol.* **2013**, *115*, 167–175. [CrossRef] [PubMed]
31. Sariyildiz, M.; Karacan, I.; Rezvani, A.; Ergin, O.; Cidem, M. Cross-education of muscle strength: Cross-training effects are not confined to untrained contralateral homologous muscle. *Scand. J. Med. Sci. Sports* **2011**, *21*, e359–e364. [CrossRef] [PubMed]
32. Hortobagyi, T.; Houmard, J.A.; Stevenson, J.R.; Fraser, D.D.; Johns, R.A.; Israel, R.G. The effects of detraining on power athletes. *Med. Sci. Sports Exerc.* **1993**, *25*, 929–935. [PubMed]
33. Shaver, L.G. Cross transfer effects of conditioning and deconditioning on muscular strength. *Ergonomics* **1975**, *18*, 9–16. [CrossRef] [PubMed]
34. Kraemer, W.J.; Fleck, S.J.; Evans, W.J. Strength and power training: Physiological mechanisms of adaptation. *Exerc. Sport Sci. Rev.* **1996**, *24*, 363–397. [CrossRef] [PubMed]
35. Staron, R.S.; Karapondo, D.L.; Kraemer, W.J.; Fry, A.C.; Gordon, S.E.; Falkel, J.E.; Hagerman, F.C.; Hikida, R.S. Skeletal muscle adaptations during early phase of heavy-resistance training in men and women. *J. Appl. Physiol.* **1994**, *76*, 1247–1255. [PubMed]

36. Enoka, R.M. Muscle strength and its development. New perspectives. *Sports Med.* **1988**, *6*, 146–168. [CrossRef] [PubMed]
37. Sale, D.G. Influence of exercise and training on motor unit activation. *Exerc. Sport Sci. Rev.* **1987**, *15*, 95–151. [CrossRef] [PubMed]
38. Moritani, T.; deVries, H.A. Potential for gross muscle hypertrophy in older men. *J. Gerontol.* **1980**, *35*, 672–682. [CrossRef] [PubMed]
39. Sale, D.G. Neural adaptation to resistance training. *Med. Sci. Sports Exerc.* **1988**, *20*, S135–S145. [CrossRef] [PubMed]
40. Ikai, M.; Fukunaga, T. A study on training effect on strength per unit cross-sectional area of muscle by means of ultrasonic measurement. *Int. Z. Angew. Physiol.* **1970**, *28*, 173–180. [CrossRef] [PubMed]
41. Kanehisa, H.; Miyashita, M. Specificity of velocity in strength training. *Eur. J. Appl. Physiol. Occup. Physiol.* **1983**, *52*, 104–106. [CrossRef] [PubMed]
42. Knight, C.A.; Kamen, G. Adaptations in muscular activation of the knee extensor muscles with strength training in young and older adults. *J. Electromyogr. Kinesiol.* **2001**, *11*, 405–412. [CrossRef]
43. Costa, P.B.; Herda, T.J.; Walter, A.A.; Valdez, A.M.; Cramer, J.T. Effects of short-term resistance training and subsequent detraining on the electromechanical delay. *Muscle Nerve* **2013**, *48*, 135–136. [CrossRef] [PubMed]
44. Van Leeuwen, D.M.; de Ruiter, C.J.; Nolte, P.A.; de Haan, A. Preoperative strength training for elderly patients awaiting total knee arthroplasty. *Rehabil. Res. Pract.* **2014**, *2014*. [CrossRef] [PubMed]
45. Rooks, D.S.; Huang, J.; Bierbaum, B.E.; Bolus, S.A.; Rubano, J.; Connolly, C.E.; Alpert, S.; Iversen, M.D.; Katz, J.N. Effect of preoperative exercise on measures of functional status in men and women undergoing total hip and knee arthroplasty. *Arthritis Rheum.* **2006**, *55*, 700–708. [CrossRef] [PubMed]
46. Topp, R.; Swank, A.M.; Quesada, P.M.; Nyland, J.; Malkani, A. The effect of prehabilitation exercise on strength and functioning after total knee arthroplasty. *PM R* **2009**, *1*, 729–735. [CrossRef] [PubMed]
47. Swank, A.M.; Kachelman, J.B.; Bibeau, W.; Quesada, P.M.; Nyland, J.; Malkani, A.; Topp, R.V. Prehabilitation before total knee arthroplasty increases strength and function in older adults with severe osteoarthritis. *J. Strength Cond. Res.* **2011**, *25*, 318–325. [CrossRef] [PubMed]

15

A Description and Comparison of Cardiorespiratory Fitness Measures in Relation to Pitching Performance Among Professional Baseball Pitchers

Javair S. Gillett [1], J. Jay Dawes [2], Frank J. Spaniol [3,*], Matthew R. Rhea [4], Joe P. Rogowski [5], Mitchel A. Magrini [6], Roberto Simao [7] and Derek J. Bunker [4]

1 Athletic Performance, Houston Rockets, Houston, TX 77002, USA; jgillett@rocketball.com
2 University of Colorado, Colorado Springs, CO 80918, USA; jdawes@uccs.edu
3 Texas A&M University-Corpus Christi, Corpus Christi, TX 78412, USA
4 A.T. Still University, Kirksville, MO 63501, USA; mrhea@atsu.edu (M.R.R.); Bunkjames7@hotmail.com (D.J.B.)
5 Athletic Heart Research Institute, Orlando, FL, 32801, USA; jrogowski@athletic-heart.com
6 Oklahoma State University, Stillwater, OK 74074, USA; mmagrini@uccs.edu
7 Federal University of Rio de Janeiro, Rio de Janeiro 21941-901, Brazil; rsimaoj@terra.com.br
* Correspondence: frank.spaniol@tamucc.edu

Academic Editor: Eling Douwe de Bruin

Abstract: The purpose of this study is to provide descriptive and comparative information regarding the cardiorespiratory fitness of professional baseball pitchers. Twenty-four (n = 24) major league (ML) baseball pitchers (starters n = 14; relievers n = 10) over seven seasons (2007–2013) were evaluated. A modified Bruce protocol and the CardioCoach™ CO_2 metabolic analyzer were used to estimate $VO_{2\,max}$ and anaerobic threshold (AT) at the beginning of each season. Performance data from each season was utilized to draw inference about pitching performance. One-way Analysis of Variance (ANOVA) was used to compare Starting (S) and Relief (R) pitchers above/below the group mean for $VO_{2\,max}$ and AT. Pearson product moment correlations were also used to examine relationships between cardiorespiratory fitness and performance. Significant differences in performance were discovered between S pitchers above/below the overall group mean for $VO_{2\,max}$. ($p \leqslant 0.05$) and for AT in Walks plus Hits per Inning Pitched (WHIP) ($p \leqslant 0.05$) and Earned Run Average (ERA) ($p \leqslant 0.05$). Significant relationships between $VO_{2\,max}$ and Walks per 9 Innings (BB/9) ($p \leqslant 0.05$), Home Runs per 9 innings (HR/9) ($p \leqslant 0.05$), Wins (W) ($p \leqslant 0.05$), Fielding Independent Pitching (FIP) ($p \leqslant 0.01$), Strikeouts (K) ($p \leqslant 0.01$), Hits per 9 innings (H/9) ($p \leqslant 0.01$), Strikeouts per 9 innings (K/9) ($p \leqslant 0.01$), ERA ($p \leqslant 0.01$), and WHIP ($p \leqslant 0.01$). Low, but significant, correlations were discovered between AT and WHIP ($p \leqslant 0.05$) and ERA ($\leqslant 0.05$). CONCLUSION: Higher aerobic capacity appears to be more influential for S than R pitchers. Strength and conditioning practitioners should ensure that pitchers, especially S pitchers at the ML level, perform sufficient and appropriate endurance training to support pitching performance.

Keywords: conditioning; endurance; pitching; performance; $VO_{2\,max}$

1. Introduction

Baseball is a sport that requires short, explosive bursts of intense effort. While the duration of each play is relatively short, a typical professional baseball game takes approximately three hours to complete [1]. During a game, only two of the nine players on the field are involved in every single play, the pitcher and catcher. While catchers perform many of their skills at submaximal intensities, pitchers are expected to deliver every pitch at maximum, or near maximum effort [2]. A starting pitcher typically delivers 80–100 pitches or more per game, whereas a relief pitcher is required to throw significantly fewer pitches per performance (40 or less). Whereas a starting pitcher is typically allowed four days between performances, a reliever might be required to throw on consecutive days.

Pitching relies heavily on the ATP-PCr system during the delivery of the pitch, followed by brief bouts (approximately 20–30 s) of aerobic recovery between pitches [3]. Subsequently, pitching appears to place a relatively low demand on the aerobic energy system [4]. In fact, Potteiger *et al.* [4] found that mean oxygen consumption ranged between 14.8–20.6 $mL \cdot kg^{-1} min^{-1}$ for pitchers pitching in a simulated game. The researchers noted that this would correspond to a continuous exercise intensity at approximately 45% of the participants mean $VO_{2\,max}$. However, since this study was performed in a laboratory setting where the pitchers did not face game competition, one may speculate that the aerobic demands may differ during actual competition.

Stockholm and Morris [5] conducted a study in which a freshman collegiate baseball pitcher's heart rate (HR) was monitored and recorded during competition (3 h and 10 min, 9 inning game) via the use of telemetry. It was discovered that the mean heart rate during the performance was approximately 87% of the player's age-predicted heart rate max (HR_{max}), with peak HR reaching 95% of the player's age-predicted HR max. This is significantly greater than HRs achieved during a laboratory study [4] and during bullpen practice sessions prior to an intra-squad game [6]. This suggests that arousal and anxiety levels may impact the physiological demands of pitching. Furthermore, being that the bulk of competitions in professional baseball occur during the summer months, greater cardiorespiratory fitness may help players better accommodate the physiological challenges and delay the onset of fatigue when playing in hot/humid environments [5–13].

Very few studies have investigated the relationship between aerobic fitness and pitching performance [4]. This may in part be due to the observations that baseball is predominantly an anaerobic sport. Ebben *et al.* [14] found that the majority of major league strength coaches do not test anaerobic capacity or aerobic endurance, which may be due to the belief that possessing a high level of aerobic fitness does not appear to limit performance amongst professional or collegiate pitchers. Furthermore, studies that have investigated aerobic fitness and pitching performance have quantified performance in terms of maintenance of ball velocity, rather than the player's actual game statistics [4]. While one may assume that the maintenance of ball velocity is an inherent predictor of performance, the art of pitching is a multifaceted and complex skill and success should not be limited to a singular variable, particularly at higher playing levels. There are other performance indicators and statistics that are more indicative of individual pitching performance and less dependent on team performance, which should be taken into consideration when seeking to evaluate or predict pitching effectiveness.

Currently, there is very little data available regarding the cardiorespiratory fitness of baseball players, especially at the professional level. Thus, the primary purpose of this investigation was to provide descriptive information regarding the cardiorespiratory fitness profiles of Major League (ML) pitchers, and compare cardiorespiratory fitness levels between starting (S) and relief (R) pitchers. A secondary purpose was to examine the relationship between cardiorespiratory fitness and selected measures of pitching performance.

2. Method, Results, Discussion

2.1. Methods

2.1.1. Experimental Approach to the Problem

The data used for this study was archival and approved by an Institutional Review Board for research with human subjects prior to data analysis. In order to compare performance between pitchers by position and fitness level and identify the relationships between cardiorespiratory fitness and pitching performance, physiological and performance statistics over seven seasons (2007–2013) for 24 ML baseball pitchers were gathered and analyzed. A correlational analysis was also performed to examine possible relationships between these variables. In addition, statistical analyses were conducted to examine the differences between S and R pitchers.

2.1.2. Subjects

Data for 24 professional pitchers, within the selected ML baseball organization, was utilized in this investigation. Only pitchers remaining within the organization throughout the entire season were included in this analysis. Since some of the subjects in this study completed multiple seasons with the organization, a total of 40 eligible cases (n = 27 S; n = 13 R) were available for evaluation. For the purpose of analysis, each case (year) was treated separately as both physiological and performance statistics are subsequent to change each season and therefore were evaluated individually. Only pitchers with 50 or more innings pitched per season were used in this study.

2.1.3. Procedures

Physiological testing was performed within the first week of spring training camp each year. All physiological tests were performed after on-field baseball practice on days in which the pitcher did not throw a bullpen session. Pitchers completed a graded, submaximal exercise test on a treadmill (Life Fitness TI, Model 97Ti/Model CLST and Woodway, Model R-DESMO, Franklin Park, IL, USA). The CardioCoach™ CO_2 metabolic analyzer and software (version 3.04.72, KORR Medical Technologies Inc., Salt Lake City, UT, USA) was used for gas analysis. This device has been found to be a valid method of assessing VO_2 at submaximal and maximal levels [15]. Subjects performed a modified Bruce protocol and were asked to complete as many stages as possible. The test was terminated when the subject requested to stop or reached volitional fatigue. Utilizing the software provided via CardioCoach™ a linear regression equation was used to predict VO_{2peak}. CardioCoach™ software was also used to identify oxygen consumption at anaerobic threshold (AT). In addition to cardiorespiratory fitness, the following anthropometric and physiological data was collected for each of the subjects: height (cm), weight (kg), percent body fat (%BF), and lean body mass (LBM). Body fat was estimated using a six-site skinfold test [16].

Performance data were accessed and gathered immediately after the season via reliable online databases [17–19]. These databases are open access sources for pitching statistics. Multiple databases were used for the purpose of comparison to ensure accuracy. The key pitching performance statistics used in this analysis included: Fielding Independent Pitching (FIP), Walks plus Hits per Inning Pitched (WHIP), and Strikeout to Walk Ratio (K/BB). These statistics were chosen because they tend to be the least influenced by uncontrollable variables (*i.e.*, team performance, defense skill, batter skill, situational hitting, stadium environment, *etc.*) and more dependent on the pitcher's overall pitching performance. Keeping this in mind additional performance statistics analyzed in this study included: Earned Run Average (ERA), Hits per 9 innings (H/9), Homeruns per 9 innings (HR/9), Strikeouts per 9 innings (K/9), and Walks per 9 innings (BB/9), Wins (W), Win/Loss Percentage (W/L%) and Strikeouts (K). Data were entered into a spreadsheet matching performance data with the physiological measures for each player for each year.

2.1.4. Statistical Analyses

A descriptive data analysis was conducted for all pitchers in the sample and by their individual positions (S or R) Comparison between fitness measures among S and R pitchers on selected fitness and performance measures was conducted via an independent samples T-test based on position. Additionally, all players were then separated into either a higher or lower cardiorespiratory fitness group within their position based on the average VO_{2peak} and AT. A one-way Analysis of Variance (ANOVA) was then utilized to examine differences between these groups. Pearson product moment correlations were then used to examine the relationship between physiological measures and performance data as a whole as well as divided by position. Data were evaluated using SPSS Statistics version 22 (SPSS, Armonk, NY, USA). Statistical significance was set at $p < 0.05$. Data are presented as means and standard deviations. Correlations were considered high (0.80–1.00), moderately high (0.60–0.79), moderate (0.40–0.59) or low (0.20–0.39) [18].

2.2. Results

Descriptive data for the entire sample is presented in Table 1. For all pitchers, average VO_{2peak} was 48.13 ± 5.30 (mL/kg/Min). For all pitchers VO_{2peak} was found to have a low-moderate relationship ($p < 0.05$) between WHIP ($r = -0.484$, $p \leqslant 0.01$), K ($r = 0.572$, $p \leqslant 0.01$) BB/9 ($r = -0.358$, $p \leqslant 0.05$) and W ($r = 0.550$, $p \leqslant 0.01$). A strong relationship ($r = 0.602$, $p \leqslant 0.01$) was found between VO_{2peak} and K/BB. Additionally, low, but significant correlations were also found between AT and K ($r = -0.328$, $p \leqslant 0.05$), K/BB ($r = -327$, $p \leqslant 0.05$) and W ($r = 0.358$, $p \leqslant 0.05$).

Table 1. Descriptive data.

Anthropometric and Fitness Variables	All Pitchers (n = 40) Mean ± SD	S Pitchers (n = 27) Mean ± SD	R Pitchers (n = 13) Mean ± SD
Age (YEARS)	28.03 ± 5.17	27.33 ± 5.46	29.46 ± 4.31
Weight (KG)	100.06 ± 6.80	99.27 ± 5.75	101.75 ± 8.59
Height (CM)	191.19 ± 5.11	192.28 ± 5.00	188.92 ± 4.80
Estimated Percent Body fat (%BF)	15.28 ± 3.45	14.21 ± 2.45	17.5 ± 4.2
Lean BODY mass (lBM) (KG)	84.63 ± 4.54	85.07 ± 3.85	83.72 ± 5.79
Estimated Max. Heart Rate (HR)	191.98 ± 5.16	192.66 ± 5.46	190.53 ± 4.31
$VO_{2\,max}$ (mL· kg^{-1}· min.)	48.13 ± 5.30	49.49 ± 4.59	45.28 ± 5.71
Anaerobic threshold (AT)	37.31 ± 7.87	38.63 ± 7.03	34.57 ± 9.06
HR at $VO_{2\,max}$	184.28 ± 9.70	182.33 ± 9.06	188.31 ± 10.09
HR at Anaerobic Threshold	162.72 ± 13.83	161.11 ± 11.97	166.08 ± 17.13

When comparing S *vs.* R pitchers there was a significant effect for position, $t = 2.50$, $p \leqslant 0.01$, with S pitchers demonstrating higher $VO_{2\,max}$ values (49.49 ± 4.59) when compared to relievers (45.28 ± 5.72) as presented in Figure 1. However, our analysis revealed no significant differences in AT between S and R.

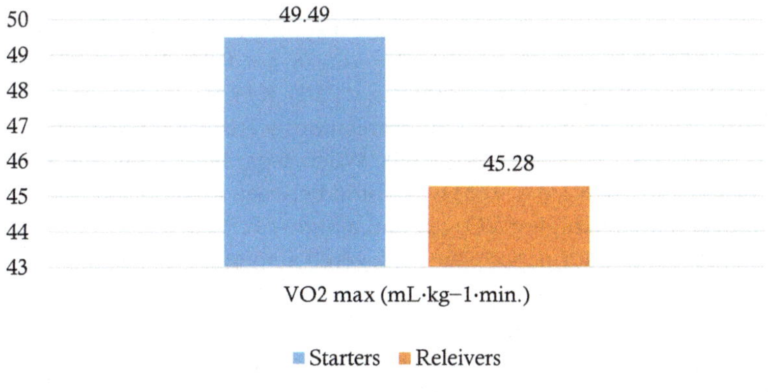

Figure 1. Differences in $VO_{2\,max}$ between Starters and Relievers.

A one-way ANOVA with pairwise comparisons revealed significantly better performance statistics among S pitchers with a VO_{2peak} above the overall group mean in FIP ($F(3,36) = 3.87$, $p \leqslant 0.01$, P), WHIP ($F(3,36) = -4.60$, $p \leqslant 0.01$), K/BB ($F(3,36) = 7.25$, $p \leqslant 0.01$), and ERA ($F(3,36) = -4.58$ $p \leqslant 0.01$). Additionally, it was discovered that S pitchers with an AT above the overall group mean demonstrated significantly better performance as measured by WHIP ($F(3,36) = 2.54$, $p \leqslant 0.05$), presented in Figure 2, and ERA ($F(3,36) = 2.52$, $p \leqslant 0.05$), presented in Figure 3. When comparing R pitchers above and below

VO_{2peak} the only significant difference discovered in measures of pitching performance was in HR/9 ($F(3,36) = 5.06, p \leqslant 0.05$).

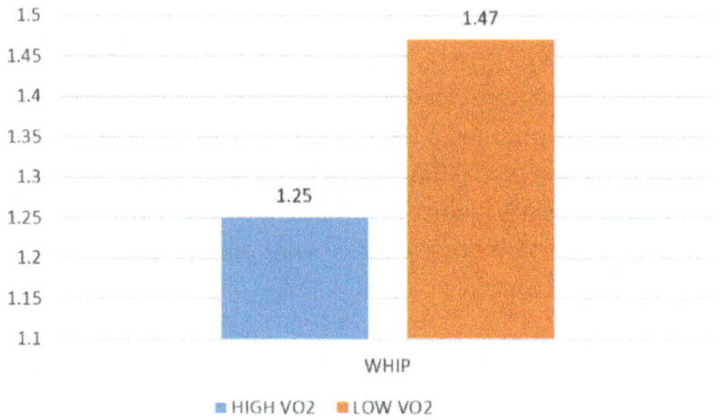

Figure 2. Differences in walks and hits per inning pitched (WHIP) amongst S pitchers with higher and lower $VO_{2\ max}$.

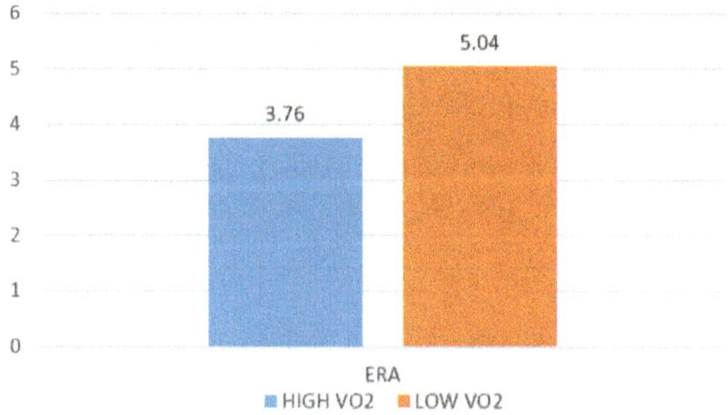

Figure 3. Differences in earned run average (ERA) amongst S pitchers with higher and lower $VO_{2\ max}$.

Among starting pitchers, Pearson product-moment correlations revealed low- high relationships between $VO_{2\ max}$ and BB/9 ($r = -0.416$), HR/9 ($r = -0.478, p \leqslant 0.05$), W ($r = 0.548$), FIP ($r = -0.567, p \leqslant 0.01$), K's ($r = 0.572, p \leqslant 0.01$), H/9 ($r = -0.589, p \leqslant 0.01$), K/9 ($r = 0.614, p \leqslant 0.01$), ERA ($r = -678, p \leqslant 0.01$), and WHIP ($r = -0.685, p \leqslant 0.01$). Low correlations were also found between AT and WHIP ($r = -431, p \leqslant 0.05$) and ERA ($r = -431, p \leqslant 0.05$). When separately analyzing R pitchers the only significant relationships ($r = 0.592, p \leqslant 0.05$) was found between FIP and $VO_{2\ max}$. This relationship indicated that R pitchers with a higher $VO_{2\ max}$ had a higher FIP. No other significant relationships between $VO_{2\ max}$ or AT and performance were discovered among R pitchers.

2.3. Discussion

The results of this study indicate that ML S pitchers are more aerobically fit than R pitchers and that several pitching performance variables appear to be related to greater $VO_{2\ max}$. For S pitchers only, there was a strong, significant correlation between $VO_{2\ max}$ and FIP, WHIP, and ERA. There was also a moderate but significant relationship between AT and both WHIP and ERA for S pitchers only. For R pitchers no significant relationships were discovered between either $VO_{2\ max}$ and AT for any of the selected measures of used in our analysis. In contrast, the sole correlation among R pitchers in this study was found when this group was subcategorized into high/low $VO_{2\ max}$. It was discovered that R pitchers with a higher $VO_{2\ max}$ actually pitched worse than those with a lower $VO_{2\ max}$ based on FIP. After analysis of R pitchers data it can be concluded that cardiorespiratory fitness may not necessarily have a positive impact on successful pitching performance among R pitchers. While the results may simply be a product of on-field demands, or due to different training and conditioning methods performed between S and R pitchers, it may also suggest that aerobic fitness has a larger impact on pitching performance for the S pitcher at the ML level.

In an attempt to identify key fitness benchmarks related to performance, further evaluations were performed on S pitchers only. The S sample was divided into higher and lower $VO_{2\ max}$ groups (greater than or less than 48.13 (mL/kg/min)) to examine differences in performance in FIP, WHIP, and ERA. The higher fitness group (n = 15, VO_2 = 50.19 $\pm$ 4.23) had an average WHIP of 1.25 $\pm$ 0.18, FIP of 3.61 $\pm$ 0.66, and average ERA of 3.77 $\pm$ 1.02. The WHIP and ERA results were significantly better ($p < 0.05$) than the lower fitness group (n = 12, VO_2 = 48.84 $\pm$ 4.97) which were found to have an average WHIP of 1.48 $\pm$ 0.17 and ERA of 5.04 $\pm$ 0.97. The higher fitness group also had a better K/9 ($p < 0.05$). In summary, S pitchers exhibiting above average $VO_{2\ max}$, pitched considerably better than S pitchers with below average $VO_{2\ max}$.

The physiological demands on S pitchers are greater than R pitchers due to the higher workload and duration of time they are expected to perform. This may result in a greater reliance on overall cardiorespiratory fitness and endurance to sustain performance throughout the duration of a game. The apparent lack of importance related to both $VO_{2\ max}$ and AT for the R pitcher is not surprising and provides additional support for constructing position or role-specific exercise programs. It makes sense that the relationship between VO_2 and AT and pitching performance measures may simply indicate the need for higher levels of endurance for S pitchers and not specific requirements for successful pitching performances for R pitchers.

The current findings support the need for personalized in-season conditioning programs dependent on the specific role a pitcher holds on their team. The S pitcher is usually on a 5 day rotation involving four days in between each pitching outing. When the major emphasis of conditioning programs is placed on minimizing reductions in power and strength over the course of the season, the use of slow, long distance runs could be counter-productive. The authors postulate that one high intensity interval training session between each pitching outing may be sufficient to help maintain aerobic fitness and maximize recovery. This approach may also serve to minimize reductions in power and strength and interference during power development and strength training sessions performed during the four days between pitching outings.

Conditioning programs for R pitchers should not mimic S pitchers, even though some R pitchers are expected to pitch multiple innings and sustain higher pitch counts. Practitioners must determine whether or not this type of R pitcher should fall under a modified conditioning program similar to a S pitcher. In this case, the R pitcher would be allowed more days to rest following an outing making it more conducive to higher intensity conditioning sessions. The day following a long outing where a R pitcher has the day off might be best to incorporate more intense conditioning sessions. It should also be noted that more extensive modifications in conditioning programs might be required to meet anthropometric needs/goals.

In summary, this is the first known study that examines aerobic capacity among ML pitchers and its potential impact on pitching performance. When interpreting the current findings it is important to realize that there are many uncontrollable variables that become more evident in field experiments. First, successful pitching performance at the professional level is certainly not identified by one single performance measure. There are many variables that lead to a positive pitching performance, making it difficult to come to precise conclusions on how much of an impact physical fitness really has on performance statistics in this analysis. In addition, pitching mechanics play an important role in successful pitching at any level. Therefore, the evaluation of the statistical findings should consider the complexity of pitching performance in general. Furthermore, it is important to note that subjects exercised to voluntary exhaustion. Subsequently, it is possible that a true $VO_{2\ max}$ may not have been reached due to lack of motivation. All of these factors should be considered when evaluating the outcomes of this study.

3. Conclusions

Practical Applications

The current data suggests that metabolic training among ML baseball starting pitchers should focus on improving both aerobic capacity and anaerobic threshold. At the higher levels of play adequate training time should be devoted to maximizing these physiological parameters to improve chances of successful performance. Concurrent training strategies should focus on maximizing both physiological variables while attempting to minimize any potential interference in maximizing power. High intensity interval training seems to be the most efficient mode of training to improve a starting pitcher's aerobic capacity. Neglecting important physiological components can have a detrimental effect on performance but athletes need evidence-based guidance to ensure productivity and a return on their training efforts.

Strength and conditioning professionals should work closely with pitchers, coaches, and organizational management to design and implement appropriate training strategies for pitchers at various levels. The reliance on research such as the current analysis ensures that training programs are evidence-based and effective. For specific examples of proposed conditioning programs for pitchers, further examination of published works are suggested [7,8,20,21].

Author Contributions: Javair S. Gillett conceived the experiment, oversaw the testing procedures, analyzed the data, and contributed in the writing and review of the manuscript; J. Jay Dawes analyzed the data and contributed in the writing and review of the manuscript; Frank J. Spaniol contributed in the writing and review of the manuscript and served as the corresponding author; Mitchel A. Magrini contributed in the writing and review of the manuscript; Matthew R. Rhea analyzed the data and contributed in the writing and review of the manuscript; Joe P. Rogowski oversaw the testing procedures and contributed in the review of the manuscript; Robert Simao contributed in the writing and review of the manuscript; and Derek J. Bunker contributed in the writing and review of the manuscript.

Conflicts of Interest: The authors declare no conflict of interest.

References

1. Baseball Prospectus. Available online: http://www.baseballprospectus.com/sortable/index.php?cid=1667158 (accessed on 6 May 2015).
2. Bradbury, J.C.; Forman, S.L. The impact of pitch counts and days of rest on performance among major-league baseball pitchers. *J. Strength Cond. Res.* **2012**, *26*, 1181–1187. [CrossRef] [PubMed]
3. Szymanski, D.J.; Fredrick, G.A. College baseball/softball periodized torso program. *Strength Cond. J.* **1999**, *22*, 42–47. [CrossRef]
4. Potteiger, J.; Blessing, D.; Wilson, G.D. The physiological responses to a single game of baseball pitching. *J. Strength Cond. Res.* **1992**, *6*, 11–18.
5. Stockholm, A.; Morris, H. A pitcher's heart rate during actual competition. *Res. Q. Am. Assoc. Health Phys. Educ. Recreat.* **1969**, *40*, 645–649.
6. Szymanski, D.J.; Myres, R.L. Heart rate responses of collegiate baseball pitchers while pitching and conditioning. *J. Strength Cond. Res.* **2007**, *21*, e28.
7. Syzmanski, D. Collegiate baseball in-season training. *Strength Cond. J.* **2007**, *29*, 68–80. [CrossRef]
8. Szymanski, D. Physiology of baseball pitching dictates specific exercise intensity for conditioning. *Strength Cond. J.* **2009**, *31*, 41–47. [CrossRef]
9. Tomlin, D.L.; Wenger, H. The relationship between aerobic fitness and recovery from high intensity intermittent exercise. *Sports Med.* **2001**, *31*, 1–11. [CrossRef] [PubMed]
10. Tripp, B.; Boswell, L.; Gansneder, B.; Shultz, S. Functional fatigue decreases 3-dimensional multi-joint position reproduction acuity in the overhead-throwing athlete. *J. Athl. Train.* **2004**, *39*, 316–320. [PubMed]
11. Tripp, B.L.; Yochem, E.M.; Uhl, T.L. Functional fatigue and upper extremity sensorimotor system acuity in baseball athletes. *J. Athl. Train.* **2007**, *42*, 90–98. [PubMed]
12. Van Wessel, T.; de Haan, A.; Van der Laarse, W.; Jaspers, R. The muscle fiber type–fiber size paradox: Hypertrophy or oxidative metabolism? *Eur. J. Appl. Physiol.* **2010**, *110*, 665–694. [CrossRef] [PubMed]

13. Yang, S.W. Assessment of professional baseball players aerobic exercise performance depending on their positions. *J. Strength Cond. Res.* **2014**, *28*, 3289–3292. [CrossRef] [PubMed]
14. Ebben, W.; Hintz, M.; Simenz, C. Strength and conditioning practices of major league baseball strength and conditioning coaches. *J. Strength Cond. Res.* **2005**, *19*, 538–546. [PubMed]
15. Dieli-Conwright, C.M.; Jensky, N.E.; Battaglia, G.; McCauley, S.; Schroeder, E.T. Validation of the CardioCoachCO_2 for submaximal and maximal metabolic exercise testing. *J. Strength Cond. Res.* **2009**, *23*, 1316–1320. [CrossRef] [PubMed]
16. Yuhasz, M.S. *Physical Fitness Manual*; University of Western Ontario: London, Canada, 1974.
17. Sports Reference, LLC, 2013. Available online: www.baseball-reference.com (accessed on 6 May 2015).
18. ESPN MLB. Available online: http://espn.go.com/mlb/ (accessed on 6 May 2015).
19. FanGraphs. Available online: www.fangraphs.com or http://www.espn.go.com/mlb/stats/pitching/_/league/nl/sort/pitches/type/expanded-2 (accessed on 6 May 2015).
20. Rhea, M.; Bunker, D. Baseball-specific conditioning. *Int. J. Sports Physiol. Perform.* **2009**, *4*, 402–407. [PubMed]
21. Rhea, M.; Oliverson, J.; Kenn, J.; Naclerio, F. Non-compatibility of power and endurance training among college baseball players. *J Strength Cond. Res.* **2008**, *22*, 230–234. [CrossRef] [PubMed]

The Effects of Mental Imagery with Video-Modeling on Self-Efficacy and Maximal Front Squat Ability

Daniel J. M. Buck, Jasmin C. Hutchinson *, Christa R. Winter and Brian A. Thompson

Springfield College, Massachusetts, MA 01109, USA; dbuck@springfieldcollege.edu (D.J.M.B.); cwinter@springfieldcollege.edu (C.R.W.); bthompson@springfieldcollege.edu (B.A.T.)
* Correspondence: jhutchinson@springfieldcollege.edu

Academic Editor: Eling Douwe de Bruin

Abstract: This study was designed to assess the effectiveness of mental imagery supplemented with video-modeling on self-efficacy and front squat strength (three repetition maximum; 3RM). Subjects (13 male, 7 female) who had at least 6 months of front squat experience were assigned to either an experimental (n = 10) or a control (n = 10) group. Subjects' 3RM and self-efficacy for the 3RM were measured at baseline. Following this, subjects in the experimental group followed a structured imagery protocol, incorporating video recordings of both their own 3RM performance and a model lifter with excellent technique, twice a day for three days. Subjects in the control group spent the same amount of time viewing a placebo video. Following three days with no physical training, measurements of front squat 3RM and self-efficacy for the 3RM were repeated. Subjects in the experimental group increased in self-efficacy following the intervention, and showed greater 3RM improvement than those in the control group. Self-efficacy was found to significantly mediate the relationship between imagery and front squat 3RM. These findings point to the importance of mental skills training for the enhancement of self-efficacy and front squat performance.

Keywords: strength and conditioning; mental skills; psychology; three repetition maximum (3RM)

1. Introduction

The front squat, which is used extensively in strength training programs at the collegiate level and higher [1], is one of the few exercises which can develop the majority of the lower body musculature as well as increase abdominal and lower back strength and stability [2]. Strength training programs are often created based on percentages of a one repetition maximum (1RM) in order to train for the desired results (e.g., hypertrophy, strength, power). The front squat is instrumental for all three aspects of training. Given the prevalence and importance of the front squat exercise in strength training programs, providing a method of increasing the load lifted during the exercise seems valuable. Increasing an athlete's 1RM shows an improvement in strength, and in the case of the squat, indicates an increased ability to produce force into the ground, increasing attributes such as vertical jump and acceleration for the enhancement of sports performance (e.g., [3]). The front squat is also a vital component of the clean, an important Olympic lift for the development of power, as the clean requires the ability to catch the bar on the shoulders in the same position as one front squats from. Achieving proper depth is also paramount when performing the clean with greater loads on the bar, as it requires the performer to drop down quickly and lower their body under the bar to catch the weight [4]. One often overlooked aspect in strength development is the use of psychological strategies, particularly more complex techniques such as mental imagery [5].

1.1. Mental Imagery

Mental imagery, defined as a cognitive process during which people use their minds to create (or recreate) experiences that are similar to real-life situations [6] has been found to enhance performance in a variety of sport settings [7]. However, the use of imagery during weight training has not been studied in great depth, to date. In early experimental studies, mental imagery was largely shown to be ineffective in enhancing the performance of strength-based tasks [8]. A meta-analysis conducted by Feltz and Landers [9] found a relatively small effect size (Cohen's d = 20) for the effects of imagery on strength tasks. However, Wright and Smith [10] point out that the majority of these studies used a traditional "visualization" imagery approach, (*i.e.*, focusing on the visual aspects of imagery) in contrast to a more comprehensive (physical, response-based) imagery approach. They argue that the "lack of functional equivalence afforded by these 'visualization'-type interventions may, therefore, explain their ineffectiveness".

Based upon the principle that imagery enhances performance because the same neurophysiological processes underlie imagery and actual movement [11,12], Holmes and Collins [13] developed the PETTLEP model. PETTLEP is an acronym for the proposed key elements to an effective imagery intervention (*i.e.*, physical, environment, task, timing, learning, emotion, and perspective components); this approach aims to maximize functional equivalence by ensuring that the imagery performed is a close representation of the actual movement. Wright and Smith [10] demonstrated the superiority of PETTLEP imagery supplemented with video over traditional (visualization) imagery in a strength task (bicep curl 1RM). In evaluating the results of their study, Wright and Smith highlighted the need for future research on the strength training effects of the PETTLEP model, and suggested that future studies focus on muscles of different sizes and on the PETTLEP imagery effects over different periods of time.

1.2. Modeling

Modeling, or observational learning, has been defined as a process in which the performer attempts to imitate an observed action or skill performed by another individual [14]. Like imagery, modeling is a cognitive process by which people can learn a variety of skills and behaviors [15]. Indeed, athletes frequently use modeling for motor skill acquisition and execution [16]. It is theorized that in doing so, an athlete symbolically encodes information about the skill as the demonstration is observed (*i.e.*, they create an internal cognitive representation of the skill), and then uses this encoded information as a guide for future action [17]. It is important to note that this need not be a deliberate process. Cross *et al.* [18], for example, provide evidence of similar neural representations for physically rehearsed and passively observed movement sequences.

Research has typically addressed modeling and imagery as separate and distinct processes, however several investigators [9,19,20] have noted that modeling and imagery are similar; both involving the use of cognitive representations and rehearsal prior to the actual physical execution of the skill [17]. During modeling, information about the skill is encoded into a cognitive representation, while during imagery a cognitive representation or image is recalled from memory; these mechanisms have been shown to have similar neural involvement [21]. While the distinction between modeling and imagery is important from an academic perspective, the effects of a combined intervention may be of greater practical interest to coaches and practitioners. Indeed, it has been suggested that, in order to optimize functional equivalence, performers can make use of pictures, sound, and/or video clips to provide stimulus and response information for imagery [22]. McCullagh, Law and Ste-Marie [23] have recently advocated for research on imagery interventions that include modeling as a component.

1.3. Self-Efficacy

Self-efficacy (SE), which is defined by Bandura [24] as "beliefs in one's capabilities to organize and execute the courses of action required to produce given attainments", is derived from four sources of information; mastery experiences (*i.e.*, past performances), vicarious experiences, verbal persuasion, and physiological states. Compared with persons who doubt their capabilities, those with high SE for accomplishing a task participate more readily, set more challenging goals for themselves, persist longer in the face of adversity, and achieve at a higher level [24]. Previous research in a strength setting has examined the effect of perceptions of goal difficulty on lower body strength performance. Participants who were misinformed during a 3RM deadlift task (*i.e.*, were unknowingly lifting 10% above their actual 3RM to create lower perceived demand), lifted a signficantly heavier load compared to participants who received correct lift information (high perceived demand) [25]. This finding highlights potential SE barriers to performance success.

Modeling and imagery are classified as similar processes within SE theory; both can serve as vicarious experiences and provide information that affects SE [17]. Imagery itself can also serve as a source of SE, as enactive mastery experience can be attained through the use of imagery [24]. Bandura has placed much emphasis on the mediating role that SE plays in the observation-behavior change relationship [24]. To date, little research has examined this mediating effect, but that which has is largely supportive of Bandura's theoretical proposition. For example, using hierarchical multiple regression analyses, Beauchamp *et al.* [26] demonstrated that pre-competition imagery use accounted for significant variance in both SE and performance in collegiate golfers. Moreover, SE was predictive of golf performance, and imagery use mediated the relationship between SE and performance. The mediating role of SE, in regards to the effects of imagery, has yet to be examined in a strength setting.

The current study was primarily designed to determine if mental imagery (using the PETTLEP model) supplemented with video-modeling, would be effective in increasing front squat 3RM. Self-efficacy was measured in order to probe the underlying mechanism by which imagery may have an effect on 3RM; that is to determine if imagery effects on front squat were mediated by SE. It was hypothesized that (1) imagery would significantly enhance SE for the front squat; (2) imagery would significantly enhance front squat 3RM; and (3) the effect of imagery on front squat 3RM would be mediated by changes in SE for the 3RM. The effect on front squat was expected to be small, given the upper limits of performance, but it is noted that even a slight trend towards a greater 3RM may still be of practical importance.

2. Materials and Methods

2.1. Experimental Approach to the Problem

The objective of this study was to determine the effects of mental imagery supplemented with video-modeling on SE and performance during the front squat exercise. Subjects were assigned to either an experimental (*i.e.*, mental imagery supplemented with video-modeling) group or a control (placebo video) group. Pre- and post-intervention measurements of front squat 3RM (lbs.) and SE for the 3RM were collected and compared using two 2 (group) $\times$ 2 (time) mixed factorial analyses of variance (ANOVAs).

2.2. Determination of Sample Size

A power analysis was conducted, using G*Power 3.1 [27], to establish appropriate sample size for a 2 (Group) $\times$ 2 (Time) mixed-factorial ANOVA. Alpha was set at 0.05 and power at 0.8 to protect beta at four times the level of alpha [28]. Predicting a moderate size effect ($f = 0.28$) of the intervention on the dependent variables [10], it was estimated that 20 subjects would be required.

2.3. Subjects

Twenty subjects (13 male, 7 female; age, 22.67 $\pm$ 1.79 years) were recruited and placed into one of two groups (experimental or control) in an alternating fashion by gender, based on the order in which each subject was recruited. There were a total of 10 subjects in the treatment group and 10 in the control group. None had any prior experience using imagery deliberately for the purpose of rehearing or improving performance on an athletic task. Inclusion criteria were that all subjects had at least 6 months of experience with the front squat exercise (*i.e.*, intermediate training status [29]) and had no recent injuries that would prevent them from effectively performing the front squat exercise. The study was approved by the Institutional Review Board, and all subjects provided written informed consent prior to testing.

2.4. Procedures

Two days of testing were required for this study. To allow for complete recovery of skeletal muscle contractility [30] and to provide adequate time for subjects to practice the imagery protocol testing sessions were separated by three days. Prior to the first test subjects were asked to refrain from any training involving the legs for two days and to refrain from all training for 24 h prior to testing. No exercise was allowed between testing sessions. The subjects were also asked to consume a similar diet before each testing session and to refrain from caffeine consumption for 6 h prior to testing. Testing sessions for each individual were conducted at the same time of day to control for any potential diurnal variation. Each session began with self-myofascial release using a foam roller followed by a series of activation exercises and static and dynamic stretches (see supplementary materials for details).

Subjects performed the front squat using a Keiser rack (Knoxville, TN, USA) and York barbell (York, PA, USA). The subject's foot position, grip width, and grip style were self-selected (all elected to use a clean grip). A 3RM test was chosen over a 1 for reasons of safety [31]. Each subject started the warm-up 5 × 60% of estimated 3RM (estimation based on recent training logs) and then progressed through the following sets: 4 × 70% estimated 3RM, 3 × 80% estimated 3RM, and 2 × 90% estimated 3RM. After these warm up sets were completed, a 3 × 100% attempt was made. If successful, the weight was increased by 10–20 lbs. per subsequent attempt until their 3RM was determined. The intervention for the experimental group consisted of a video-enhanced imagery protocol. Each subject was recorded using a Samsung Schneider Kreuznach Camcorder (Taegu, Korea) during their 3RM front squat on Day 1. Recording took place slightly forward of the subject's right side for the entire three repetitions in order to be able to determine proper squat depth (*i.e.*, femur parallel to the ground). If the subject was able to successfully complete a subsequent 3RM with a greater load, only the highest successful 3RM video was saved.

Following completion of the 3RM protocol, subjects viewed their own video, and were provided with a corresponding imagery script. Subjects were then sent an e-mail with a copy of their video as well as a video of one of two individuals (one male, one female) completing the front squat with excellent technique. As perceived similarity to models is an important attribute for maximizing SE [24], the models were the same age range as the subjects, and subjects were each sent a video-model matching their identified gender. Subjects were asked to view both videos six times between testing sessions (twice each day), and to use the script provided to image themselves performing the front squat with the same technique as the model lifter. Reminder texts were sent to the subjects once each day between testing days in order to remind them to watch the videos. The imagery script followed PETTLEP guidelines; subjects were directed to visualize the front squat in their usual lifting environment and to visualize the movement in real time, paying particular attention to the technical aspects of the movement (e.g., head, spine and hip alignment) using the model as a guide. They were also directed to exert emotional control and to feel their muscles activate as if they were physically performing the exercise. Subjects kept an imagery log in which they recorded the time and date of their imagery sessions; this log was checked prior to the second session to ensure adherence to the protocol. The control group received a placebo video, a video of a baby squatting, which they were asked to view the same number of times (*i.e.*, twice a day for three days) as the experimental group. This video was intended to parallel the videos seen by the experimental group by providing similar visual material, but no usable information.

On Day 2, following all warm-up procedures and prior to beginning the testing set, experimental subjects viewed the model video as well as their own 3RM video from Day 1. After viewing the videos, subjects were guided through the imagery protocol by the researcher. Particular emphasis was placed on kinesthetic elements and imagining the lift at the speed at which it would occur. Subjects were told that they may view either video again prior to the testing set if they desired (two subjects elected to do so). Control group subjects viewed the placebo video prior to beginning the testing set.

Subjects' SE for the 3RM was assessed immediately prior to each testing set using a task-specific SE scale, which was constructed according to Bandura's guidelines [32]. Bandura asserts that "scales of perceived self-efficacy must be tailored to the particular domain of functioning that is the object of interest", therefore subjects were asked to rate their confidence in their ability to perform the front squat with maximal weight (*i.e.*, the weight currently being attempted) and proper technique on a scale ranging from 0 (cannot do at all) to 100 (highly certain I can do). If a subsequent set of three repetitions was completed successfully, this measurement process was repeated. Only the SE data associated with the highest successful 3RM was saved and used for data analysis.

2.5. Statistical Analysis

Two 2 × 2 mixed factorial ANOVAs were conducted to analyze the SE and 3RM data; the independent groups factor was group (experimental/control) and the repeated measures factor was time (pre/post). The significance level for each ANOVA was set at 0.05. Additional post-hoc tests were conducted using independent as well as paired samples t-tests; the Bonferroni adjusted significance level for the t-tests was set at 0.00625. Cohen's effect size d was also computed for all post hoc comparisons relying on pooled standard deviations when appropriate.

Where interaction effects were significant, regression analyses [33] were conducted to investigate the hypothesis that SE mediates the effect of mental imagery on 3RM performance. To facilitate this analysis, change scores (*i.e.*, pre intervention—post intervention) were calculated for SE and 3RM. The first step of the analysis was to regress the dependent variable (3RM change) on the independent variable (group) in order to confirm that the independent variable was a significant predictor of the dependent variable. Following this the mediator (SE change) was regressed on the independent variable (group) to confirm that the independent variable was a significant predictor of the mediator. Finally, the dependent variable (3RM change) was regressed on both the mediator (SE change) and independent variable (group) in order to confirm that the mediator was a significant predictor of the dependent variable, while controlling for the independent variable. IBM SPSS version 21 was used for data analysis.

3. Results

The current study was designed to determine if mental imagery supplemented with video-modeling was effective in increasing self-efficacy and 3RM in the front squat. Twenty subjects (n_{exp} = 10 and n_{ctrl} = 10) completed the study. 3RM tests were separated by 3 days to allow for full recovery and to provide time for subjects to practice the imagery protocol. Descriptive statistics for the dependent variables are presented in Table 1.

Table 1. Descriptive statistics and effect sizes for experimental and control groups.

Variable	Pretest		Posttest		Cohen's d
	Mean	*SD*	Mean	*SD*	
3RM (lbs.)					
Experimental	183.00	61.92	191.50	62.41	−2.52
Control	179.00	36.04	181.50	37.57	−0.35
Self-Efficacy					
Experimental	82.40	6.75	90.10	7.85	−1.49
Control	83.50	11.10	76.70	11.27	+0.40

Analyzing the SE data, a significant group x time interaction was revealed, $F(1, 18) = 6.65, p = 0.019, \eta^2 = 0.27$. Follow-up post-hoc tests indicated no significant difference in SE scores between groups pre intervention, $t(18) = 0.27, p = 0.792, d = 0.12$; however, a significant difference was determined post intervention with the experimental group reporting higher SE scores, $t(18) = 3.08, p = 0.006; d = 1.40$. In addition, no significant difference in SE scores of the control group was found from pretest to posttest, $t(9) = 1.26, p = 0.238, d = 0.40$, while the SE scores of the experimental group increased significantly from pretest to posttest, $t(9) = -4.71, p = 0.001, d = -1.49$.

The analysis of the 3RM strength data also revealed a significant group by time interaction, $F(1,18) = 5.73, p = 0.028, \eta^2 = 0.24$. Follow-up post-hoc tests indicated no significant difference in 3RM strength between groups pre, $t(18) = 0.18, p = 0.862, d = 0.08$, and post intervention, $t(18) = 0.43, p = 0.669, d = 0.20$. The experimental group, however, showed a significant increase (Mdiff = 8.5 lbs.) in 3RM strength from pretest to posttest, $t(9) = -7.97, p = .000, d = -2.52$. The pre- to posttest increase for the control group (Mdiff = 2.5 lbs.) was not significant, $t(9) = -1.10, p = 0.299, d = -0.35$.

Given the significant group by time interactions for both dependent variables, linear regression was used to investigate the hypothesis that SE mediates the effect of video-supplemented mental imagery on 3RM performance. Regression results indicated that Group was a significant predictor of SE change, $\beta = 0.532, p = 0.016$, and that SE change was a significant predictor of 3RM change, $\beta = 0.654, p = 0.002$. These results support the mediational hypothesis. Experimental group initially predicted 3RM change (step one of the analysis; $\beta = 0.492, p = 0.028$), but was not a significant predictor of 3RM change after controlling for change in SE, $\beta = 0.250, p = 0.257$, consistent with partial mediation. Approximately 46% of the variance in 3RM change was accounted for by change in SE ($R^2 = 0.457$).

4. Discussions

The results of this study indicate that a mental imagery protocol supplemented with video-modeling is one mechanism by which SE might positively influence front squat 3RM.

Subjects who followed the video-imagery protocol showed a 10.7% increase in SE while subjects in the control group decreased in SE by a similar amount (12.3%). It is unknown why SE would decrease in the control group. It could be speculated that, without any meaningful intervention, the control subjects may have lacked motivation to repeat the task in such a short time-frame. Given the proposed bidirectional relationship between SE and motivation [24], this could account for the decline in SE.

Overall, our findings are in agreement with Silbernagel *et al.* [9] who found a positive association between imagery use and SE. This notion is of importance to strength coaches because SE is significantly and positively related to athletic performance [34,35]. Moreover, previous research has shown SE to have greater influence on performance in non-continuous sport conditions (consisting of discrete trials) when compared to continuous, dynamic sports [36], suggesting that strength and conditioning settings may be optimal for implementing this type of intervention. Future research involving elements of strength training other than 3RM would be valuable.

It has previously been reported [6] that athletes who were more confident in their ability to use imagery used it more often, creating a positive cycle of imagery use and SE. Although pre-task imagery use was found to influence SE and performance in the present study, future research should consider the theorized bidirectional relationship between SE and imagery use and examine the interplay of these variables in greater depth.

According to SE theory [14,24], enhanced SE should lead athletes "to set higher goals, exert more effort and persist resiliently in the face of adversity, all of which are likely to contribute to improved performances" [26]. In this study, there was a significantly greater increase in 3RM for the experimental group than for the control group. These findings are in line with those previously reported by Wright and Smith [10] who observed superior strength gains following a video-supplemented PETTLEP imagery program compared to other conditions (*i.e.*, traditional imagery, physical practice, and control). Thus, the results of the study provide additional empirical support for the use of comprehensive, video-supplemented imagery in strength tasks. This study extends previous findings [11,12] by demonstrating the mediating role of SE in the imagery-performance relationship in a strength task.

While the results of the present study are encouraging, some methodological limitations should be noted. The completed imagery logs suggest that participants attempted to complete the intervention task as instructed, but without a direct measure of imagery success we can only infer that they indeed used an imagery strategy. It is possible that the experimental subjects used a declarative observational strategy instead of (or in addition to) imagery, wherein they made visual comparisons between their performance and that of the model and subsequently changed certain aspects of their technique to match the model lifter. Further, despite the use of a control group, it is not possible to rule out potential effects of subject expectations. While neither group was explicitly advised that the intervention was designed to improve performance, it is more likely that the experimental group considered that the intervention might improve their 3RM. Perhaps a more effective control, for future studies seeking to replicate these findings, might be to use the same videos as for the experimental group but assign a different task (one that precludes the explicit use of imagery; e.g., making verbal descriptions of what they see).

No attempt was made to control for individual differences in modelling or imagery ability. As with any skill, imagery may be more effective for some individuals than others, depending on their ability to utilize imagery effectively [35]. Future studies might be conducted over a longer time period in order to develop imagery skills before posttest data are recorded. Such research may also be beneficial to better understand how imagery affects maximal lifting over time, as subtle changes in technique may require more time to translate into improved 3RM scores. Bandura advocates that gradations of challenge [32] be built into efficacy scales. In the present study we adopted the staggered approach described as 3RM values were not known at the first trial. Studies taking a more longitudinal approach could make use of a graded SE scale, specific to each individual's previous 3RM (*i.e.*, subjects' efficacy to achieve a 3RM that is 3%, 6%, 9%, *etc.* greater than before). A baseline trial to establish 3RM could also be used to achieve this.

Subjects' current athletic status or background was not considered in the current study, thus a comparison of competitive vs. recreational athletes may be a worthwhile future endeavor. It might also be interesting to explore the effects of mental imagery with video-modeling in less-trained populations, particularly as neuroimaging studies have shown that the neural networks activated by mental imagery differ between novices and experts [37]. Another valuable extension of the present study might be to couple mental imagery with movement sequences (*i.e.*, dynamic imagery). Recent research indicates dynamic imagery may be superior in terms of enhancing technical efficacy and temporal congruence between imagery and performance [38].

The present study did not separate the effects of self- and other-modeling. Thus, it is unclear whether vicarious experience (viewing others) or personal accomplishment (viewing self) combined with mental imagery was more enhancing to SE and/or 3RM. Future research that endeavors to disentangle these effects is warranted and may further our understanding of the effects of imagery and video-modeling in a strength and conditioning setting.

5. Conclusions

The use of mental imagery with video-modeling appears to be an effective intervention to enhance SE for the front squat and front squat 3RM. Specifically, the current study demonstrates that front squat SE and 3RM are significantly ($p < 0.001$) increased following a brief (3-day) video-supplemented imagery intervention. As far as a contribution to theory, the results of the mediational analysis predicting performance are consistent with theorizing by Bandura [24] and point to mental imagery with video-modeling as a factor through which SE influences performance.

The application of mental skills, such as imagery, in the strength and conditioning field is growing but remains under-utilized at present [5]. Mental skills are an important aspect of athletic development and, like physical skills, should be practiced often and with purpose. One benefit to mental imagery is that, once learned, it can be practiced anywhere at any time, moreover recent advances in technology have made digital recording more accessible than ever before and video can be easily distributed to athletes to supplement their mental skills training.

Video-supplemented imagery may be particularly useful for athletes who have difficulty in generating, maintaining, and controlling mental images. For college/university strength coaches who generally have athletes over a 4 to 5 year span, the opportunity exists to develop a comprehensive program of mental imagery supplemented with video-modeling which may be very helpful for assisting in athlete learning and development, potentially leading to improved SE and performance in the weight room as well as in athletic competition. In sum, mental imagery should be considered as a part of strength and conditioning programs with a goal to improve athletic performance and team success.

Author Contributions: D.J.M.B., J.C.H. and B.A.T. conceived and designed the experiments; D.J.M.B. and J.C.H. performed the experiments; C.R.W., D.J.M.B. and J.C.H. analyzed the data; D.J.M.B. and J.C.H. wrote the paper.

Conflicts of Interest: The authors declare no conflict of interest.

Abbreviations

The following abbreviations are used in this manuscript:

3RM	Three repetition maximum
1RM	One repetition maximum
PETTLEP	Physical, environment, task, timing, learning, emotion, and perspective components (elements of an effective imagery intervention)
SE	Self-efficacy

References

1. McKean, M.R.; Dunn, P.K.; Burkett, B.J. The lumbar and sacrum movement pattern during the back squat exercise. *J. Strength Cond. Res.* **2010**, *24*, 2731–2741. [CrossRef] [PubMed]
2. Gullett, J.C.; Tillman, M.D.; Gutierrez, G.M.; Chow, J.W. A biomechanical comparison of back and front squats in healthy trained individuals. *J. Strength Cond. Res.* **2009**, *23*, 284–292. [CrossRef] [PubMed]
3. Wisløff, U.; Castagna, C.; Helgerud, J.; Jones, R.; Hoff, J. Strong correlation of maximal squat strength with sprint performance and vertical jump height in elite soccer players. *Br. J. Sports Med.* **2004**, *38*, 285–288. [CrossRef] [PubMed]
4. Hori, N.; Newton, R.U.; Andrews, W.A.; Kawamori, N.; McGuigan, M.R.; Nosaka, K. Does Performance of Hang Power Clean Differentiate Performance of Jumping, Sprinting, and Changing of Direction? *J. Strength Cond. Res.* **2008**, *22*, 412–418. [CrossRef] [PubMed]
5. Radcliffe, J.N.; Comfort, P.; Fawcett, T. The perception of psychology and the frequency of psychological strategies used by strength and conditioning practitioners. *J. Strength Cond. Res.* **2013**, *27*, 1136–1146. [CrossRef] [PubMed]
6. Silbernagel, M.S.; Short, S.E.; Ross-Stewart, L.C. Athletes' use of exercise imagery during weight training. *J. Strength Cond. Res.* **2007**, *21*, 1077–1081. [CrossRef] [PubMed]
7. Driskell, J.E.; Copper, C.; Moran, A. Does mental practice enhance performance? *J. Appl. Psychol.* **1994**, *79*, 481–492. [CrossRef]
8. Tenenbaum, G.; Bar-Eli, M.; Hoffman, J.R.; Jablonovski, R.; Sade, S.; Shitrit, D. The effect of cognitive and somatic psyching-up techniques on isokinetic leg strength performance. *J. Strength Cond. Res.* **1995**, *9*, 3–7. [CrossRef]
9. Feltz, D.L.; Landers, D.M. The effects of mental practice on motor skill learning and performance: A meta-analysis. *J. Sport Psychol.* **1983**, *5*, 25–57.
10. Wright, J.; Smith, D. The effect of PETTLEP imagery on strength performance. *Int. Rev. Sport Exerc. Psychol.* **2009**, *7*, 18–31. [CrossRef]
11. Decety, J.; Jeannerod, M. Mentally simulated movements in virtual reality: Does Fitts's law hold in motor imagery? *Behav. Brain Res.* **1996**, *72*, 127–134. [CrossRef]

12. Fox, P.T.; Pardo, J.V.; Petersen, S.E.; Raichle, M.E. Supplementary motor and premotor responses to actual and imagined hand movements with positron emission tomography. *Soc. Neurosci. Abstr.* **1987**, *13*, 1433.
13. Holmes, P.S.; Collins, D.J. The PETTLEP approach to motor imagery: A functional equivalence model for sport psychologists. *J. Appl. Sport Psychol.* **2001**, *13*, 60–83. [CrossRef]
14. Bandura, A. *Social Foundations of Thought and Action: A Social Cognitive Theory*; Prentice-Hall: Englewood Cliffs, NJ, USA, 1986.
15. McCullagh, P.; Weiss, M.R.; Ross, D. Modeling considerations in motor skill acquisition and performance: An integrated approach. In *Exercise Sports Sciences Reviews*; Pandolf, K.B., Ed.; Williams & Wilkins: Baltimore, MD, USA, 1989; pp. 475–513.
16. Cumming, J.; Clark, S.E.; Ste-Marie, D.M.; McCullagh, P.; Hall, C. The functions of observational learning questionnaire (FOLQ). *Psychol. Sport Exerc.* **2005**, *6*, 517–537. [CrossRef]
17. SooHoo, S.; Takemoto, K.Y.; McCullagh, P. A comparison of modeling and imagery on the performance of a motor skill. *J. Sport Behav.* **2004**, *27*, 349–366.
18. Cross, E.S.; Kraemer, D.J.; Hamilton, A.F.; Kelley, W.M.; Grafton, S.T. Sensitivity of the action observation network to physical and observational learning. *Cereb. Cortex* **2009**, *19*, 315–326. [CrossRef] [PubMed]
19. McCullagh, P.; Weiss, M.R. Modeling: Considerations for motor skill performance and psychological responses. In *Handbook of Research on Sport Psychology*; Singer, R.N., Hasenblaus, H.A., Janelle, C.M., Eds.; Wiley & Sons: New York, NY, USA, 2001; pp. 205–238.
20. Vogt, S. On relations between perceiving, imagining, and performing in the learning of cyclical movement sequences. *Br. J. Psychol.* **1995**, *86*, 191–216. [CrossRef] [PubMed]
21. Clark, S.; Tremblay, F.; Ste-Marie, D. Differential modulation of corticospinal excitability during observation, mental imagery and imitation of hand actions. *Neuropsychologia* **2003**, *42*, 105–112. [CrossRef]
22. Cumming, J.; Williams, S.E. The role of imagery in performance. In *Handbook of Sport and Performance Psychology*; Murphy, S., Ed.; Oxford University Press: New York, NY, USA, 2012; pp. 213–232.
23. McCullagh, P.; Law, B.; Ste-Marie, D. Modeling and performance. In *The Oxford Handbook of Sport and Performance Psychology*; Murphy, S., Ed.; Oxford University Press: New York, NY, USA, 2012; pp. 250–272.
24. Bandura, A. *Self-efficacy: The Exercise of Control*; Freeman: New York, NY, USA, 1997.
25. McMahon, J.J.; Thomasson, M.; Barnes, J.; Graber, S.; Fawcett, T.; Comfort, P. Manipulation of perception of goal difficulty in weightlifting performance. The performance inhibition effect of precise goal difficulty on weightlifting performance. *J. Sports Sci.* **2002**, *27*, S118–S119.
26. Beauchamp, M.R.; Bray, S.R.; Albinson, J.G. Pre-competition imagery, self-efficacy and performance in collegiate golfers. *J. Sports Sci.* **2002**, *20*, 697–705. [CrossRef] [PubMed]
27. Faul, F.; Erdfelder, E.; Buchner, A.; Lang, A.G. Statistical power analyses using G*Power 3.1: Tests for correlation and regression analyses. *Behav. Res. Methods* **2009**, *41*, 1149–1160. [CrossRef] [PubMed]
28. Cohen, J. *Statistical Power Analysis for the Behavioral Sciences*, 2nd ed.; Lawrence Earlbaum Associates: Hillsdale, NJ, USA, 1988.
29. Baechle, T.R.; Earle, R.W. *Essentials of Strength Training and Conditioning*; Human Kinetics: Champaign, IL, USA, 2008.
30. Raastad, T.; Hallén, J. Recovery of skeletal muscle contractility after high- and moderate-intensity strength exercise. *Eur. J. Appl. Phys.* **2000**, *82*, 206–214. [CrossRef] [PubMed]
31. Brzycki, M. Strength testing—Predicting a one-rep max from reps-to-fatigue. *J. Phys. Educ. Recreat. Dance* **1993**, *64*, 88–90. [CrossRef]
32. Bandura, A. Guide for constructing self-efficacy scales. In *Self-efficacy Beliefs of Adolescents*; Pajares, F., Urdan, T.C., Eds.; Information Age Publishing: Charlotte, NC, USA, 2006.
33. Baron, R.M.; Kenny, D.A. The moderator–mediator variable distinction in social psychological research: Conceptual, strategic, and statistical considerations. *J. Pers. Soc. Psychol.* **1986**, *51*, 1173–1182. [CrossRef] [PubMed]
34. Moritz, S.E.; Feltz, D.L.; Fahrbach, K.R.; Mack, D.E. The relation of self-efficacy measures to sport performance: A meta-analytic review. *Res. Q. Exerc. Sport.* **2000**, *71*, 280–294. [CrossRef] [PubMed]
35. Woodman, T.; Hardy, L. The relative impact of cognitive anxiety and self-confidence upon sport performance: A meta-analysis. *J. Sports Sci.* **2003**, *21*, 443–457. [CrossRef] [PubMed]
36. Short, S.E.; Tenute, A.; Feltz, D.L. Imagery use in sport: Mediational effects for efficacy. *J. Sports Sci.* **2005**, *23*, 951–960. [CrossRef] [PubMed]

37. Debarnot, U.; Sperduti, M.; Di Rienzo, F.; Guillot, A. Experts bodies, experts minds: How physical and mental training shape the brain. *Front. Hum. Neurosci.* **2014**, *9*. [CrossRef] [PubMed]
38. Guillot, A.; Moschberger, K.; Collet, C. Coupling movement with imagery as a new perspective for motor imagery practice. *Behav. Brain Funct.* **2013**, *9*, 146–151. [CrossRef] [PubMed]

17

A Comparison between Chocolate Milk and a Raw Milk Honey Solution's Influence on Delayed Onset of Muscle Soreness

Andrew Hatchett *, Christopher Berry, Claudia Oliva, Douglas Wiley, Jacob St. Hilaire and Alex LaRochelle

Health Sciences, Department of Biology, Franklin Pierce University, Rindge, NH 03461, USA;
Berrycl1@live.franklinpierce.edu (C.B.); Olivacl2@live.franklinpierce.edu (C.O.);
drwilley@email.uark.edu (D.W.); St.Hilairej12@live.franklinpierce.edu (J.S.H.);
Larochellea12@live.franklinpierce.edu (A.L.)
* Correspondence: Hatchetta@franklinpierce.edu

Academic Editor: Beat Knechtle

Abstract: This investigation sought to examine the effect that a chocolate milk solution (CMS) and a raw milk solution (RMS) had on lower extremity induced delayed onset of muscle soreness (DOMS). Twenty trained male participants completed a set of questionnaires, prior to completing a lower extremity DOMS protocol, to determine the level of discomfort and functional limitations. Once the DOMS protocol was completed, participants were randomly assigned to either the CM or RM group. Once assigned, participants ingested 240 mL of the respective solution and completed the same set of questionnaires immediately post, 24-, 48- and 72-h post DOMS protocol. Additionally, for 10 days post-ingestion participants were contacted to learn if any negative effects were experienced as a result of ingesting either solution. Both groups reported an increase in lower extremity discomfort at each data collection interval post-DOMS protocol (post, 24-, 48- and 72-h). Participants assigned to the RM group reported high discomfort post and a relative decline in discomfort from immediately post-DOMS protocol to 72-h post. The RMS group reported substantially less discomfort at 72-h when compared to the CMS group. Ingestion of a raw milk solution immediately post strength exercise can substantially reduce the level of self-reported discomfort associated with DOMS.

Keywords: DOMS; chocolate; milk; raw; recovery; soreness; honey; strength; exercise

1. Introduction

Delayed onset of muscle soreness (DOMS) is an outcome often associated with exercise-induced muscle damage (EIMD) [1]. DOMS usually occurs after an increase in intensity or volume of training or when the schedule of exercise is altered [2–4]. The classical symptoms of DOMS include strength losses, pain, swelling, tenderness or stiffness, loss of full range of motion, flexibility, force production and mobility [2,5,6]. It is known that delayed onset muscle soreness increases the intensity of pain within 24 h after exercise, reaches a peak between 24 h and 48 h, disappears within 5–7 days after exercise [7]. A number of modalities have been investigated in the search for a treatment that may reduce the effects of EIMD and/or accelerate recovery [1,8].

A typical method athletes and active persons attempt to aid this process is through the use of dietary supplementation via post-exercise protein drinks [9]. Chocolate milk has also been observed to be an effective recovery aid after exercise. For instance, Karp *et al.* [10] observed similar increases in time to exhaustion and total work for individuals that consumed chocolate milk when compared to a traditional electrolyte replenishing drink subsequent to exhaustive exercise [9]. Evidence continues to emerge in support of chocolate milk, a cocoa-based beverage, as an effective recovery aid due to its optimal carbohydrate to protein ratio [10–15].

Heat treatments, such as those used in pasteurization, are generally assumed to impair protein quality [16]. The cocoa found in chocolate milk has gone through the alkalization process therefore reducing the antioxidant potential [11,17]. Recently, unpasteurized raw milk consumption has increased in popularity and emerged into a nationwide movement despite the acknowledgement of risks associated with foodborne pathogens [18,19]. Raw milk, or unpasteurized milk, is fresh and has not undergone heat treatment (pasteurization). Proponents of raw milk believe that due to the fact it has not been pasteurized, it contains greater amounts of and higher quality nutrients, enzymes and bacteria [20]. Honey has been used for its healing, nutritional and therapeutic properties since ancient times. It possesses anti-bacterial, anti-inflammatory and anti-oxidant properties that may be beneficial for preventing inflammatory processes [21]. Perhaps due to the controversial nature of raw milk, limited research has been conducted with raw milk.

With chocolate milk being a processed food commonly used and researched as a recovery aid from intense physical activity and raw milk being a relatively novel product, especially when combined with honey for the same purpose a comparison between the two has yet to be conducted. Therefore, this study examined the effects of a chocolate milk solution (CMS) and a raw milk and honey solution (RMS) on delayed onset muscle soreness.

2. Materials and Method

2.1. Study Design

This study was designed to investigate if participants reported a difference in delayed onset of muscle soreness after ingesting a chocolate milk solution or a raw milk and honey solution. Participants reported to the Functional Movement Laboratory (FML) at Franklin Pierce University on six different occasions (T1–T6) during the study. T1 consisted of a study briefing designed to inform the participants of the study protocol, obtain completed informed consent agreements, record anthropomorphic measurement and to establish a one repetition maximal load (1RM) of a barbell back squat. Seventy-two hours post-T1 participants reported to the FML for T2. T2 consisted of participants completing the DOMS measure, followed by the completion of the DOMS protocol. T3 occurred immediately after the participant completed the DOMS protocol, where the randomly assigned milk solution was offered and the DOMS measure was completed. Each of the following data collection periods the DOMS measure was completed: T4 (24 h post), T5 (48 h post) and T6 (72 h post). Following the T6 face-to-face data collection each participant was contacted each day for seven days to determine if they were experiencing any abnormal effects due to their participation in the study. This study was approved by the Franklin Pierce University Rindge Institutional Review Board Sub-Committee.

2.2. Participants

Twenty healthy male collegiate sprint football players participated in this study. Subjects had a mean age of 20.00 $\pm$ 0.85 years. (mean $\pm$ SD), a height 174.69 $\pm$ 1.68 cm, a mean weight of 79.37 $\pm$ 1.52 kg, a mean 1RM back squat of 126.55 $\pm$ 3.62 kg and a mean 80% of their individual 1RM back squat of 102.51 $\pm$ 2.77. All subjects were informed of the study protocol and potential negative side effects associated with participation prior to providing their written consent.

2.3. Experimental Trial

Participants reported to the FML on six different occasions (T1–T6) during the study. T1 consisted of a study briefing designed to inform the participants of the study protocol, obtain completed informed consent agreements, record anthropomorphic measurements and to establish a one repetition maximal load (1RM) of a barbell back squat. During this initial meeting it was stressed to the participants the unique nature of the study and the potential side effects associated with the ingestion of raw milk. The participants were also offered detailed information regarding raw milk both verbally and in hardcopy form. It was further stressed to the participants that once they have listened to and read the information regarding raw milk that their participation was completely voluntary and they could withdraw at any time during the study with no negative consequences.

Seventy-two hours post-T1 participants reported to the FML for T2. T2 consisted of participants completing the measure of DOMS. The measure was a FPS-R (Face Pain Scale—Revised) prior to the next phase of the study to determine level of lower extremity discomfort prior to participating in the second phase of T2. The second phase of T2 involved the participants completing four sets of 10 repetitions of 80% of their previously obtained 1RM after a sufficient warm up. Participants were monitored by trained research assistants for complete range of motion, accuracy of amount of weight lifted, and accuracy of repetitions completed, as well as for safety of the participant. Once the participant completed the fourth set of 10 repetitions, they were guided to another member of the research team to be randomly assigned to either the chocolate milk (CM) group or the raw milk (RM) group.

When group assignment was made the participant completed the DOMS questionnaire. Once the questionnaire was completed, the participant was offered approximately 240 mL of either beverage and asked to consume the beverage promptly (within 5 min post DOMS protocol completion). Participants were then asked to report to the FML 24 (T4), 48 (T5) and 72 (T6) hours post T3 for completion of the FPS-R.

Additionally, a member of the research team contacted each participant in order to determine if they were experiencing any internal discomfort attributed to the ingestion of either beverage immediately after consumption and once per day for10 days following consumption. If any ill effects were reported a negative side effect protocol was prepared for implementation.

2.4. DOMS Measures

Delayed onset of muscle soreness (DOMS) was assessed with two independent instruments. One instrument was a visual analog scale.

FRP-S: Participant's perceived pain discomfort level was assessed using a standardized protocol. Assessments of discomfort were performed with a blank FRP-S for each assessment to minimize bias from previous reporting. The FPS-R is a 6-point scale, with 6 different faces that represent increasing levels of pain intensity. Participants were asked to select the one expression that best characterized his pain intensity, from the left-most face ("No pain"), to the right-most face ("Very much pain"). Each illustration corresponded to a numeric score (0, 2, 4, 6, 8, or 10). Research supports the validity of this pain measure [22].

2.5. Statistical Analysis

To calculate the chances of benefit and harm, the smallest worthwhile or important effect for each dependent variable was the smallest standardized (Cohen) change in the mean −0.2 times the between subject SD for baseline values of all participants [23]—which has been used in similar investigations [23]. Practical inferences were drawn using the approach identified by Hopkins (2006) and utilized by Cockburn, 2010. Quantitative chances of benefit and harm were assessed qualitatively: <1% indicated almost certainly none; 1% to 5% indicated very unlikely; 5% to 25% indicated unlikely; 25% to 75% indicated possibly; 75% to 95% indicated likely; 95% to 99% indicated very likely; and >99% indicated almost certainly [23,24]. This method provides a way to qualify clear outcomes with a descriptor that represents the likelihood that the true value will have the observed magnitude. They are also free of the burden of Type I and Type II errors because they are probabilistic rather than definitive statements [24] Because of the large number of comparisons that could be reported, we only reported changes from baseline to 24, 48 and 72 h. Previous research has shown that the point at which milk-based carbohydrate-protein supplements become beneficial is 48 h after muscle-damaging exercise [25].

3. Results

Physical characteristics of both groups were similar. The mean age of participants was 20 years, mean height 68.775 inches and mean weight 175.89 pounds. Also similar between each group were the strength measures: mean 1RM back squat was 279 pounds and the mean value for 80% of each respective 1RM back squat was 226 pounds. (Table 1).

Table 1. Participant characteristics mean values (pooled and sorted by group assignment) $N = 20$ (Raw Milk Solution (RMS) $n = 10$, Chocolate Milk Solution (CMS) $n = 10$).

Variable	Pooled	RMS	CMS
Age (years)	20	19.9	20.1
Height (cm)	174.70	172.72	176.66
Weight (kg)	79.78	77.14	82.43
1RM (kg)	126.55	127.46	125.66
RM% (kg)	102.51	102.51	102.51

Both groups showed an increase in DOMS as a result of the assigned and completed protocol. Reported lower extremity soreness peaked at 48 h for the CM group and immediately after completing the DOMS protocol for the RM group. Both groups reported similar levels of discomfort 24 h post DOMS protocol with an increase in discomfort from 24 to 48 h post DOMS protocol.

At 72 h post-DOMS protocol, both groups reported a lower level of discomfort trending to baseline values.

Each dependent variable was analyzed, using a published spreadsheet [23], to determine the effect of the respective solution as the difference in the change between each group. Participant descriptive data and muscle soreness data are presented as absolute means + SD (Figure 1).

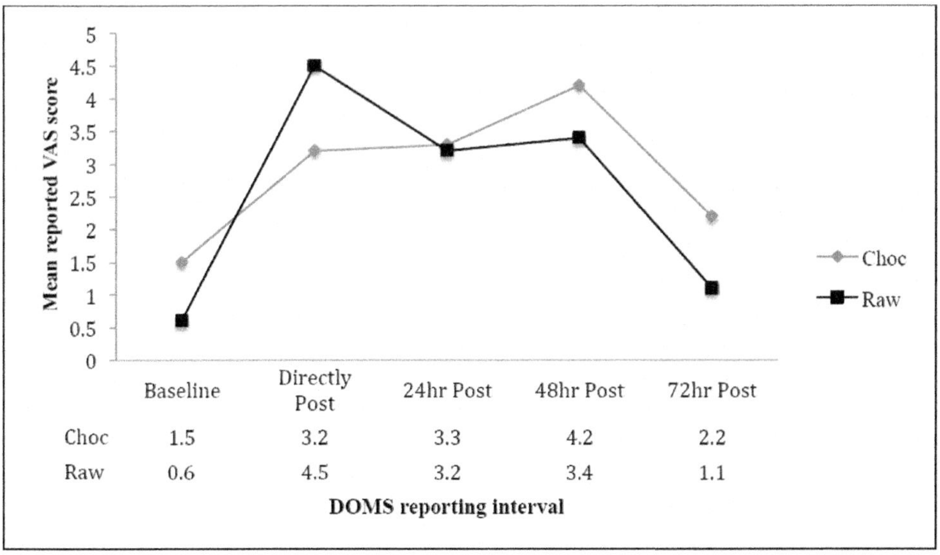

Figure 1. Changes in reported visual acuity scale (VAS) score regarding lower extremity muscle soreness pre-exercise induced muscle soreness (EIMS) protocol, directly post EIMS, 24 h, 48 h and 72 h post-EIMS for both the Raw Milk Solution (RMS) group and the Chocolate Milk Solution (CMS) group.

There was a likely benefit to the ingestion of the RMS at 48 (0.8 ± 2.55) and 72 h (1.1 ± 1.68) post-EIMS protocol. The difference between the CMS group and the RMS was unclear at baseline (0.1 ± 1.35) and 24 h post-EIMS (0.1 ± 1.69) (Table 2).

Table 2. Effect of solution timing on the changes between groups in muscle soreness following muscledamaging exercise.

Comparison	Mean Effect ± 90% CI	Qualitative Inference
Baseline	0.1 ± 1.35	Unclear
24 h	0.1 ± 1.69	Unclear
48 h	0.8 ± 2.55	Increase likely
72 h	1.1 ± 1.68	Increase likely

4. Discussion

This study investigated how a raw milk and honey solution would compare to a chocolate milk solution in the attenuation of lower extremity DOMS. The primary finding of this study was that the consumption of a raw milk and honey solution immediately following relatively aggressive lower extremity exercise reduced reported muscle soreness to a greater extent when compared to chocolate milk over a 72-h time frame. Secondary findings indicate that the consumption of a raw milk and honey solution elicited no reported negative side effects up to 10 days post consumption.

Participants for this study were members of a small University's Sprint Football team. This particular group was chosen to participate due to the fact that the members of this team had recently (within the past seven days) finished their spring training cycle in which each of the athletes completed the same program during this cycle allowing for a very similar training state among participants. Additionally, the Sprint Football is unique when compared to traditional football in that the athletes must maintain a body weight of 172 pounds and a minimum of 5% body fat during the football season [24]. This requirement has lead to the athletes being of very similar size and capacity.

Delayed Onset of Muscle Soreness and milk products.

The reasons behind DOMS have been a steady interest for many sports scientists for a long time. Although several factors including lactic acid, connective tissue damage surrounding muscles, muscle temperature, muscle spasm, inflammatory responses, free radicals, and nitric oxides have been suggested for causing DOMS, there is no clear explanation [26–28]. Previous literature has speculated that the cause of DOMS is due to structural muscle damages and perturbation of calcium homeostasis or acute inflammatory responses to exercise [28–30].

Consistent with previously reported results, the consumption of a milk-based solution with an elevated carbohydrate level reduces the DOMS [23]. However, what has not been reported prior to this study is the difference between a raw milk solution and a commercially available milk solution with elevated carbohydrate levels. Advocates for raw milk have made the case that the pasteurization process denatures the macronutrients and many of the micronutrients present in the milk.

In a recent review of nutritional interventions on delayed onset muscle soreness Kim and Lee (2014) presents information regarding the influence of polyphenol. The major biological functions of polyphenol are antioxidant capacity and anti-inflammation. According to previous studies, a potential mechanism for reducing DOMS by ingestion with polyphenol is its action on membrane stability and reduced lipid peroxidation by inhibiting peroxyl radical activation [28]. Honey contains a number of antioxidants from a variety of sources, including polyphenolics. The antioxidant components found in varieties of honey have been associated with improving vasodilation and conditions associated with inflammatory response [31].

In should be noted, the small independent dairy farm that the raw milk was obtained for this study undergoes laboratory testing to determine the safety of the milk it offers on a monthly basis. Prior to this research being conducted, the researches obtained a copy of the most recent laboratory results. The samples used in the laboratory tests were collected two days before the dairy collected the milk used in the study. Independent laboratory results indicated that the milk used in this study was safe for human consumption. The storage and distribution of the milk during this study was also consistent with appropriate food hygiene practices, thus limiting the opportunity for food-borne illness.

The exact mechanism for the greater decrease in DOMS when athletes consumed the RMS is unclear. Perhaps, as postulated by Cockburn *et al.* [23], this difference is due to limiting increases in protein degradation and stimulating protein synthesis of the polyphenol content of the honey used. Additionally, it may be possible that micronutrient denaturing through the process of pasteurization influenced the CMS. The fat content of the RMS was higher than that of the CMS, this may be associated with the difference in reported soreness. Further studies should expand on this research to explore different combinations of carbohydrate, milk type and fat content.

5. Conclusions

We have demonstrated that consuming a raw milk and honey solution immediately after muscle damaging exercise can increase the recovery rate substantially when compared to the consumption of chocolate milk, a commonly accepted recovery drink. Further research should be conducted examining the relationship between the unique nutrient combination found in a raw milk and honey solution.

Author Contributions: A.H. conceived the experiment. A.H., C.B., D.W., C.O., A.L. and J.S.H. designed and conducted the experiment. A.H. analyzed the data and wrote the paper.

Conflicts of Interest: The authors declare no conflict of interest.

References

1. Hill, J.; Howatson, G.; van Someren, K.; Leeder, J.; Pedlar, C. Compression garments and recovery from exercise-induced muscle damage: A meta-analysis. *Br. J. Sports Med.* **2014**, *48*, 1340–1346. [CrossRef] [PubMed]
2. Veqar, Z.; Imtiyaz, S. Vibration therapy in management of delayed onset muscle soreness (DOMS). *J. Clin. Diagn. Res.* **2014**, *8*, LE01–LE04. [CrossRef] [PubMed]
3. Gulick, D.T.; Kimura, I.F. Delayed onset muscle soreness: What is it and how do we treat it? *J. Sport Rehabil.* **1996**, *5*, 234–243.
4. Wessel, J.; Wan, A. Effect of stretching on the intensity of delayed-onset muscle soreness. *Clin. J. Sport Med.* **1994**, *4*, 83–87. [CrossRef]
5. Cheung, K.; Hume, P.A.; Maxwell, L. Delayed onset muscle soreness: Treatment strategies and performance factors. *Sports Med.* **2003**, *33*, 145–164. [CrossRef] [PubMed]
6. Veqar, Z. Causes and management of delayed onset muscle soreness: A review. *Elixir Hum. Physiol.* **2013**, *55*, 13205–13211.
7. Lee, J.; Kang, J.; Park, S.; Yoon, S.; Jeong, S.; Heo, M. Effects of inter-electrode distance on delayed onset muscle soreness in microcurrent therapy. *J. Phys. Ther. Sci.* **2013**, *25*, 1451–1454. [CrossRef] [PubMed]
8. Howatson, G.; van Someren, K. The prevention and treatment of exercise induced muscle damage. *Sports Med.* **2008**, *38*, 483–503. [CrossRef] [PubMed]
9. McBrier, N.M.; Vairo, G.L.; Bagshaw, D.; Lekan, J.M.; Bordi, P.L.; Kris-Etherton, P.M. Cocoa-based protein and carbohydrate drink decreases perceived soreness after exhaustive aerobic exercise: A pragmatic preliminary analysis. *J. Strength Cond. Res. Assoc.* **2010**, *24*, 2203–2210. [CrossRef] [PubMed]
10. Karp, J.; Johnston, J.; Tecklenburg, S.; Mickleborough, T.; Fly, A.; Stager, J. Chocolate milk as a post-exercise recovery aid. *Int. J. Sport Nutr. Exerc. Metab.* **2006**, *16*, 78–91. [PubMed]
11. Peschek, K.; Pritchett, R.; Bergman, E.; Pritchett, K. The effects of acute post exercise consumption of two cocoa-based beverages with varying flavanol content on indices of muscle recovery following downhill treadmill running. *Nutrients* **2013**, *6*, 50–62. [CrossRef] [PubMed]
12. Gilson, S.F.; Saunders, M.J.; Moran, C.W.; Moore, R.W.; Womack, C.J.; Todd, M.K. Effects of chocolate milk consumption on markers of muscle recovery following soccer training: A randomized cross-over study. *J. Int. Soc. Sports Nutr.* **2010**, *7*, 19. [CrossRef] [PubMed]

13. Pritchett, K.; Bishop, P.; Pritchett, R.; Green, M.; Katica, C. Acute effects of chocolate milk and a commercial recovery beverage on post exercise recovery indices and endurance cycling performance. *Appl. Physiol. Nutr. Metab.* **2009**, *34*, 1017–1022. [CrossRef] [PubMed]
14. Spaccarotella, K.J.; Andzel, W.D. The effects of low fat chocolate milk on post exercise recovery in collegiate athletes. *J. Strength Cond. Res.* **2011**, *25*, 3456–3460. [CrossRef] [PubMed]
15. Thomas, K.; Morris, P.; Stevenson, E. Improved endurance capacity following chocolate milk consumption compared with 2 commercially available sports drinks. *Appl. Physiol. Nutr. Metab.* **2009**, *34*, 78–82. [CrossRef] [PubMed]
16. Sarwar, G.; Peace, R.W.; Botting, H.G. Differences in protein digestibility and quality of liquid concentrate and powder forms of milk-based infant formulas fed to rats. *Am. J. Clin. Nutr.* **1989**, *49*, 806–813. [PubMed]
17. Miller, K.B.; Hurst, W.J.; Payne, M.J.; Stuart, D.A.; Apgar, J.; Sweigart, D.S.; Ou, B. Impact on alkalization on the antioxidant and flavanol content of commercial cocoa powders. *J. Agric. Food Chem.* **2008**, *56*, 8527–8533. [CrossRef] [PubMed]
18. Mummah, S.; Oelrich, B.; Hope, J.; Vu, Q.; Gardner, C.D. Effect of raw milk on lactose intolerance: A randomized controlled pilot study. *Ann. Fam. Med.* **2014**, *12*, 134–141. [CrossRef] [PubMed]
19. Oliver, S.P.; Boor, K.J.; Murphy, S.C.; Murinda, S.E. Food safety hazards associated with consumption of raw milk. *Foodborne Pathog. Dis.* **2009**, *6*, 793–806. [CrossRef] [PubMed]
20. Raw Milk *vs.* Pasteurized Milk. Available online: http://www.realmilk.com/health/raw-milk-vs-pasteurized-milk/ (accessed on 11 December 2015).
21. Vallianou, N.G.; Gounari, P.; Skourtis, A.; Panagos, J.; Kazazis, C. Honey and its anti-inflammatory, anti-bacterial and anti-oxidant properties. *Gen. Med.* **2014**, *2*. [CrossRef]
22. Ferreira-Valente, M.A.; Pais-Ribeiro, J.L.; Jensen, M.P. Validity of four pain intensity rating scales. *Pain* **2011**, *152*, 2399–2404. [CrossRef] [PubMed]
23. Cockburn, E.; Robson-Ansley, P.; Hayes, P.R.; Stevenson, E. Effect of volume of milk consumed on the attenuation of exercise-induced muscle damage. *Eur. J. Appl. Physiol.* **2012**, *112*, 3187–3194. [CrossRef] [PubMed]
24. Hopkins, W.G. A Spreadsheet for Analysis of Straightforward Controlled Trials. Available online: http://www.sportsci.org/jour/03whgtrials.htm.25 (accessed on 11 December 2015).
25. Collegiate Sprint Football League Information. Available online: http://www.sprintfootball.com/p4_league_information.jsp (accessed on 11 December 2015).
26. Cockburn, E.; Hayes, P.R.; French, D.N.; Stevenson, E.; St Clair Gibson, A. Acute milk-based protein-CHO supplementation attenuates exercise-induced muscle damage. *Appl. Physiol.* **2008**, *33*, 775–783. [CrossRef] [PubMed]
27. Close, G.L.; Ashton, T.; McArdle, A.; MacLaren, D.P. The emerging role of free radicals in delayed onset muscle soreness and contraction-induced muscle injury. *Comp. Biochem. Physiol. A Mol. Integr. Physiol.* **2005**, *142*, 257–266. [CrossRef] [PubMed]
28. Radak, Z.; Naito, H.; Taylor, A.W.; Goto, S. Nitric oxide: Is it the cause of muscle soreness? *Nitr. Oxide* **2012**, *26*, 89–94. [CrossRef] [PubMed]
29. Kim, J.; Lee, J. A review of nutritional intervention on delayed onset muscle soreness. *Part I J. Exerc. Rehabil.* **2014**, *10*, 349–356. [CrossRef] [PubMed]
30. Armstrong, R.B. Mechanisms of exercise-induced delayed onset muscular soreness: A brief review. *Med. Sci. Sports Exerc.* **1984**, *16*, 529–538. [CrossRef] [PubMed]
31. Khalil, M.I.; Sulaiman, S.A. The potential role of honey and its polyphenols in preventing heart diseases: A review. *Afr. J. Tradit. Complement. Altern. Med.* **2010**, *7*, 315–321. [CrossRef] [PubMed]

18

The Acute Effects of Heavy Deadlifts on Vertical Jump Performance in Men

Jerry C. Arias, Jared W. Coburn *, Lee E. Brown and Andrew J. Galpin

Center for Sport Performance, Department of Kinesiology, California State University, Fullerton, CA 92831, USA; titanedgeathletics@gmail.com (J.C.A.); leebrown@fullerton.edu (L.E.B.); agalpin@fullerton.edu (A.J.G.)
* Correspondence: jcoburn@fullerton.edu

Academic Editor: Eling Douwe de Bruin

Abstract: The purpose of this study was to investigate the effects of deadlifts as a postactivation potentiation stimulus on vertical jump performance. Fifteen men (age, 23.9 $\pm$ 4.2 years; height, 176.3 $\pm$ 8.6 cm; mass, 76.1 $\pm$ 16.3 kg) participated in the study. Participants visited the lab for three sessions, each separated by at least 48 h. One repetition maximum (1RM) in the deadlift was measured during the first visit. For Visit 2, participants performed one of two experimental sessions: a deadlift session or a control session. Participants performed a single maximal vertical jump (VJ; counter movement jump without an arm swing), then either performed five repetitions of the deadlift using 85% 1RM (deadlift session) or were told to stand still for ten seconds (control). Following either condition, participants performed single VJ at 15 s, 2, 4, 6, 8, 10, 12, 14, and 16 min post condition. Peak VJ height and peak ground reaction forces (pGRF) were measured using a force plate. For Visit 3, whatever condition was not administered at Visit 2 was performed. The results showed that VJ height was significantly lower 15 s following deadlifting (36.9 $\pm$ 5.1 cm) compared to the control condition (40.1 $\pm$ 4.6 cm). In addition, VJ height 15 s after the deadlift was lower than VJ height measured at minutes 2–16 following the deadlift. Performance of five repetitions of deadlifting did not affect pGRF. These results suggest that performing five repetitions of the deadlift exercise at 85% 1RM does not induce a postactivation potentiation (PAP) effect, and may in fact cause an acute reduction in VJ performance.

Keywords: postactivation potentiation; PAP; power

---

1. Introduction

Postactivation potentiation (PAP) is defined as an increase in muscle twitch and low-frequency tetanic force after a "conditioning" contractile activity [1]. It is believed that the potentiating effect from the conditioning activity may be due to phosphorylation of the myosin regulatory light chains, or increased excitability of alpha motor neurons in the spinal cord [2]. The "conditioning" activity that has been used in past research to evoke PAP has included both dynamic [3–5] and isometric [6,7] muscle actions. Past research has shown PAP to be effective in producing greater performance in high intensity activities such as jumping and sprinting [8–11]. However, there is also evidence to suggest that PAP has no significant effect on performance variables [4,12–15] or may actually impair performance [16,17]. The latter may result when fatigue from the conditioning activity is greater than the potentiating effect [2].

Differences between studies, such as exercise selection, intensity, type of muscle contraction, rest periods following the potentiating activity, subject characteristics (age, strength, sex), and the variables being measured may all contribute to such variability in results. For example, it has been demonstrated that trained individuals may be more responsive to a potentiating stimulus than untrained individuals [18], at least partly due to differences in absolute and/or relative strength.

The time from the PAP stimulus until performance is assessed has also affected the interpretation of the effectiveness of PAP stimuli. For example, some studies have reported positive effects 4 to 12 min following the PAP stimulus [9], but no positive effect at 10 [4] or 15 s [9]. However, at least one other study did report increases in jump performance 20 s and four minutes following isometric squats in adult male participants [19]. Thus, further research into the timing of an optimal PAP effect is warranted.

When selecting an exercise to induce a PAP stimulus, it is important to select one that is both effective and practical to use. While previous studies have examined the use of exercises such as the back squat to elicit a PAP effect [3,4,9,20], there may be similar but more effective exercises. The deadlift exercise was chosen for the present study because it is a relatively simple exercise to perform, and requires similar muscle actions to that of a vertical jump (hip and knee extension). From a practical standpoint, it requires minimal equipment. If an athlete wanted to take advantage of a PAP response out on the field or court prior to competition, all that would be needed would be a heavy object to lift off the ground. Therefore, the purpose of this study was to investigate the effects of heavy deadlifts on vertical jump (VJ) and ground reaction forces (GRF) in resistance trained men.

2. Methods

2.1. Participants

Fifteen (age = 23.9 $\pm$ 4.2 years; height = 176.3 $\pm$ 8.6 cm; body mass = 80.1 $\pm$ 10.2 kg; deadlift 1RM = 152.4 $\pm$ 27.9 kg; relative deadlift 1RM = 1.9 $\pm$ 0.2 $kg \cdot kg^{-1}$) men volunteered to participate in this study. Prior to testing, participants signed a statement of informed consent approved by the University Institutional Review Board. All participants met the following inclusion criteria: male between 18 and 35 years, performed at least one lower body resistance exercise session per week for the past six months, and free of injuries that would limit their ability to perform maximal deadlifts or jumping exercises. Participants were instructed to refrain from any type of resistance training that involved the lower body 48 h prior to testing, maintain a normal diet, and drink half a liter of water on test day to ensure proper hydration.

2.2. Experimental Design

Three laboratory sessions, separated by at least 48 h, were required for each participant. The first session was an orientation/familiarization visit. During the orientation session, participants were asked to complete the following: informed consent, measurements of height and weight, maximum vertical jump height, and 1RM testing in the deadlift. The other two sessions were either the deadlift or control session. During these two sessions, participants were required to do a countermovement jump for determination of VJ height, followed by either the treatment (85% 1RM deadlift for five repetitions) or control (no deadlift). The order of these sessions were randomized for the first participant and counterbalanced for each remaining participant. These sessions began with a dynamic warm-up, which included twenty jumping jacks, ten walking T-Dives, ten walking lunges, and ten repetitions of the deadlift with a 45 lb. Olympic bar. The warm-up was followed by five minutes of sitting rest. Following the brief rest period, subjects either completed the control or treatment protocol. This was followed by single countermovement jumps at 15 s, 2, 4, 6, 8, 10, 12, 14, and 16 min post deadlift or control period. Participants were resting in a sitting position between the jumps. The use of an 85% 1RM load in the deadlift was chosen because it had previously been shown that the use of maximal or near maximal intensity (>80%) has greater effects at inducing PAP when followed by an explosive activity such as jumping [10,21].

2.3. 1RM Testing

The 1RM testing procedure began with a warm up of five to ten repetitions at 40% to 60% of estimated 1RM. After a one minute rest, the participant performed three to five repetitions at 60%–80%

of perceived maximum (moderate-to-hard exertion). The participant then attempted a 1RM lift. If the lift was successful, a rest period of 3–5 min was provided before attempting a heavier weight. The goal was to find the 1RM within three to five maximal efforts. The process of increasing the weight was continued by increments of approximately 7.5 to 15 kg, until the participant was able to only complete one repetition successfully. If the participant was not able to execute the lift successfully, the weight was reduced by 2.2 to 4.5 kg. A Certified Strength and Conditioning Specialist certified through the National Strength and Conditioning Association oversaw each attempt. A deadlift 1RM attempt was deemed successful if at the end of the ascent phase the participant stood erect with knees and hips extended, the torso upright, and the should girdle retracted.

2.4. Vertical Jump and Ground Reaction Force Testing

Subjects performed countermovement jumps on a force platform. The countermovement jumps were performed in accordance with Young *et al.* [22] and similar to the procedures to that of Till & Cook [12]. Participants began in a standing position with hands positioned on their hips, then flexing the hips and knees, and immediately jumping vertically as high as possible. The force plate was used to estimate VJ height (cm) using the time in the air equation: distance = $(1/2\ gt^2)/2$, where g is gravity at 9.81 $m \cdot s^2$ and t is the flight time. Measurements of VJ height (primary outcome variable) and peak ground reaction forces (pGRF; secondary outcome variable) were collected immediately following each jump. VJ height and pGRF were measured on a force plate (AMTI force platform, Advanced Mechanical Technology, Inc., Watertown, MA, USA). Data were collected at a sampling frequency of 1000 Hz using a computer and custom LabVIEW version 7.1 software (National Instruments Corporation, Austin, TX, USA). Verbal encouragement was given during both conditions to encourage maximal performance.

2.5. Statistical Analyses

All statistical analyses were conducted using IBM SPSS Statistics 20.0 (IBM Corporation, Somers, NY, USA). A 2 × 10 (condition × time) repeated measured analysis of variance (ANOVA) was performed for each dependent variable (VJ height and pGRF). Significant interactions were followed up with one-way repeated measures ANOVAs, Tukey post hoc tests, and paired *t*-tests as appropriate. Alpha was set at 0.05. Effect sizes were calculated by SPSS as partial eta squared ($\eta_p{}^2 = SS_{effect}/(SS_{effect} + SS_{error})$.

3. Results

For VJ height, there was a significant 2-way (treatment × time) interaction ($p < 0.05$). For the deadlift condition, follow-up tests indicated VJ height at 15 s post deadlift was significantly ($p < 0.05$) lower than VJ height at 2, 4, 6, 8, 10, 12, 14, and 16 min (Figure 1). For the control condition, there was no significant main effect for time ($p > 0.05$). In addition, VJ height at 15 s was significantly lower for the deadlift condition compared to the control condition.

For pGRF, there was no significant ($p > 0.05$) two-way (treatment × time) interaction or main effects for time (Figure 2). Effect sizes for VJ height and pGRF were interpreted as trivial to small effects (Table 1).

Table 1. Effect sizes (calculated as partial eta squared) for the dependent variables.

Variable	Effect Size (Partial Eta Squared)
VJ Height (deadlift condition)	0.226
VJ Height (control condition)	0.153
pGRF (deadlift condition)	0.067
pGRF (control condition)	0.025

Effect sizes for dependent variables. The numbers represent the proportion of the total variance that was due to the treatment (either deadlift or control condition). pGRF = peak ground reaction forces.

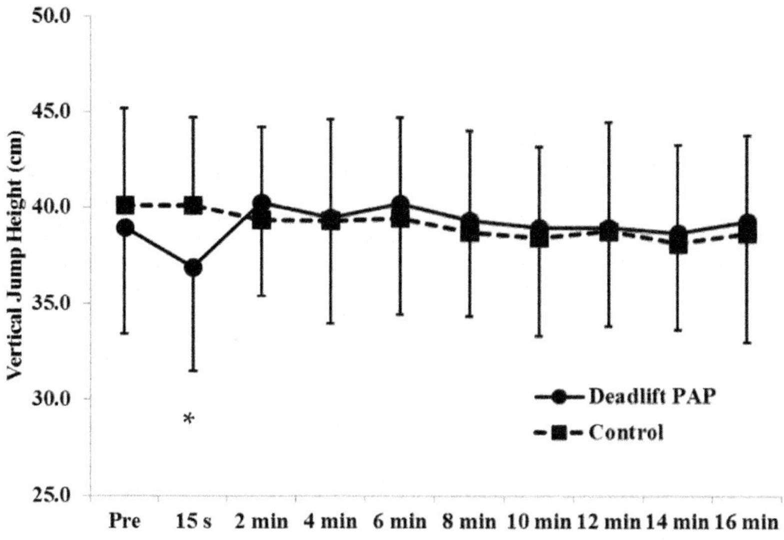

Figure 1. Vertical jump (VJ) height (mean ± SD). There was a significant 2-way (treatment × time) interaction ($p < 0.05$). The deadlift condition led to a significant decrease in vertical jump height 15 s after deadlifting compared to subsequent time periods. * = less than 2, 4, 6, 8, 10, 12, 14, and 16 min. In addition, VJ height at 15 s was significantly lower for the deadlift condition compared to the control condition.

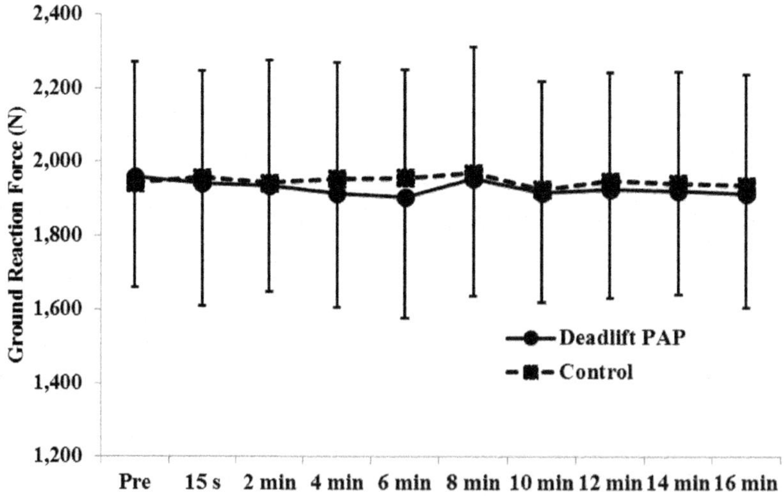

Figure 2. Ground reaction force (mean ± SD). There was no significant interaction or main effects ($p > 0.05$).

4. Discussion

The purpose of this study was to determine the potentiating effects of heavy deadlifts on VJ height and pGRF. It was hypothesized that VJ height and pGRF would both improve following the deadlifts compared to the control condition. However, heavy deadlifts decreased VJ height 15 s post lifting compared to subsequent time periods. Furthermore, there were no significant effects of heavy deadlifts on pGRF.

Although the movement patterns during the deadlift exercise are similar to the VJ (extension of the hip, knee, and ankle joints), they are different with regard to joint ranges of motion. To our knowledge, only one other study has used the deadlift exercise as a conditioning stimulus to achieve a PAP effect [12]. They had subjects perform the deadlift for five repetitions at their 5RM. They did not find any significant improvements in either sprint times or vertical jump performance measures. Although they used different methodologies than the present study, both studies failed to find improved performance. Previous research has shown that the biomechanics of vertical jumping are altered in different ways by Olympic weightlifting, plyometrics, and a combination of the two [23]. This may also be true when considering the acute effects of heavy deadlifts, as used in the present study, compared to various forms of squatting as used in most other studies examining PAP. Thus, exercise selection may influence the effectiveness of the conditioning stimulus. Future studies should directly compare various PAP exercises, including the deadlift and back squat variations, to determine their relative effects on the PAP response.

Previous studies have shown improvements in vertical jump performance following back squats [5,22,24]. For example, Young *et al.* [22] examined the effects of using 5RM half-squats on loaded counter-movement jumps (LCMJ), and found that the LCMJ was 2.8% higher following half-squats. Lowery *et al.* [20] also reported significant increases in vertical jump four minutes following moderate (70% 1RM) and high intensity (93% 1RM), but not low intensity (56% 1RM), back squat loads. Vertical jump height was reported to have returned to baseline by minutes 8 and 12. Furthermore, they reported decreases in vertical jump height when measured immediately following the back squats using the moderate and high intensity loads. These studies are in contrast to the findings of Mangus *et al.* [3], who found no potentiating effects of half and quarter-squats on vertical jump performance. Although the results of our study may have been attributed to the use of the selected exercise (deadlift), the literature suggests that even when the same exercise is used in different studies, the results are inconsistent.

The timing of the jumps after the attempted PAP stimulus may also have contributed to the findings of the present study. There is evidence to suggest that fatigue and potentiation can coexist in skeletal muscle [25]. It has been suggested that fatigue may be dominant in the early stages of recovery, and thus, may hinder performance of subsequent voluntary activity [26]. In the present study, jumps were performed at 15 s, 2, 4, 6, 8, 10, 12, 14, and 16 min after the potentiating stimulus. Our finding of a reduction in VJ at 15 s suggests that fatigue was dominant immediately following the deadlift. Jensen and Ebben [4] also found no significant improvements in VJ height with similar rest periods (10 s, 1, 2, 3, and 4 min) following a 5RM back squat. Crewther *et al.* [9] examined the acute potentiating effects of back squats on the CMJ, sprint performance, and horizontal sled pushes. Their results indicated a significant reduction in CMJ height at 15 s, followed by improvements at 4, 8, and 12 min, and then a further decrease in CMJ performance at 16 min. Thus, performance may be significantly hindered when jumps are performed immediately after the potentiating stimulus. Arabatzi *et al.* [19], however, found that squat jump performance was enhanced both 20 s and four minutes following the performance of 3×3 maximal isometric squats. This was true only for the adult male participants, however. Preadolescent and adolescent males and females, and adult females, did not demonstrate a PAP effect during the squat jumps. While the higher absolute loads used by stronger individuals might allow the PAP effect to last for a longer period of time, it would also likely cause greater fatigue to be evident during the early phase of recovery following the PAP stimulus [20]. In our study, the 85% 1RM load used for the PAP stimulus may have induced significant fatigue, but was not enough to induce a PAP effect sufficient to lead to increases in VJ performance as the fatigue subsided. Once again, these studies illustrate the complex interplay of age, sex, type of conditioning stimulus, absolute and relative strength, and timing of assessment in determining the effectiveness of a conditioning stimulus at inducing a PAP effect [20].

Interestingly, both the Crewther *et al.* [9] and Jensen and Ebben [4] studies measured jumps at the four minute interval, yet only Crewther *et al.* showed significant improvements. Jensen and Ebben [4] measured consecutive jumps in one minute intervals, while our study used two minute intervals, and both failed to show significant improvements. However, Crewther *et al.* [9] allowed 4 min to pass between jumps and found significant improvements in jump height at 4, 8, and 12 min. This indicates there may be an ideal time, somewhere between 4 and 12 min, in which fatigue dissipates enough to allow the potentiation response to be evident. With regard to the present study, perhaps we would have observed a potentiating effect if we had begun vertical jump testing at four minutes after the conditioning activity, rather than including prior test jumps at 15 s and 2 min following the deadlifts. The jumps prior to the 4 min time period may have further fatigued, or delayed the recovery of, our subjects, masking the PAP response. This evidence supports the hypothesis that fatigue and potentiation can coexist, and in order to induce PAP, one must allow enough time to elapse to see any performance enhancement.

The strength level of the subjects may also have affected the PAP response [26]. Subjects who are stronger have been shown to have a greater potentiation response when compared to weaker individuals [22,27]. Chiu *et al.* [27] investigated the response to postactivation potentiation between athletes involved in sports requiring explosive strength, and recreationally trained subjects. Their results showed that athletes exhibited greater potentiation compared to recreationally trained individuals. Likewise, Young *et al.* [22] showed that subjects who had the greatest increase in mean jump height following the squat set, also achieved the greatest 5RM. They concluded that the stronger the individual, the greater the gain in power through PAP. It is possible that because we used recreationally trained men, and not athletes, the participants may not have been strong enough to benefit from the PAP stimulus (mean 5RM load, 129.7 $\pm$ 23.5 kg.; mean deadlift 1RM, 152.4 $\pm$ 27.9 kg; relative deadlift 1RM = 1.9 $\pm$ 0.2 $kg \cdot kg^{-1}$). The importance of absolute *vs.* relative strength must also be considered. Although few studies have reported relative strength values for their subjects, it seems reasonable that this may be at least as important as absolute strength in determining the effectiveness of a PAP stimulus on vertical jump height and power [28].

5. Conclusions

In conclusion, the lack of a positive PAP effect of deadlifts on VJ height or pGRF may be attributed to three main findings. First, the deadlift exercise may not have had enough specificity to the CMJ. Perhaps the back squat or jump squat would have yielded improvements in performance. Secondly, our results may have been affected by the recovery time chosen. The present study allowed 2 min in between jumps, and just 15 s following the PAP stimulus. It is possible that this was not enough time to recover and allow fatigue to dissipate. We can infer that if more time was given prior to the first jumps performed after the deadlifts, potentiation may have been evident and subsequent performance might have increased. Lastly, using only recreationally trained subjects, and not a stronger population of athletes, may have contributed to the lack of PAP response. In the present study, the subjects were required to have performed only one lower body resistance exercise session per week for the past six months. Therefore, our participants may not have been strong enough (absolute or relative strength) or trained enough to be able to induce the PAP response necessary to achieve an increase in vertical jump performance. The evidence from previous studies supports the contention that stronger individuals will benefit more from PAP methods than recreationally trained individuals.

Based on these results, the use of heavy deadlifts, as performed in this study, may not be sufficient to induce PAP in recreationally trained individuals, and may in fact reduce performance for several minutes due to fatigue. However, the present study also used relatively short rest periods following the PAP stimulus. If strength and conditioning practitioners wish to use deadlifts as a PAP stimulus to increase their athlete's performance, they may want to allow somewhere between 4 and 12 min between the conditioning stimulus and the performance activity before assessing their effects.

Author Contributions: Jerry C. Arias, Jared W. Coburn, Lee E. Brown, and Andrew J. Galpin conceived and designed the study. Jerry C. Arias performed all data collection. Jerry C. Arias and Jared W. Coburn analyzed and interpreted the data and wrote the paper.

Conflicts of Interest: The authors declare no conflict of interest.

References

1. Sale, D.G. Postactivation potentiation: Role in human performance. *Exerc. Sport Sci. Rev.* **2002**, *30*, 138–143. [CrossRef] [PubMed]
2. Hodgson, M.; Docherty, D.; Robbins, D. Post-activation potentiation: Underlying physiology and implications for motor performance. *Sports Med.* **2005**, *35*, 585–595. [CrossRef] [PubMed]
3. Mangus, B.C.; Takahashi, M.; Mercer, J.A.; Holcomb, W.R.; McWhorter, J.W.; Sanchez, R. Investigation of vertical jump performance after completing heavy squat exercises. *J. Strength Cond. Res.* **2006**, *20*, 597–600. [CrossRef] [PubMed]
4. Jensen, R.L.; Ebben, W.P. Kinetic analysis of complex training rest interval effect on vertical jump performance. *J. Strength Cond. Res.* **2003**, *17*, 345–349. [CrossRef] [PubMed]
5. Gourgoulis, V.; Aggeloussis, N.; Kasimatis, P.; Mavromatis, G.; Garas, A. Effect of a submaximal half-squats warm-up program on vertical jumping ability. *J. Strength Cond. Res.* **2003**, *17*, 342–344. [CrossRef] [PubMed]
6. Rixon, K.P.; Lamont, H.S.; Bemben, M.G. Influence of type of muscle contraction, gender, and lifting experience on postactivation potentiation performance. *J. Strength Cond. Res.* **2007**, *21*, 500–505. [CrossRef] [PubMed]
7. French, D.N.; Kraemer, W.J.; Cooke, C.B. Changes in dynamic exercise performance following a sequence of preconditioning isometric muscle actions. *J. Strength Cond. Res.* **2003**, *17*, 678–685. [CrossRef] [PubMed]
8. McCann, M.R.; Flanagan, S.P. The effects of exercise selection and rest interval on postactivation potentiation of vertical jump performance. *J. Strength Cond. Res.* **2010**, *24*, 1285–1291. [CrossRef] [PubMed]
9. Crewther, B.T.; Kilduff, L.P.; Cook, C.J.; Middleton, M.K.; Bunce, P.J.; Yang, G.Z. The acute potentiating effects of back squats on athlete performance. *J. Strength Cond. Res.* **2011**, *25*, 3319–3325. [CrossRef] [PubMed]
10. Saez Saez de Villarreal, E.; Gonzalez-Badillo, J.J.; Izquierdo, M. Optimal warm-up stimuli of muscle activation to enhance short and long-term acute jumping performance. *Eur. J. Appl. Physiol.* **2007**, *100*, 393–401. [CrossRef] [PubMed]
11. Weber, K.R.; Brown, L.E.; Coburn, J.W.; Zinder, S.M. Acute effects of heavy-load squats on consecutive squat jump performance. *J. Strength Cond. Res.* **2008**, *22*, 726–730. [CrossRef] [PubMed]
12. Till, K.A.; Cooke, C. The effects of postactivation potentiation on sprint and jump performance of male academy soccer players. *J. Strength Cond. Res.* **2009**, *23*, 1960–1967. [CrossRef] [PubMed]
13. Scott, S.L.; Docherty, D. Acute effects of heavy preloading on vertical and horizontal jump performance. *J. Strength Cond. Res.* **2004**, *18*, 201–205. [CrossRef] [PubMed]
14. Hrysomallis, C.; Kidgell, D. Effect of heavy dynamic resistive exercise on acute upper-body power. *J. Strength Cond. Res.* **2001**, *15*, 426–430. [CrossRef] [PubMed]
15. Behm, D.G.; Button, D.C.; Barbour, G.; Butt, J.C.; Young, W.B. Conflicting effects of fatigue and potentiation on voluntary force. *J. Strength Cond. Res.* **2004**, *18*, 365–372. [CrossRef] [PubMed]
16. Tsolakis, C.; Bogdanis, G.C.; Nikolaou, A.; Zacharogiannis, E. Influence of type of muscle contraction and gender on postactivation potentiation of upper and lower limb explosive performance in elite fencers. *J Sports Sci. Med.* **2011**, *10*, 577–583. [PubMed]
17. Witmer, C.A.; Davis, S.E.; Moir, G.L. The acute effects of back squats on vertical jump performance in men and women. *J Sports Sci. Med.* **2010**, *9*, 206–213. [PubMed]
18. Berning, J.M.; Adams, K.J.; DeBeliso, M.; Sevene-Adams, P.G.; Harris, C.; Stamford, B.A. Effect of functional isometric squats on vertical jump in trained and untrained men. *J. Strength Cond. Res. Natl. Strength Cond. Assoc.* **2010**, *24*, 2285–2289. [CrossRef] [PubMed]
19. Arabatzi, F.; Patikas, D.; Zafeiridis, A.; Giavroudis, K.; Kannas, T.; Gourgoulis, V.; Kotzamanidis, C.M. The post-activation potentiation effect on squat jump performance: Age and sex effect. *Pediatr. Exerc. Sci.* **2014**, *26*, 187–194. [CrossRef] [PubMed]
20. Lowery, R.P.; Duncan, N.M.; Loenneke, J.P.; Sikorski, E.M.; Naimo, M.A.; Brown, L.E.; Wilson, F.G.; Wilson, J.M. The effects of potentiating stimuli intensity under varying rest periods on vertical jump performance and power. *J. Strength Cond. Res.* **2012**, *26*, 3320–3325. [CrossRef] [PubMed]
21. Rahimi, R. The acute effects of heavy *versus* light-load squats on sprint performance. *Phys. Educ. Sport* **2007**, *5*, 163–169.
22. Young, W.B.; Jenner, A.; Griffiths, K. Acute enhancement of power performance from heavy load squats. *J. Strength Cond. Res.* **1998**, *12*, 82–84. [CrossRef]

23. Arabatzi, F.; Kellis, E.; Saez-Saez De Villarreal, E. Vertical jump biomechanics after plyometric, weight lifting, and combined (weight lifting + plyometric) training. *J. Strength Cond. Res.* **2010**, *24*, 2440–2448. [CrossRef] [PubMed]
24. Kilduff, L.P.; Bevan, H.R.; Kingsley, M.I.; Owen, N.J.; Bennett, M.A.; Bunce, P.J.; Hore, A.M.; Maw, J.R.; Cunningham, D.J. Postactivation potentiation in professional rugby players: Optimal recovery. *J. Strength Cond. Res.* **2007**, *21*, 1134–1138. [CrossRef] [PubMed]
25. Rassier, D.E.; Macintosh, B.R. Coexistence of potentiation and fatigue in skeletal muscle. *Braz. J. Med. Biol. Res.* **2000**, *33*, 499–508. [CrossRef] [PubMed]
26. Tillin, N.A.; Bishop, D. Factors modulating post-activation potentiation and its effect on performance of subsequent explosive activities. *Sports Med.* **2009**, *39*, 147–166. [CrossRef] [PubMed]
27. Chiu, L.Z.; Fry, A.C.; Weiss, L.W.; Schilling, B.K.; Brown, L.E.; Smith, S.L. Postactivation potentiation response in athletic and recreationally trained individuals. *J. Strength Cond. Res.* **2003**, *17*, 671–677. [CrossRef] [PubMed]
28. Duthie, G.M.; Young, W.B.; Aitken, D.A. The acute effects of heavy loads on jump squat performance: An evaluation of the complex and contrast methods of power development. *J. Strength Cond. Res.* **2002**, *16*, 530–538. [CrossRef] [PubMed]

PERMISSIONS

All chapters in this book were first published in Sports, by MDPI; hereby published with permission under the Creative Commons Attribution License or equivalent. Every chapter published in this book has been scrutinized by our experts. Their significance has been extensively debated. The topics covered herein carry significant findings which will fuel the growth of the discipline. They may even be implemented as practical applications or may be referred to as a beginning point for another development.

The contributors of this book come from diverse backgrounds, making this book a truly international effort. This book will bring forth new frontiers with its revolutionizing research information and detailed analysis of the nascent developments around the world.

We would like to thank all the contributing authors for lending their expertise to make the book truly unique. They have played a crucial role in the development of this book. Without their invaluable contributions this book wouldn't have been possible. They have made vital efforts to compile up to date information on the varied aspects of this subject to make this book a valuable addition to the collection of many professionals and students.

This book was conceptualized with the vision of imparting up-to-date information and advanced data in this field. To ensure the same, a matchless editorial board was set up. Every individual on the board went through rigorous rounds of assessment to prove their worth. After which they invested a large part of their time researching and compiling the most relevant data for our readers.

The editorial board has been involved in producing this book since its inception. They have spent rigorous hours researching and exploring the diverse topics which have resulted in the successful publishing of this book. They have passed on their knowledge of decades through this book. To expedite this challenging task, the publisher supported the team at every step. A small team of assistant editors was also appointed to further simplify the editing procedure and attain best results for the readers.

Apart from the editorial board, the designing team has also invested a significant amount of their time in understanding the subject and creating the most relevant covers. They scrutinized every image to scout for the most suitable representation of the subject and create an appropriate cover for the book.

The publishing team has been an ardent support to the editorial, designing and production team. Their endless efforts to recruit the best for this project, has resulted in the accomplishment of this book. They are a veteran in the field of academics and their pool of knowledge is as vast as their experience in printing. Their expertise and guidance has proved useful at every step. Their uncompromising quality standards have made this book an exceptional effort. Their encouragement from time to time has been an inspiration for everyone.

The publisher and the editorial board hope that this book will prove to be a valuable piece of knowledge for researchers, students, practitioners and scholars across the globe.

LIST OF CONTRIBUTORS

Carol Hall and Rachel Kay
School of Animal, Rural and Environmental Sciences, Nottingham Trent University, Southwell, Nottinghamshire, United Kingdom

Ian Varley
School of Science and Technology, Nottingham Trent University, Nottingham, Nottinghamshire, United Kingdom

David Crundall
School of Social Sciences (Psychology), Nottingham Trent University, Nottingham, Nottinghamshire, United Kingdom

Valentín E. Fernández-Elías and Ricardo Mora-Rodriguez
Exercise Physiology Laboratory, University of Castilla-La Mancha, Toledo, Spain

Alberto Martínez-Abellán, José María López-Gullón, Ricardo Morá n-Navarro and Ernesto De la Cruz-Sánchez
Department of Physical Activity and Sport, University of Murcia, Murcia, Spain

Jesús G. Pallarés
Exercise Physiology Laboratory, University of Castilla-La Mancha, Toledo, Spain
Department of Physical Activity and Sport, University of Murcia, Murcia, Spain

Kathryn R. Martin
Epidemiology Group, School of Medicine and Dentistry, University of Aberdeen, Aberdeen, United Kingdom
Medical Research Council Unit for Lifelong Health and Ageing at University College London, London, United Kingdom
Laboratory of Epidemiology and Population Sciences, National Institute of Aging, National Institutes of Health, Bethesda, Maryland United States of America

Rachel Cooper, Rebecca Hardy and Diana Kuh
Medical Research Council Unit for Lifelong Health and Ageing at University College London, London, United Kingdom

Tamara B. Harris
Laboratory of Epidemiology and Population Sciences, National Institute of Aging, National Institutes of Health, Bethesda, Maryland United States of America

Soren Brage
Medical Research Council Epidemiology Unit, School of Clinical Medicine, Institute of Metabolic Science, University of Cambridge, Cambridge, United Kingdom

Nikolaos E. Koundourakis
Department of Clinical Chemistry, School of Medicine, University of Crete, Heraklion, Greece

Nikolaos E. Androulakis
Department of Laboratory Haematology, University Hospital, Heraklion, Crete, Greece

Niki Malliaraki and Andrew N. Margioris
Departments of Clinical Chemistry, University of Crete, School of Medicine, and University Hospital, Heraklion, Greece

Nadine Hummel and Virginia L. Flanagin
German Center for Vertigo and Balance Disorders, University Hospital Munich, Campus Grosshadern, Munich, Germany
Graduate School of Systemic Neurosciences, Ludwig-Maximilians University, Planegg-Martinsried, Germany

Katharina Hüfner and Olympia Kremmyda
German Center for Vertigo and Balance Disorders, University Hospital Munich, Campus Grosshadern, Munich, Germany

Department of Neurology, University Hospital Munich, Campus Grosshadern, Munich, Germany

Thomas Stephan
German Center for Vertigo and Balance Disorders, University Hospital Munich, Campus Grosshadern, Munich, Germany
Graduate School of Systemic Neurosciences, Ludwig-Maximilians University, Planegg-Martinsried, Germany
Department of Neurology, University Hospital Munich, Campus Grosshadern, Munich, Germany
Institute for Clinical Neurosciences, University Hospital Munich, Campus Grosshadern, Munich, Germany

Jennifer Linn
Department of Neuroradiology, University Hospital Munich, Campus Grosshadern, Munich, Germany

Thomas Brandt
German Center for Vertigo and Balance Disorders, University Hospital Munich, Campus Grosshadern, Munich, Germany
Institute for Clinical Neurosciences, University Hospital Munich, Campus Grosshadern, Munich, Germany

Nabangshu S. Das
Department of Biomedical Engineering, Faculty of Engineering, University of Malaya, Kuala Lumpur, Malaysia

Juliana Usman and Noor Azuan Abu Osman
Department of Biomedical Engineering, Faculty of Engineering, University of Malaya, Kuala Lumpur, Malaysia
Centre of Applied Biomechanics, University of Malaya, Kuala Lumpur, Malaysia

Dipankar Choudhury
Faculty of Mechanical Engineering, Brno University of Technology, Brno, Czech Republic
CEITEC-Central European Institute of Technology, Brno University of Technology, Brno, Czech Republic

Antonius Rohlmann, Thomas Zander, Friedmar Graichen, Hendrik Schmidt and Georg Bergmann
Julius Wolff Institute, Charitú-Universitätsmedizin Berlin, Berlin, Germany

Espen Tønnessen, Thomas A. Haugen and Erlend Hem
The Norwegian Olympic Federation, Oslo, Norway

Øystein Sylta and Stephen Seiler
Faculty of Health and Sport Sciences, University of Agder, Kristiansand, Norway

Ida S. Svendsen
School of Sport, Exercise and Health Sciences, Loughborough University, Leicestershire, United Kingdom

Vikram Puvenna and Nicola Marchi
Cerebrovascular Research, Cleveland Clinic Lerner College of Medicine, Cleveland, Ohio, United States of America
Department of Neurosurgery, Cleveland Clinic Lerner College of Medicine, Cleveland, Ohio, United States of America
Department of Molecular Medicine, Cleveland Clinic Lerner College of Medicine, Cleveland, Ohio, United States of America

Chanda Brennan
Cerebrovascular Research, Cleveland Clinic Lerner College of Medicine, Cleveland, Ohio, United States of America
Department of Molecular Medicine, Cleveland Clinic Lerner College of Medicine, Cleveland, Ohio, United States of America
Department of Clinical-Bioanalytical Chemistry, Cleveland State University, Cleveland, Ohio, United States of America

Gerald Shaw and Cui Yang
Department of Neuroscience, University of Florida, Gainesville, Florida, United States of America

Jeffrey J. Bazarian and Kian Merchant-Borna
Departments of Emergency Medicine and Neurosurgery, University of Rochester Medical Center, Rochester, New York, United States of America

Damir Janigro
Cerebrovascular Research, Cleveland Clinic Lerner College of Medicine, Cleveland, Ohio, United States of America
Department of Neurosurgery, Cleveland Clinic Lerner College of Medicine, Cleveland, Ohio, United States of America
Department of Molecular Medicine, Cleveland Clinic Lerner College of Medicine, Cleveland, Ohio, United States of America
Department of Clinical-Bioanalytical Chemistry, Cleveland State University, Cleveland, Ohio, United States of America

Jochen Mayer and Ansgar Thiel
Institute of Sports Science, University of Tübingen, Tübingen, Germany

Karen Hind
Carnegie Research Institute, Leeds Metropolitan University, Leeds, West Yorkshire, United Kingdom

Fraser Birrell
Institute of Cellular Medicine, Newcastle University, Newcastle upon Tyne, United Kingdom

Belinda Beck
School of Rehabilitation Sciences, Griffith University, Gold Coast, Australia

Cornelia Frank
Neurocognition and Action - Biomechanics Research Group, Faculty of Psychology and Sports Science, Bielefeld University, Bielefeld, Germany
Cognitive Interaction Technology - Center of Excellence (CITEC), Bielefeld University, Bielefeld, Germany

William M. Land
Department of Kinesiology, Health, & Nutrition, University of Texas at San Antonio, San Antonio, Texas, United States of America

Carmen Popp
Neurocognition and Action - Biomechanics Research Group, Faculty of Psychology and Sports Science, Bielefeld University, Bielefeld, Germany

Thomas Schack
Neurocognition and Action - Biomechanics Research Group, Faculty of Psychology and Sports Science, Bielefeld University, Bielefeld, Germany
Cognitive Interaction Technology - Center of Excellence (CITEC), Bielefeld University, Bielefeld, Germany
Research Institute for Cognition and Robotics (CoR-Lab), Bielefeld University, Bielefeld, Germany

Eric Luis Uhlmann
Management and Human Resources Department, HEC Paris, Jouy-en-Josas, France

Christopher M. Barnes
Department of Management and Organization, Foster School of Business, University of Washington, Seattle, Washington, United States of America

Jeffrey J. Bazarian, Kian Merchant-Borna and Beau Abar
Emergency Medicine, University of Rochester School of Medicine and Dentistry, Rochester, New York, United States of America

Tong Zhu
Imaging Sciences, University of Rochester School of Medicine and Dentistry, Rochester, New York, United States of America

Jianhui Zhong
Imaging Sciences, Biomedical Engineering, and Physics, University of Rochester, Rochester, New York, United States of America

Damir Janigro
Cleveland Clinic Lerner Research Institute, Cleveland, Ohio, United States of America]

Eric Rozen
Athletics and Recreation, University of Rochester, Rochester, New York, United States of America

Andrew Roberts
University of Rochester, Rochester, New York, United States of America

Hannah Javien
Hamilton College, Clinton, New York, United States of America

Eric G Blackman
Physics and Astronomy, University of Rochester, Rochester, New York, United States of America

Michael D. Lee, Mark Steyvers and Brent Miller
Department of Cognitive Sciences, University of California Irvine, Irvine, California, United States of America

Ruud J. R. Den Hartigh
Department of Psychology, University of Groningen, Groningen, The Netherlands
Epsylon Laboratory, Faculty of Sport and Physical Education Sciences, Montpellier 1 University, Montpellier, France

Christophe Gernigon
Epsylon Laboratory, Faculty of Sport and Physical Education Sciences, Montpellier 1 University, Montpellier, France

Nico W. Van Yperen and Paul L. C. Van Geert
Department of Psychology, University of Groningen, Groningen, The Netherlands

Ludovic Marin
Movement to Health Laboratory (M2H), Faculty of Sport and Physical Education Sciences, Montpellier 1 University, Montpellier, France

Daniel Mon
Universidad Politécnica de Madrid. Sports Department, Madrid, Spain

Maria S. Zakynthinaki
Applied Mathematics and Computers Laboratory, Technical University of Crete, Greece

Carlos A. Cordente
Universidad Politécnica de Madrid. Sports Department, Madrid, Spain

Antonio Monroy Antón
Universidad Francisco de Vitoria. Sports Department. Madrid, Spain

David López Jiménez
Universidad Autónoma de Chile. Profesor investigador. Santiago de Chile, Chile

Rebecca M. Stanley and James Dollman
Exercise for Health and Human Performance Group, School of Health Sciences, University of South Australia, Adelaide, South Australia, Australia

Kate Ridley
Sport, Health and Physical Education Group, School of Education, Flinders University, Adelaide, South Australia, Australia

Timothy S. Olds
Health and Use of Time Group, School of Health Sciences, University of South Australia, Adelaide, South Australia, Australia

Esther Kristina Diekhof, Susanne Wittmer and Luise Reimers
University of Hamburg, Biocenter Grindel and Zoological Museum, Institute for Human Biology, Neuroendocrinology Unit, Hamburg, Germany

Hugo Folgado
Department of Sport and Health, Universidade de Évora, Évora, Portugal
Research Center for Sports Sciences, Health and Human Development (CIDESD), Universidade de Trás-os-Montes e Alto Douro, Vila Real, Portugal

Ricardo Duarte
Interdisciplinary Center for the Study of Human Performance (CIPER), Faculdade de Motricidade Humana, Universidade de Lisboa, Lisboa, Portugal

Orlando Fernandes
Department of Sport and Health, Universidade de Évora, Évora, Portugal

Jaime Sampaio
Research Center for Sports Sciences, Health and Human Development (CIDESD), Universidade de Trás-os-Montes e Alto Douro, Vila Real, Portugal

Diana A. Santos, Catarina N. Matias, Cláudia S. Minderico, Luís B. Sardinha and Analiza M. Silva
Exercise and Health Laboratory, CIPER, Faculdade de Motricidade Humana, Universidade de Lisboa, Cruz-Quebrada, Portugal

John A. Dawson and David B. Allison
Office of Energetics, Nutrition Obesity Research Center, School of Public Health, University of Alabama at Birmingham, Birmingham, Alabama, United States of America

Paulo M. Rocha
Exercise and Health Laboratory, CIPER, Faculdade de Motricidade Humana, Universidade de Lisboa, Cruz-Quebrada, Portugal
Sport Medicine and Training Control Unit, Portuguese Institute of Sport and Youth, Cruz-Quebrada, Portugal

Michael Mäs
ETH Zurich, Chair of Sociology, in particular of Modeling and Simulation, Zurich, Switzerland

Jacob Dijkstra
Department of Sociology/ICS, University of Groningen, Groningen, The Netherlands

Tao Cheng and Thomas Wicks
SpaceTimeLab, Department of Civil, Environmental and Geomatic Engineering, University College London, London, United Kingdom

Adeilton dos Santos Gonzaga, Maicon Rodrigues Albuquerque and Israel Teoldo da Costa
Physical Education Departament - Universidade Federal de Viçosa, Viçosa, Minas Gerais, Brazil

Leandro Fernandes Malloy-Diniz
Mental Health Department, Universidade Federal de Minas Gerais, Belo Horizonte, Minas Gerais, Brazil

Pablo Juan Greco
Sports Departament - Universidade Federal de Minas Gerais, Belo Horizonte, Minas Gerais, Brazil

J. Matias Kivikangas and Simo Järvelä
Department of Information and Service Economy, Aalto University School of Business, Helsinki, Finland

Jari Kätsyri
Department of Media Technology, Aalto University School of Science, Espoo, Finland

Niklas Ravaja
Department of Information and Service Economy, Aalto University School of Business, Helsinki, Finland
Department of Social Research and Helsinki Institute for Information Technology, University of Helsinki, Helsinki, Finland

Youneés Hachana, Ghada Ben Rajeb, Riadh Khlifa and Ridha Aouadi
Research Unit: Analyse et Évaluation des Facteurs Affectant la Performance Sportive, Institut Supérieur du Sport et de l'Éducation Physique, Ksar Said, Tunisia. Université de la Manouba, Tunis, Tunisia

Helmi Chaabéne
School of Exercise Science, Australian Catholic University, Brisbane, Australia

Karim Chamari
Athlete Health and Performance Research Centre, ASPETAR, Qatar Orthopaedic and Sports Medicine Hospital, Doha, Qatar

Tim J. Gabbett
Tunisian Research Laboratory "Sport Performance Optimization," National Centre of Medicine and Science in Sports (CNMSS), Tunis, Tunisia
School of Human Movement Studies, the University of Queensland, Brisbane, Australia

Olivier Galy
Laboratory ACTES, (EA 3596: Department of Physiology), Faculty of Physical Activity and Sports, University of Guadeloupe, Pointe á Pitre, France
Laboratory CNEP (EA4242), University of New Caledonia, Nouméa, New Caledonia

Christelle Peyreigne
Laboratory INSERM (U 1046), University of Montpellier 1 and 2, Montpellier Hospital, France
Faculty of Physical Activity and Sports (EA 2991), University of Montpellier 1, Montpellier, France

Jacques Mercier
Laboratory INSERM (U 1046), University of Montpellier 1 and 2, Montpellier Hospital, France

Olivier Hue
Laboratory ACTES, (EA 3596: Department of Physiology), Faculty of Physical Activity and Sports, University of Guadeloupe, Pointe á Pitre, France

Index

A
Acceleration, 10-13, 24, 26, 85, 176
Acute Effects, 53, 192-193, 195, 197, 199-200
Adolescence, 90-91, 93, 95-97, 111-113, 116-117, 119
Amateur Swimming Association's (asa), 91
Anaerobic Threshold (at), 168, 170
Analysis of Variance (anova), 168, 170, 195
Arterial Stiffness, 99, 105, 107, 109

B
Bioenergetics, 91

C
Cardiac Autonomic, 44-45, 47, 49, 51-57
Cardiorespiratory, 27, 32, 104, 168-173, 175
Chocolate Milk, 186-192
Clinical Assessment, 34-35, 37, 39, 41-43
Cognitive Differences, 1
Conscientiousness, 27-28, 30-31
Cross-sectional Data Analysis, 120, 142

D
Decision-making, 1-5, 7-9, 73
Delayed Onset of Muscle Soreness (doms), 186, 188
Dominant Limb, 34, 38
Dynamic Constant External Resistance (dcer), 158-159
Dynamic Perception, 58-59, 61-63

E
Elite Swimmers, 41, 44, 55-56, 91, 95, 97, 111, 116, 118-119, 145
Emotional Stability, 27-28, 31
Energetic Substrates, 66
Exercise-induced Muscle Damage (eimd), 186
External Resistance Training, 158-161, 163, 165, 167
Extroversion, 27-28, 31
Eysenck's Theory, 28

F
Fitness Measures, 88, 109, 168-171, 173, 175
Freshmen Field Players, 10-11, 13, 17, 19, 21, 25
Functional Movement Laboratory (fml), 187
Fundamental Movement Skills, 76, 80-83, 87-89
Fundamental Movement Skills (fms), 76, 80-83

G
Game Intelligence, 2, 8
Glycemic Control, 99-100, 105, 107
Ground Reaction Forces (grf), 194

H
Health-related Quality of Life (hr-qol), 100
Heart Rate (hr), 45, 67-68, 169
Heart Rate Variability, 44-45, 49, 51, 55-57
Heavy Deadlifts, 193-199
High-intensity Running, 10-11, 23-24

I
Institutional Ethics, 12, 112

M
Martial Arts, 99-100, 103-105, 107, 109
Maximal Front Squat Ability, 176
Maximal Speed, 10
Mental Imagery, 176-185
Metabolic Diseases, 99-100, 102-105, 107, 109
Metabolic Equivalents (mets), 99
Mixed Linear Models, 90-91, 111
Modelling, 89-91, 93, 95, 97, 111-113, 117-119, 182
Modelling Female, 90-91, 93, 95, 97
Moderate-vigorous Pa (mvpa), 77
Multi-level Modelling (mlm), 113
Multilayer Perceptron (mlp), 120, 122, 124
Muscle Soreness, 186-192

N
Neuromuscular Adaptation, 158
Non-dominant Limb, 34, 38

O

Olympic Games, 98, 120-125, 139-140, 142, 157
One Repetition Maximum (1rm), 176, 193
Optimal Preparation, 58, 63

P

Paralympic Swimmers, 34, 38, 41-42, 44
Paralympics, 44
Physical Activity, 27-33, 52, 76-77, 79-81, 83, 85-89, 98-100, 102, 105, 107-108, 147, 156, 187
Physical Activity Intervention, 76
Physical Education (pe), 76-77, 85
Physical Self-perception, 76-77, 81, 84, 87
Physiological Characteristics, 10-11, 13, 17, 19, 21, 25, 97
Pitching Performance, 168-173
Postactivation Potentiation, 193, 198-200
Professional Baseball Pitchers, 168
Progression, 90-91, 96-97, 111-113, 116-119, 141

Q

Quadratic Functions, 90, 94-96, 111, 113-114

R

Rating of Perceived Exertion (rpe), 67, 160
Raw Milk Honey Solution, 186-187, 189, 191
Reactive Agility, 1-5, 7-9
Recovery Duration, 66-67, 69, 71, 73-75
Repeated Training Bout, 44-45, 47, 49, 51, 53, 55, 57
Root Mean Square of Successive Differences (rmssd), 44

S

Salivary Responses, 44-45, 47, 49, 51-53, 55, 57
Scapula Motion, 34-35, 37, 39, 41, 43
Scapula Upward Rotation, 34-35, 37-43
Self-determination Theory, 27, 32
Self-efficacy, 81, 176-181, 183-185
Sex Difference, 119-120, 123, 140, 145
Short-term Dynamic Constant, 158-159, 161, 163, 165, 167
Skill Development, 8, 58-59, 63, 89
Small Sided Games (ssg), 66-67
Standard Deviation (sd), 122
Static Perception, 58-61, 63
Strength Gains, 158-159, 163-165, 181
Sub-elite Swimmer, 111, 117
Subsequent Detraining, 158-160, 167
Swimming Performance, 90-91, 93, 95, 97, 120, 122-123, 133, 136, 139-142, 145-146

T

Talent Development, 58-59, 62-65, 96-97, 111, 117-118, 145
Talent Identification (ti), 111
Technical Proficiency, 66-67, 69, 73, 75
Technical Skills (ts), 66
Three Repetition Maximum (3rm), 176
Triple Hop (th), 10, 13,17-18

V

Vertical Jump Performance, 193, 195, 197-199
Video-based Visual Training, 1-3, 5, 7, 9
Video-modeling, 176-183, 185
Visual Perception, 1-2, 8-9

W

World Championships, 120-123, 125, 127, 129, 131, 133, 135, 137, 139-143, 145

Y

Youth Sports, 58

CPSIA information can be obtained
at www.ICGtesting.com
Printed in the USA
BVOW07*1013061117
499663BV00004B/26/P

9 781682 864982